to Rena

Arc *of* Interference

Warm wishes,

Medical Anthropology
for Worlds on Edge

Arc *of*

Critical Global Health: Evidence, Efficacy, Ethnography
A SERIES EDITED BY VINCANNE ADAMS AND JOÃO BIEHL

Interference

João Biehl & Vincanne Adams EDITORS

DUKE UNIVERSITY PRESS DURHAM AND LONDON 2023

© 2023 Duke University Press. All rights reserved
Printed in the United States of America on acid-free paper ∞
Project Editor: Jessica Ryan | Designed by Aimee C. Harrison
Typeset in Portrait Text, Helvetica Neue Condensed, and
Happy Times at the IKOB (Lucas Le Bihan) by Westchester Publishing

Library of Congress Cataloging-in-Publication Data
Names: Biehl, João Guilherme, editor. | Adams, Vincanne,
[date] editor.
Title: Arc of interference : medical anthropology for worlds on
edge / João Biehl and Vincanne Adams, editors.
Other titles: Critical global health.
Description: Durham : Duke University Press, 2023. | Series:
Critical global health | Includes bibliographical references and
index.
Identifiers: LCCN 2022043178 (print)
LCCN 2022043179 (ebook)
ISBN 9781478019800 (paperback)
ISBN 9781478017097 (hardcover)
ISBN 9781478024378 (ebook)
Subjects: LCSH: Medical anthropology. | Social medicine. |
Discrimination in medical care. | Public health—Anthropological
aspects. | BISAC: SOCIAL SCIENCE / Anthropology / Cultural &
Social | MEDICAL / Public Health
Classification: LCC GN296 .A725 2023 (print) | LCC GN296 (ebook) |
DDC 306.4/61—dc23/eng/20221202
LC record available at https://lccn.loc.gov/2022043178
LC ebook record available at https://lccn.loc.gov/2022043179

To our mentor Arthur Kleinman
And in memory of Paul Farmer

CONTENTS

Against the Grain

Medical Anthropology in the Anthropocene

THE TRICK OF THE WORLD—its secret and its truth—is that it is the fountain of all things. The analytic task before medical anthropology is to contain at least the most important parts of that messy complexity and contingency, the pain and the pleasures, the sorrows and joys, the desires and remembrances, and, sometimes, the catastrophe.

The challenge of translating into words the world's seemingly effortless trick—which means fixing the flux into local and time-bound descriptions and understanding—includes, as it ever has in our best accounts of it, an awareness of power and privilege. These shield some and expose others, and this is largely a book about the exposed. If João Biehl, an editor of this volume, writes not of fountains but of "life's onslaught," it's because many would speak of raging torrents rather than of refreshing wellsprings.

It is the experience of this flow that emerges here as the primary source for medical anthropology and for anthropology writ large. Because whether our local moral worlds are perceived as fountain or flood, the way we know them most intimately—even as they lurch toward an imperiled and perhaps finite future—is through lived experience. What could be more mundane, more worldly, than the fate of each of us when faced with the truly universal (anthropologists don't use this word often, and with reason) fact of our own mortality? (We do perseverate on that one.) Medical anthropology serves, in this work, as a stern reminder that life's currents include, for all of us and unequally, illness, injury, and a shared fate of finitude.

This is a book about life and death and about the aftermath of death. That alone makes it relevant to our species and to others, but *Arc of Interference* is also a book about the possibility of something more and something wonderful: across the continents, people struggle to care for one another and to make sense of suffering. Making such sense was the task of a now obscure branch of theology known as theodicy. That term may have largely disappeared, but each of this book's chapters reminds us that making sense of fate, and altering its horizons, is a task taken up in urgently in extraordinary and ordinary times, to invoke terms from the liturgical calendar, in at least some religious traditions, which Davíd Carrasco (reviving an anthropological tradition, and also with good reason) warns are neglected at our analytic peril.

In the face of suffering, regardless of its cause, there is nonetheless relief and comfort from family, friends, and even strangers. The "care-ful ethnography" pioneered here suggests this happens after death, as well. In the land of the living, sick or injured people seek care, and caregiving is central to the journey between birth and death. As a number of these chapters show, caregiving begins before death and reliably extends well beyond it. It is, Arthur Kleinman has argued in his beautiful and (for me, at least) devastating *The Soul of Care*, "the invisible glue that holds society together."

For the injured or ill, the search for succor occurs not before meaning making but is central to it. The quest for care, like giving or receiving it, is a fundamentally social process, as anthropologists have long maintained and as the contributors to this book show us in vivid manner. So why do we see attempts, in so many scholarly accounts of sickness and suffering, to reduce personal experience to chaff to be discarded? Why do we desocialize the obviously irreducible sociality of sickness?

I'm not referring primarily, as many revanchist (and sometimes simply resentful) medical anthropologists once did, to papers published in leading medical journals. I'm referring to the analyses proffered by many trained in psychology, sociology, demography, epidemiology, and biostatistics. I'm thinking, too, of current strains of history, political economy, and philosophy. Forget about economics, which is classed as a social science in most US universities but often reads, when it reads at all, like amateur mathematics.

If the desocialization of social science is a development profoundly to be rued—or, at least, to be recognized and named—it's also a trend long countered by Kleinman, whose radically humanist work *Arc of Interference* honors. For decades, as this book shows, he has deplored the stripping away of context, which means not only the social milieu of local moral worlds but the history that underpins them. His plangent critique has been laid out in an oeuvre that has restored the social to our understanding of many misfortunes—and to the search for an ethical or moral perch in a world on the edge.

Human experience, even at its most interior, is social experience, lived out within local worlds enmeshed not only in physical bodies but also in broader and cosmopolitan social webs, themselves spun into global assemblages. It's *all* social, which is why desocialization of analyses of health and sickness does violence to any shared understanding of those worlds. If at first Kleinman chafed against the category fallacies of psychiatry, he soon lifted his eyes to the desocialized social sciences, genetics, epidemiology, and the rising host of those contemplating health disparities with little attention to lived experience. Many in these traditions were looking, he and his wife and collaborator Joan Kleinman once wrote, "at anything but experience."

The implications of this critique and of Kleinman's written work—and of this book—are nothing short of vast, as would be evident without my own admiring comments. *Arc of Interference* interrogates a number of framing binaries that continue to chafe. In her contribution, Margaret Lock situates hers (and Kleinman's career) in the old and fraught debate about nurture versus nature, noting that, "with the consolidation of the discipline of genetics, and the gradual formation of deterministic neo-Darwinism over the course of the twentieth century, a separation of the social and biological sciences became even more marked." It is impossible not to think of another psychiatrist, Frantz Fanon, who sought to link the "interior" psychological worlds of colonial subjects with the degrading and degraded French colonial rule he labored to end. But Kleinman's key contributions are more numerous than efforts to bridge this ancient gap between the personal and ostensibly impersonal.

The ethics of attending to suffering, in this book sometimes termed *arts of care*, require intimate knowledge of experience. For some, those with the ability to sustain reverent attention, this is often easy to glean. All you have to do, at least to start, is ask what really matters, and surely anyone with a modicum of curiosity and empathy and persistence might cull important insights. But the aftermath of sickness reveals that many forms of expertise are marshaled to explain away, rather than to grasp, intimate experience. When we fail to faithfully echo and amplify the demands of the afflicted, it's small wonder many are mistrustful of expertise and academics.

There are, these days, plenty of reasons to restore that trust through what is termed in these pages *care-ful ethnography*. A long-prophesied pandemic of a respiratory virus is upon us. As the hammer of COVID-19 falls unevenly across the globe, this brand of medical anthropology might itself constitute a form of care. As Carrasco has it, echoing Kleinman, ethnography itself, and even humanitarian forensics engaged in bringing up the bodies, can constitute a form of caregiving in the face of affliction.

Fear, Flood, Fire, Foe

Unsurprisingly, given such arguments, this collection is focused on experience. It is, of course, the contributors' intention to theorize social experience, which is inevitably personal or interior—internalized and relational—as well.

The experience examined in these pages is rarely of the joyful kind. But it's important to note that the individual chapters here are the fruit of decades of work, and they tell us what really matters to these scholars. War and famine in German-blockaded Holland. Racism of varied forms. Colonial predations, including the sack of the environment, the thinning or destruction of indigenous communities and the historical trauma (and massive displacement) that ensued, sparking enduring pathologies, including depression, suicide (including even self-immolation), domestic violence, substance abuse. The degradation of the planet and epidemics and pandemics hitherto unknown or taking on new and more virulent forms.

This grim list goes on. Then again, these chapters are a tribute to a medical anthropologist whose books included subtitles such as "living a moral life amidst uncertainty and danger." But *Arc of Interference* is no jeremiad, no catalog of wrongs. Nor is it only what Robert Desjarlais, taking a tender and philosophical turn, terms *demise writing*. There is within it much demise, and many funerals, but these chapters bring to mind smoothed bits of sea glass. Taken together, assembled, they constitute a treasure.

The pounding of sand and shards into sea glass worthy of a crown might not be a welcome metaphor for the radically egalitarian, but the reader—at least, this one—can almost see the book's contributors bent over their forges. A prime example of this patient reviewing for me, and of the value of the metaphor, is Vincanne Adams's elegant reflection on a dreadful if ontologically entrancing topic that has troubled her for years and that few other writers could render in respectful and evocative prose. Each of these contributions surely required intense heat and years of polishing, and we're left with a gem that's both easy and difficult to read.

Easy because these chapters each condense long years of work into essays that draw on Kleinman's insights and on his decades of engagement with and in China. (Other volumes, crafted largely with his former students in China, pay more focused tribute to his work there). These chapters, these bits of sea glass, glitter with propulsive force, throwing off lessons through narrative ("A guru got up to speak to the assembled transgender women"; "Here is where the artist comes into the picture"). The heat of these narratives might make some readers shrink back in dismay, and that's why the book is hard.

In addition to the brute force of events such as wildfires, self-immolations in Tibet, and scorching deaths in the Sonoran Desert are intimate but no less molten stories about, say, the loss of the father of one of this book's contributors; he was so horrified by the indignities meted out to the bodies of his Mexican American students, who, after perishing in a car accident, were so unceremoniously piled in a frigid morgue that he took his own life.

Unlike the ahistorical accounts of early twentieth-century ethnography, these chapters are firmly rooted in time, even to the point of creating new verbs, such as *futuring* and *horizoning*, which further unmoor the notion of the ethnographic present. Jean Comaroff reminds us, in her reliably felicitous way, that anthropology "has echoed the Romantic strain inherent in Euro-modernity itself, its enduring obsession with certainties lost, with time 'lapsing,' ever receding into history." A corrective, she continues, is to be found in "a commitment to take seriously the temporal understandings of others, the distinct ontological realities they live by."

The reader knows, early on, that we are deep within the Anthropocene, with (to cite the troubling reflections of Adriana Petryna) its "epic storms from warming oceans, wildfires burning with unprecedented intensity, rising sea levels, massive crop failures, extreme heat, prolonged droughts." Many horizons are obscured in smoke and flame, but not all is lost. The "vast abrupt of climate change," she continues in considering a ballooning future of wildfires in the United States, reminds us that the "permutations of an absent horizon concept include futility and hope, as well as curiosity."

The value of this brand of anthropology should be obvious, surely, in the Anthropocene, when, as Comaroff writes, there's an "ominous sense of dread as the birds fly off and calamity seems imminent." Who among us doesn't see the future as different from the past? Who among us isn't called, or simply able, to peer toward the horizon? Who doesn't have to?

Arc of Interference

These chapters don't need a foreword or an afterword to tie them together; they are already linked to Kleinman's work, and that (with apologies for another shiny metaphor) is golden thread enough. But it's important, at least to me, to say a few words about the individual contributions, their complementarity, their vast abrupts, their ties to the thread.

It's important to me because I know the work of these scholars well and have been engaged in some of it. Yet within their contributions—already classed as jewels—are surprises for even the most well-versed practitioners of medical anthropology. Some of the surprises, such as Petryna's work of horizoning, are novel concepts; some are fruitful reworkings of old concepts, and still others include felicitous turns of phrase.

In each chapter we find twists in the narrative that hadn't previously been shared. Many introduce new characters, who are, by definition, unique and important regardless of how commonly encountered their views may be. Most of all, though, I found myself marking "things you want to know" in each and every chapter. These, too, are situated in the flux of time. To give a few examples, and in no particular order: of wildfires in the United States, Petryna reminds us that the hour is late and some switches may well be irrevocably flipped. Desjarlais informs the reader that, in Nepal, the Buddhist Hyolmo people know that a good death "helps them to achieve liberation or a good rebirth." The period after death and before life, in the liminal realm known as the *bardo*, can last up to forty-nine days—a relief to some raised on the related notion of limbo, even though, we learn, a good rebirth requires the help of the living. (The contrast offered by the accounts of Adams and Desjarlais, working in more or less the same region, is another strength of this volume.) Carrasco, speaking from the US-Mexico border, shows how central religious readings are to the lived experience of those seeking to cross it, not only for these pilgrims, but for their transnational social networks. This set of chapters speaks explicitly to partnerships between the living and the dead, as Carrasco reminds us.

Other contributions build on understanding likely out of grasp just a generation earlier. Lock explains that the Japanese word *jibun*, "translated into English as 'self,'" implies that the "concept cannot be separate from the social realm" and that "humans have approximately 20,000 genes, and not 100,000, as had been predicted." Lock then takes her knowledge of this subject to interrogate the emerging field of molecular epigenetics.

Salmaan Keshavjee reminds us that one of the masterminds of the United Nations was Jan Smuts, an architect of apartheid in his home country. João

Biehl relates, in an altogether new fashion, the dolorous aftermath of his rapport with Catarina, the main character of his book *Vita*; she died almost twenty years ago. (All long-term ethnographers know this pain, although too few write about it as beautifully and generously as Biehl.) Janis H. Jenkins asserts, unsurprisingly to those in the trenches of care delivery, that many psychiatrists take cultural relativism much farther than do psychiatric anthropologists. (She goes further, arguing that "a sustained ethnographic approach to the experience of mental illness should productively focus on engaged processes of struggle rather than symptoms.") Marcia Inhorn, in her study of twenty-first-century quests for conception, describes an expanding practice of "reprotravel" that links India to China (and, in her report, forty-eight other countries) to global Dubai, where, right now, more than half of all residents are from India. Lawrence Cohen writes of the experience of trans- and third-gendered people in India, whose fates, we hope, were not shortened by COVID-19 as the hammer falls with terrible force across the subcontinent, which is also the locus of David S. Jones's reminders that we don't fully understand either the dynamics of cardiac disease there or the cardiotravel that echoes Inhorn's insights as much as, or more than, Cohen's.

The *ethnographic open* of this book is one of its greatest charms. Cohen—like me, one of Kleinman's students lucky enough to pursue degrees in both medicine and anthropology—also brings forth the ethnographer's own vacillation between certainty and uncertainty, the sort of confession we feared to make as students. "I asked his cousin what she meant," he confides to the reader, "more or less knowing." Anthropology as an aspirational project is, as Kleinman reminded us decades ago, almost always about moving from knowing less to knowing more.

This stumbling march forward, toward knowing more, offers another reason to appreciate the treasure assembled here, scored by the filigreed detail of all extravagant ornaments. These details are important. In moments of immodesty, some anthropologists refer to this as "ethnographic detail" to trundle out the tired vignette, the vestigial exoticism, the curated conversations, the arcana, the labored reveal. But in truth, such detail may often be found in even newspaper articles about any of the topics at hand. What lends it force, in this book, are the analyses in which the specific is enmeshed—that and conversations and rumors and acknowledgment of the ethnographer's uncertainty in moving from knowing less to knowing more while aware, as Cohen and others observe, that it's sometimes best to ask less. Reverent listening inevitably requires silence.

Another beauty of this book is that its constituent pieces come from the borderland (in Kleinman's term, but others here speak of flux, junctures, crossroads, or a nexus) between more than one discipline. Some, like those of Jenkins and Desjarlais and Kleinman himself, emerge from among psychiatry, psychology, and anthropology. Others draw on anthropology and environmental science. Jones, a physician-historian, is also an anthropologist, whether he says so or not, and his work picks apart category fallacies while offering surprising ethnographic detail from the practice of cardiology in India. All of them link the large-scale to the local, the outside to the inside, the past to the present, and the present to our uncertain future.

What, then, of caregiving and the arts of care, which several of these chapters show to continue beyond death? If social science is a blood sport, and at times readily mocked as the arena of low-stakes and absurdly bitter feuds, a focus on caregiving and care-ful ethnography lends humility to our proceedings. And that kind of work helps preclude the notion that all ethnographic work might qualify as care-ful, in itself an adequate response to suffering. For a responsible alternative to the latter, one need only read the elegiac chapter by Carrasco. It was his father, who spent decades assisting migrants to and around El Paso, Texas, who took his life after bearing witness to too much indignity, too much grisly loss.

Carrasco's stories—of his father and of the bodies in the desert and of the *retablos* linking all of it to the world of the saints—call to mind not so much the fate of Catarina as, more precisely, Biehl's beautiful attempt to honor her posthumously with a memorial. She died not in the desert but in a place meant to be an oasis, as disheveled and confining as she found it. There, we learn, she one night called out for her mother and died. What American reader doesn't read this and think of George Floyd? Biehl's account is intergenerational, since he knew Catarina and her children, but we didn't get a chance to know Floyd in this way. If the struggle for racial justice in the United States doesn't figure prominently in this volume, there's reason to hope that this will continue to be rectified by scholars who are also writing within this broader tradition of care-ful ethnography.

This is not, as noted, a cheerful book. Although the care and caregiving of the Hyolmo Buddhists strike a merciful note, there's a dark side of caregiving, too. Care, as Biehl observes, is often "an act of frustration, a behind-the-scenes affective grappling by gendered bodies in complicity, love, and aggression, in the face of political disregard and a battered history."

A number of old dichotomies beyond nature-nurture, including the alleged distinction between communicable and noncommunicable diseases, are exploded here. It's simply not true, as Keshavjee shows, that the former receive warranted attention while the latter do not. (Jones, too, explodes some of these myths.) Perhaps a fifth of all cancer diagnoses, and many more in some settings, are likely caused by infectious pathogens, which suggests another category fallacy to explore.

Much of the current debate about decolonizing global health has neglected to mention caregiving even in passing, which, one suspects, would have disappointed Fanon. Caregiving has been largely stripped out of public health, and nowhere is this more true than in the postcolony. Call this the myopia of the healthy and well placed, a staple of our current iterations of global health. Disease control is not at all the same as caring for those afflicted by pathogens, which like other pathogenic forces—here, climate change, migration, growing inequality itself—strike some while others are spared. The vast abrupt of the current pandemic, which has left millions dead in the space of a year, has no doubt fueled new forms of structural violence and (one fears) too many old ways of explaining it away.

The COVID-19 pandemic emerged as this book was being edited and is a reminder of the perils of such suffering sweepstakes, in which one pressing concern is pitted against another. But if there's a reason I don't have a chapter in this volume, it's Ebola, which drives home several of the points made by Jones and in Keshavjee's chapter on tuberculosis. As in South Africa, so, too, across a continent under colonial rule, which was when control-over-care paradigms arose. They persist in current discussions of "health security" and are made manifest in our current status quo of COVID-vaccine nationalism, which has led so far to vaccine apartheid. Jan Smuts might not have approved, since workers are essential to the political economy he helped to usher in.

Critical Medical Anthropologist in the Anthropocene

Arc of Interference, drawing on Kleinman's many arcs, reveals an astoundingly generative mind and what's at stake in fields as disparate as psychiatry, environmental science, medical anthropology, social medicine, and even philosophy and social theory.

Future biographers and historians of medical anthropology and social medicine (to say nothing of Chinese studies) will no doubt attempt to carve Kleinman's long and rich career into distinct periods. It would be easy to do by simply attending to his written work, with attention to chronology. But what strikes me, as his student and friend, is that the long arc of his interference has focused his attention on a fairly small number of matters. These are precisely those captured in this book.

I wouldn't have asserted as much even a decade ago. I might instead have marveled at the differences between *Patients and Healers in the Context of Culture* (1980) and, say, *Writing at the Margins* (1997). But instead of seeing an arc from narrowly focused medical ethnography to structural violence, it's really his ability to elicit what really matters in diverse settings and, as anthropologist and clinician, to respond. These gifts were themselves crowned by turning to his own experience in *The Soul of Care*. The golden thread of his work is less demise writing than sober reflection about what really matters, and that is often to allay suffering while confronting the fears of our own, and others', finitude.

If there's something I wish to add to this already glittering arrangement, it's a final word about Kleinman as doctor and teacher. As Biehl notes, his ethnographic corpus is "colored by his simultaneous commitments as a clinician and an anthropologist." And here, with the indulgence of the editors, I swerve to the personal, as Cohen does in describing the anxious back-and-forth between green student and exacting mentor. Familiarity with that anxiety is surely one reason I found his essay so affecting, and why many former students and trainees will smile in reading that "Kleinman's provocation, and it is never an easy one to bear, is to work toward a mode of interference of one's own."

Most of the people contributing to this collection have been, formally, students or trainees of Kleinman. (I count a few physician-anthropologists who might stake that claim.) I'd wager that a good number have also been his patients or benefited from his compassion and clinical skills, as have thousands of others, from Boston to Beijing.

And I'd like him to smile when I note that what underpins the heat that forged the jewel and the glass, and even the sea that battered the glass, is also in that borderland between encompassing devotion and respect and love. I want to express a conviction that it is love and kindness and fellow feeling that underpins Kleinman's work more than any analytic framework, ideology, or training ever could. The reader can sense that appreciation surging forth in these pages.

Of course, I know this claim wouldn't likely be encountered in a scholarly journal; it can barely fit in a book published by a university press. But it is true, and worth saying: Kleinman is a great doctor and teacher because he is, however transformed by his own experience, a loving and caring person. We knew that well before his wife, Joan Kleinman, first exhibited signs of the early-onset dementia that would finally claim her life. *The Soul of Care* taught others what we already knew: that Arthur Kleinman would rise to the task. And that the task was sure to be hard.

And so, in the end, Kleinman's arc bends toward both justice and mercy. As seas rise, glaciers melt, and forests burn, we will all need to follow this lead. And as his students know, that will lead us not to certain places and topics, but to a full embrace of what really matters to all of us, well before we reach the *bardo*.

The book's polished gems, like Kleinman's work, stand alone and confer beauty on the journey's arc. What more fitting tribute to a physician and scholar who has devoted himself to his fellow travelers, and especially those pushed and shoved in their travails across our beautiful and riven world.

Arc of Interference

A deadly pestilence is in our town, strikes us and spares not, and the house of Cadmus is emptied of its people while Black Death grows rich in groaning and lamentation. . . . Raise up our city, save it and raise it up. . . . If you rule this land . . . better to rule it full of people than empty. For neither tower nor ship is anything when . . . none live in it together.—SOPHOCLES, *OEDIPUS THE KING*

Me and you, we got more yesterday than anybody. We need some kind of tomorrow.
—TONI MORRISON, *BELOVED*

Our time is specialized in producing absences. . . . My provocation about postponing the end of the world is exactly to always be able to tell one more story.—AILTON KRENAK, *IDEAS TO POSTPONE THE END OF THE WORLD*

THAT WE LIVE IN WORLDS ON EDGE has served as a premise for much of the past decades of anthropology, in which inequality, violence, and uncertainty have been pervasive, exhausting social lives but still sometimes harboring visions of surprising escapes. Anxiety and anomie have been deeply felt on the edges of autocracy and predatory capitalism, of disintegrating cultures and forced migration, of infrastructural breakdown and abrupt climate change—mediated by extreme populism, war, disinformation, and state and corporate efforts to dismantle piecemeal, though meaningful, agendas of socioeconomic rights. Meanwhile, the "ethnographic sensorium" has also kept eliciting peoples' plasticity and desires for self-determination and things to be otherwise.[1]

Today, we find ourselves past that stage of foreboding, and this writing, too, takes place at an edge of calamity's unfolding. While Russia wages a brutal neocolonial war against Ukraine and democracy itself, the COVID-19 pandemic continues to rage across the world, undoing taken-for-granted ways of knowing and acting and revealing the thorough impotence of social safety nets, health-care systems, and hoped-for bonds of solidarity.

Amid rippling health, economic, and political damage we are forced to reckon with the deadly impact of environmental decline; the utter fragility of our systems of preparedness; and the entrenched forms of structural violence that exacerbate vulnerability, mortality rates, mental illness, and disparities in care. These collective disasters affect and kill unevenly along the vectors of race, gender, class, nation and region.[2]

Social media-saturated and divided as ever, necropolitical scenarios ask us to put what remains of our faith in the virologists, epidemiologists, vaccine developers, climate planners, governments, nonprofit organizations, and other technocratic solutions to restore some sense of normality to social and economic life. But these, too, may fall short, reconfiguring and reinforcing inequities and control systems even after stimulus packages are unleashed and anticipated lifesaving technologies become available.[3]

Meanwhile, Black Americans have reached a tipping point brought on by the white supremacy and systemic racism that, for centuries, have constrained their lives and foreclosed the life chances of people of color, often under the guise of a liberal political order, humanism, and fallacious systems of accountability. The police violence that has brutally marked the daily experiences of entire communities is, at long last, at the fore of political discourse around the world. The horrors of the killing of George Floyd on May 25, 2020, have also prompted a recalling of generations of murdered Black citizens and unprecedented displays of activism and imagination for what could replace unjust modes of governance and oppressive dynamics of inclusion and exclusion, here and elsewhere.[4]

Amid this general sense of vertigo and facing the fleeting promise of repair and abolition, we know that the pandemic, planetary demise, injustice, inequality, and health collapse are connected: not wanting to discount one as the product of any other, we can still see how the cumulative effects give rise to a sense of possibility for a refashioned world in their wake. What, then, does the present moment ask of anthropology—of our listening and evidence making and of our own "response-ability" toward practical solidarity in the face of so much that is on edge?[5] How do we write about these times and thus take a leap toward interfering in their course, attentive not only to the massive scale of vulnerability, affliction, and death that has come into view but also to the "active will to [create] community" and insurgencies therein?[6]

Alternative forms of intentionality and conviviality emerge alongside newfangled scales of harm and caregiving. People the world over are propelled by this unparalleled state of urgency into rethinking the architectures and assumptions of medical capitalism, political power, and social and economic life. And we, too, are thrust into recasting our disciplinary bequest, research foci, and public roles as scholars.

As we ponder what and who needs our work, we must appraise with humility anthropology's origins and entanglements in colonialism, environmental imperialism, and systemic racism. But we also must maintain a commitment to the empirical potentials that interlocution opens up and to learning from human ingenuities, plasticities, and fugitivities in the face of death in all its forms. For the discipline has also thrived from relational and situated knowledge making that has tried to destabilize hierarchies of expertise; from historically attuned analysis and an openness to insurgent archives; and from reflexive engagement as diverse practitioners have sought to unsettle hierarchies in the category of the human and established forms of thought about the ethical and the political.

If *intervention* signifies a mode of technical and political fix, constrained by certain temporalities and geographies of scope and scale, anthropology, at best, should afford alternate modes of *interference*: interrupting ideals of naturalness, breaking open commonsense understandings and technical assessments that inform "which kinds of lives societies support," and summoning intellectual and political engagements and a "will to live" that go beyond one-off humanitarian rescues tethered to supposedly isolated events.[7] Through all this, *interference* calls for a disrupting and moving along the discipline's taken-for-granted concepts and commitments. Attentive to both the longue durée of chronic precariousness (aggravated by emergencies) and the unanticipated dynamisms and trajectories of local worlds, we can collaborate in opening up new vistas into today's shifting grounds of the biosocial, the material, and the politico-economic. In the process, ethnographic creations may themselves emerge along *arcs of interference*—conceptual and political projects whose endpoints remain always out of view, but which, in beckoning us to intellectual work, solidarity, and commitments to justice, may enlarge our sense of what is possible and activate a sharper "horizoning" capacity, as Adriana Petryna puts it.

Against the backdrop of tipping points and the heightened struggle against systemic racism, we thus ask: How can anthropology track the circuitous pathways—the arcs of historical and political possibilities that remain ever in view—that may guide us as we find ourselves refashioning a world not just in COVID-19's wake but in the wake of the multiple precipitous worlds on edge that we have created?[8] How can we best approximate the ruinations, survivals, and technological reinventions of today's lifeworlds—these ongoing worldly fabrications and the unresolved lives therein? How might the *ethnographic open* animate the imagination of new worlds and possibilities of justice, equality, and freedom?

The challenge is to work toward an attuning of the social sciences to the restlessness and sense of moral purpose that animate critical thought and social action in the local worlds that we learn from, write about, and think with. As Angela Davis powerfully says, "The refusal or inability *to do something, say something,* when a thing needed doing or saying, [is] unbearable."[9] To calibrate our efforts might mean to embrace silence as much as the demand to speak, to sit with our interlocutors in solidarity, not always knowing for certain how exactly to act.

Our effort in *Arc of Interference* emanates from a shared trust that critical medical anthropology might be uniquely equipped to interfere in our embattled present, given its long-standing and particular commitments to ethnographic engagement with the distinct human conditions of our times and to the articulation of theoretical and practical contributions to health and care, as well as to the ways these core subjects are, for better or worse, studied. The work of ethnography pushes us to think against the grain, with and through difference, attentive to the nonteleological ways that social and political forces unfold, the uncertain and unexpected in the world, and to care for the as-yet-unthought that keeps modes of existence and knowledge making open to extemporization and constant recalibration.

In trespassing disciplinary boundaries and challenging methodologically authorized analytical distance among medicine, health, and the social, the field of medical anthropology has long illuminated the dynamic interplay of the human and the material, the cultural and the biological, technology and affect, the clinic and the home, and the local and the planetary. Medical anthropologists have, almost routinely, demonstrated how local and global studies can rise above their delineated confines to create a stronger kind of hybrid, crossover knowledge. All the while, scholars have striven to balance critical social inquiry and critiques of knowledge with a responsiveness (with all its double binds and limits) to the lived experience of affliction and an attentiveness to the micro, meso, and macro ways suffering and injustice are resisted.[10]

The COVID-19 pandemic and the turbulent forces unfolding as a result have shown the marked relevance of central medical anthropological insights and concepts today. Just as *structural vulnerability* is a critical lens to explain why a respiratory virus so disproportionately spreads among minority groups and along other lines of social stratification, so, too, is *racialization* key to making sense of inequities in death rates and their codification in medical literature and, in so doing, breaking open regimes of systemic violence, invisibilization, and disregard.[11] Reigning paradigms for fragmented public health systems are revealed as wholly inadequate to handle the many facets of an epidemic response—logistics, contact tracing, outreach, and community engagement, not to mention surge hospital capacity for supportive care—and yet a *pharmaceuticalized pandemic-industrial complex* capitalizes from the chaos with salvific promises of unleashing economies of technocratic, market-based, magic-bullet solutions—even while, from other sites, the neoliberal biopolitical order seems increasingly called into question.[12] At the same time, timeworn concepts such as structure are shown to be more complex in the present than their past uses allowed, beckoning for new models such as toxicity, the commons, speculation, and multispecies cohabitation.

Importantly, medical anthropologists have also concerned themselves with the everyday, lived effects of these political-economic decisions. Their work has been attuned, for instance, to the labor regimes that subtend normative conceptions of health, determining what is deemed essential to life, whose lives are paramount to save, and who is destined to die, in hospitals or at home. Ethnographic care and attention to the making and remaking of lifeworlds under these conditions has thus revealed many novel attempts at living and "house-ing" under duress that can take center stage and speak back to policy and public debates.[13] At a more personal level, reflecting on the possibilities of care in this bizarre, atomized, and constrained present, we see how contemporary crises can serve as renewed opportunities for each one of us to "learn how to endure with purpose and make this a period of emotional and moral transformation," in Arthur Kleinman's words.[14]

As the movements of the day and the senses of dread and foreboding— but also hope that comes with them—grab our attention, we find ourselves asking: What space remains for considering the work of the anthropological imagination that predates the moment we live in? How might medical anthropological engagements with other worlds, and other problems, be brought along in this work and still speak in potent ways to current urgencies?

––––––––––––––––   ✎

Arc of Interference is a stocktaking of contemporary, humanist medical anthropology: its influence on ethical debates and social theory and the ways it is continuously transforming the stakes of critique and public discourse in our times. It is guided by a return to the work and legacies of Arthur Kleinman, one of the most important figures in medical anthropology.[15] We find *arc* an appropriate term to evoke Kleinman's influence on the field, as his seminal contributions to cultural psychiatry, social medicine, global health, medical humanities, Asian studies, and many intersecting fields continue to inspire students, conceptual and empirical work, and critical political and intellectual debates in medical anthropology today. Kleinman's specific modes of inquiry are, of course, one among many critical approaches to medical anthropology, but his commitments to questions of experience and intersubjectivity amid accelerated social and politico-economic transformation and to envisioning ethnographic engagement as a work of care have served as conceptual springboards for the vibrant and diverse debates, methods, orientations, and theoretical commitments that continue to define the field.[16]

We are inspired by Lawrence Cohen's insight about Kleinman's career and relentless studying, theorizing, and reflecting on care as itself one of *interfering* in both commonsense and technical expertise at various levels: "from the enactment of a form of clinical practice that works otherwise to the production of a form of speech or writing that does not complain (and thus merely reinstantiate competing moral demands as an unending contest) but interferes in this oppositional terrain" (see chapter 7).

The term *arc of interference* thus evokes the intellectual and professional tasks that have guided Kleinman's career since the early 1970s, when, as a young physician just out of public health service and research in Taiwan, he came to Harvard University to work across history of science and anthropology on the comparative study of medical systems. In 1973, Kleinman published a set of essays that contained the ethnographic seeds of the concepts he would continue to trace over his fifty-year career.[17] The most seminal of these articles, "Medicine's Symbolic Reality," probed the philosophy of medicine and questioned how biomedical knowledge was culturally constructed. Another essay pointed out the blindness of public health when it came to modeling health care in society. Left out of these analyses were family relations and nonprofessional healing, Kleinman noted, the most important source of caregiving (both personally and quantitatively) for many patients. In an additional text, Kleinman drew from his pioneering ethnographic work in China and Taiwan and critiqued scholars of China for effacing questions of health, emotions, and values. In contrast, Kleinman indicated how a study of medicine and health more generally were crucial to understanding the historical transformation China was experiencing at the time.

In these essays and the many that would follow, Kleinman would bring ethnographic knowledges and sensibilities to bear on various aspects of biomedicine's commonsense orientations to illness and disease, health systems, and mental illness and care and unsettled them, modeling a kind of productive interference that in turn shaped his own theory-making within anthropology. For instance, *Patients and Healers in the Context of Culture*, Kleinman's first single-authored ethnography, set out to articulate an approach to medical anthropology that would emphasize the work of caregivers and privilege people-centered ethnography as a mode of theory making. The book offered a new way to conceive of the field that until then had been closely linked to public health, with its temporal and epistemological commitments to certain kinds of intervention. He would go on to call for an ethnographic approach centered on the human experience of suffering as a means of liberating ethnographic subjects from the reductive and dominant medical and social-welfare categories of analysis; to study the cross-cultural experience of bereavement and depression in ways that challenged psychiatric categories of mental illness; and to write about illness narratives as entry points into the primary grounds of care and caregiving.

Through the arc of his work, Kleinman would keep social experience and the question of the moral ever in view. Indeed, his career has been shaped by the visceral desire to fashion a more resonantly human understanding of the experiences of illness and treatment, cultural and socioeconomic influences on therapeutic relationships and outcomes, the construction (and limitations) of bioethics, and the social processes that underlie biomedical knowledge production. These commitments to comparative work on the place of values in professional practice and in everyday life—always attentive to *category fallacies, illness narratives, social suffering*, and the *arts of caregiving*—arrived at a critical juncture in anthropology. As poststructuralist and postmodern critiques were chiefly redirecting anthropologists' attention to destabilizations of truth and power, Kleinman's work would inspire the discipline to maintain an ethnographic practice attuned to diverse institutional realities and intellectual traditions and to the personal stakes of these endeavors.

This is the central argument in Kleinman's more recent book, *A Passion for Society* (coauthored with Iain Wilkinson), which explored a longer lineage of critical thinkers, such as Max Weber and Hannah Arendt, whose *life of the mind* and *amor mundi* rejected the idea of "objective" social science divorced from practical solidarities. Throughout his career, Kleinman has consistently advanced this commitment to ethnography as much as an art of living as a vehicle for knowledge production: "What really matters" is the exercise of "presence, openness, listening, doing, enduring, and the cherishing of people and memories" and the enduring social bonds of care that hold things together.[18]

The essays in *Arc of Interference* continue to engage these central concerns. The chapters open up Kleinman's enduring influences through the lens of ethnographic and theoretical engagements with issues of key social, medical, and political import in the context of the far-right turmoil and inequality we see across the planet. An agonistic critique pulsating through all of Kleinman's work also permeates the chapters in this book, grappling not only with how geopolitical structures of violence, impoverishment, ecocide, and affliction actually work, but also with new ways to break open the political imagination through ethnographic storytelling.

What does it mean to interfere in the medical and political realms of today's preposterous social orders, when ethnographic insights bring into view, with increasing nuance, the displacement of taken-for-granted subject positions and the ambiguities of moral calculations? What opportunities for clinical and policy engagement remain as the horizons of calculability disappear and ethnographic evidence continues to both displace and inform them? And how can this productive tension that ethnography generates when put into conversation with other forms of social-science expertise and knowledge disrupt and refigure our intellectual and political responses to contemporary predicaments, from the COVID-19 pandemic and its aftermath to ongoing racialized violence and the multiple fiscal and environmental crises that loom ahead?

Arc of Interference frames Kleinman's work (and, by extension, medical anthropology) as a means to a situated practice of critical thinking and engagement with the actual and the otherwise in three senses. The first is vis-à-vis the ethnographic, capturing the longevity of the anthropologist's contributions that have opened up space for exploring health as a construction and a contested way of being, local moral worlds and human conditions, and the arts of caregiving. The second is conceptual, as an intellectual practice that interferes with or bends our thinking about what remains as a concern for (and means of attending to) "modes of being human" and the ethical, and the political amid all kinds of posthuman turns in anthropology and critical theory.[19] And the third is vis-à-vis the possibilities for a publicly engaged anthropology: innovating new spaces for scholarship, calling on social scientists to seek broader audiences, and working to transcend the gaps between positions of empirical rigor and critique—spaces of interference—to cultivate what Kleinman calls a moral movement for social change that can inspire new arts of living.

As scholars aware of the limits of reasoned discourse in interfering in profiteering machineries and exclusionary worldviews, yet also inspired by emancipatory ideas, we wonder for whom we should be writing and the forms of understanding and doing our storytelling might unleash. Facing unmoored social and ever more complex human health predicaments, how might a *care-ful* anthropology encompass radically divergent forms and definitions of living and dying? And how might a concern with "what really matters" to peoples attend to issues in beyond-human, beyond-material realms (ecological, religious, and so on)?[20]

Ethnographically attentive to the interdependence and plasticity of lifeforms across scales, the contributors to this volume place themselves in dialogue with Kleinman's multiple interferences by weaving together the affective trajectories of singular lives and "tiny solidarities" with large-scale political-economic, technological, medical, and environmental dynamics.[21] As Judith Butler notes, "Perhaps the human is the name we give to this very negotiation that emerges from a living creature among creatures and in the midst of forms of living that exceed us."[22] But tracking such negotiations over the figuring, disfiguring, and refiguring of human conditions is never only the prerogative of the social scientist.

Throughout *Arc of Interference*, we engage and write *with* people and their beleaguered lifeworlds. Aware that "history is literally present in all that we do" (in the words of James Baldwin), we seek to learn how vulnerable peoples understand and conceptualize their plight and do the work of scaling, healing, and inventing in everyday interactions.[23] People, the worlds they navigate, and the outlooks they articulate are more compounding, incomplete, and multiplying than dominant analytical schemes tend to account for, or are even capable of conceptualizing. These essays offer a thought space for their survivals and horizon making and for a theorizing that is never detached from praxis.

Arc of Interference is organized into four parts, each clustered around a concept, theory, or problem space addressed by Arthur Kleinman over his professional and intellectual arc. The ethnographic foci of these chapters span histories to the present and engage Kleinman's work with various degrees of explicitness while cross-pollinating multiple intellectual traditions. These encounters with Kleinman's empirical and theoretical contributions circumvent reification and, instead, attend to their open-endedness and ongoing influences on medical anthropology.

In "Part I: Traversing Imperiled Worlds and Envisaging Human Futures," we are immersed in a series of dystopic worlds marked by uncontrolled wildfires, border violence, and suicide by self-immolation. These are contexts in which the reconsideration of the prospects for survivability and caregiving feel more urgent than ever, but where the moral certainty that could drive that survival and care has become inextricably entwined with racial and nationalist politics, a grievous politics of exclusion, and the onset of paralysis in the face of environmental destruction by an overheating planet and the demise of conventional forms of expertise.

The chapters by Vincanne Adams, Davíd Carrasco, and Adriana Petryna bring into stark relief the question of what prospects remain for the figure of the human and for action under these conditions of duress. How might an anthropology that is committed to the work of rectifying social suffering, moral clarity, and care—themes for which Kleinman was a trailblazer throughout his career—best attend to the specter and evidence of demise? How, in other words, might our very assumptions about how best to do a contemporary moral anthropology be shaped by sustained ethnographic immersion in how people the world over are reckoning with the possibilities of interference, even as moral certainty and imaginable futures increasingly recede from view?

In "Part II: The Category Fallacy and Care amid the Experts," we are asked to consider how the ethnographic archive might serve as a critical interference in the field of medical innovation and in improving forms of clinical care. Kleinman's extensive legacy sits squarely in this terrain, where the insights of the anthropological imagination recalibrate, or even unseat, presumed architectures of diagnosis and response. Early on, Kleinman noted that cross-cultural health researchers must keep in mind that culture does more than merely color the experience of illness; it actually informs the very categories by which illness is understood and through which certain forms of intervention are deemed possible. Kleinman termed the failure to recognize the foundationally cultural constructions of illness as the "category fallacy."[24] Initially levied at transcultural psychiatry, this critique has shaped an entire school of thought in medical anthropology.

Here, Salmaan Keshavjee, David S. Jones, and Janis H. Jenkins draw from their inceptions in the worlds of global health, social medicine, anthropology, and the history of science to reveal how the social construction of diagnostic categories and therapeutic possibilities for tuberculosis, heart disease, and mental health across diverse settings—from India to the American Southwest—can have profound implications for health policy and caregiving, caught as they are between injunctions to amplify the realm of the possible and to settle for the "appropriate" or "sustainable." Interference here takes the form of decolonizing global health via unsettling its most common senses, highlighting the fallibility of assumptions surrounding scarcity and the affliction and death those assumptions ensure and calling to task regimes of care that are premised on institutionalized inequities.

In "Part III: Worlds of Biotechnological Promise and the Plasticity of Self and Power," Lawrence Cohen, Marcia C. Inhorn, and Margaret Lock explore the possibilities and perils of new regimes of knowledge and care that are emerging around biometrics, reproductive health, and epigenetics as they impinge on self-fashioning, the body politic, and "the art of living socially."[25] Their essays consider the world-making capacities of technological innovations in computer science, experimental medicine, and the life sciences and their multifarious impacts on vulnerable human populations. We see these projects and their ambivalent effects at play in the promises of biometrics to maximize welfare and health-care inclusion in India; the use of reproductive technologies as inter-Asian opportunities for family making; and the use of epigenetic technologies to map human life under conditions of environmental decline and historical trauma vis-à-vis settler colonialism.

Collectively, the chapters in part III show how science and technology are integral to the restructuring of power relations and bodily experience. Highlighting the plasticity of both biopolitical governance and human aspiration, the authors refute tacit and coherent notions of the self, biology, and the social. All the while, they remind us that the stakes of categories such as "progress" and "innovation" in times of such accelerated technocapitalist reformulations are not just alignments of culture and expectation, but also a consideration of technologies' moral and political wakes. Interference here comes not in the form of directing clinical care, but in recalibrating our certainty around who the figure of the self or human is at the center of technological progress and in crafting an ethnographic sensibility that is closely attentive to peoples' own "bricolage."[26]

In "Part IV: Tracing Arts of Living (or, Anthropologies after Hope Has Departed)," Robert Desjarlais, João Biehl, and Jean Comaroff reflect on caregiving, anthropological thought, and writing in the face of death and the world's fundamental contingency. Drawing from their long-term relations with their ethnographic interlocutors in Nepal and Brazil, respectively, Desjarlais and Biehl explore the moral and emotional dynamics and mutual gift giving at work in caring for the afflicted—the relational "now of cognizability," in Walter Benjamin's words—and think through the spectral care for those absent or faintly present, pondering how these memorials both inform and exceed peoples' ongoing arts of existence.[27] Comaroff extends these intimate meditations by brainstorming the role of social thought "on borrowed time." Taking into account anthropology's historical reckonings with the figure of the human, as well as core insights from this volume's critical essays, she offers us a newly humanist ethical compass in the midst of the Anthropocene.

These meditations on the practical wisdom of caregiving and healing that traverses and transcends individual lives, symptoms and their schemes, and the chaotic present, then, also provoke a more nuanced way to understand the simultaneous relationship of the anthropologist—as caregiver, as scholar, as activist, as storyteller—to broader arcs of history and the unknown. Here the authors find common ground on the idea of the *ethnographic open*, which forces us to think about the human figures that are crafted, persist, and reemerge through multigenerational bonds of affect, love, and ethnographic relationality—call it ethical immanence.

In an afterword to the volume, Arthur Kleinman reflects on the preceding chapters in relation to his own experiences as an anthropologist and caregiver, particularly for his late wife and lifelong collaborator, Joan Kleinman.

"The soul of care," as he poignantly notes, lies in its irreducible sociality, efforts at presence, and persistent moral obligations.

———

And so we return to the imperiled present and the particular ethics of care to which we are called. For it may be this *ethnographic open* that will enable us to remain attuned to the overwhelming forces of inequality, structural violence, and myopic politics that have now accumulated to what seems a breaking point, but also to the plasticity of people enacting moments of transformation and to the unfinished nature of what may yet unfold—to what may transcend this vertiginous moment and our social ills.

There is indeed a great deal of demise going on, from the utter impotence of dismantled welfare systems to new scales of police brutality and health inequities, cultures and discourses of appalling exclusion and silencing—but there is also a great deal of envisaging and working for; of tinkering, creativity, and previously unimagined coalitions of solidarity emerging.[28] New conceptions of and modes of engendering security proliferate; new systems of mutual aid abound in communities; and efforts to secure some basic universal access to care seem more urgent, as well as more possible, than ever before.

How we maintain a state of wonder at the radical unpredictability of social and political trajectories while calling to account that which must be named is the question at hand. It resembles the intentionalities and commitments not unlike that of ethnographic research with its perils (the foreclosure of analytic opportunities under the weight of already sedimented theory) and possibilities (interfering with new forms of thinking, acting, politics and caring emerging from the lifeworlds and imagination of real people navigating fraught conditions).[29] Wonder, after all, is not just wishful thinking. It has its etymological roots in astonishment, suggesting an unfamiliar orientation to social and political realities and to ideals of well-being. To be committed to this astonishment is to invite, as ethnography does, contradictions and unknowns as interferences in our everyday knowledge and practice. In considering and advancing medical anthropology's long *arc of interference*, the essays assembled here provide us with a provisional map of dispositions to adopt as we live, study, write about, and interfere always open to both what is immanent and unthought within and what may be beyond these worlds on edge.

Notes

1 | Biehl and Locke, "Ethnographic Sensorium." See also Adams, *Markets of Sorrow, Labors of Faith*; Allison, *Precarious Japan*; Garcia, *The Pastoral Clinic*; Livingston, *Improvising Medicine*; Malabou, *Plasticity at the Dusk of Writing*; Miyazaki, *The Method of Hope*; Pandian, *A Possible Anthropology*; Povinelli, "The Will to Be Otherwise/The Effort of Endurance"; Simpson, *Mohawk Interruptus*; Stewart, *Ordinary Affects*; Thomas, *Political Life in the Wake of the Plantation*.

2 | Biehl and Günay, "How to Teach Anthropology in a Pandemic?"

3 | Greene and Vargha, "How Epidemics End."

4 | Campt, *Listening to Images*; Davis, *Are Prisons Obsolete?*; Gilmore, *Golden Gulag*; Glaude, *Begin Again*; Ralph, *The Torture Letters*; Shange, *Progressive Dystopia*; Taylor, *From #BlackLivesMatter to Black Liberation*; Vitale, *The End of Policing*; Williams, *The Pursuit of Happiness*.

5 | Haraway, *When Species Meet*, 89.

6 | Mbembe, *Out of the Dark Night*, 2.

7 | Biehl, *Will to Live*; Biehl and Petryna, *When People Come First*; Geertz, "Common Sense as a Cultural System"; Mbembe, *Out of the Dark Night*.

8 | Petryna, "Horizoning"; Petryna, "Wildfires at the Edges of Science."

9 | Davis, *With My Mind on Freedom*, 93–94.

10 | See, for example, Bourgois and Schonberg, *Righteous Dopefiend*; Briggs and Mantini-Briggs, *Tell Me Why My Children Died*; Farmer, *Pathologies of Power*; Fassin, *When Bodies Remember*; Holmes, *Fresh Fruit, Broken Bodies*; Knight, *Addicted. Pregnant. Poor*; Whyte, *Second Chances*.

11 | On structural vulnerability, see, for example, Farmer, "Never Again?"; Metzl and Hansen, "Structural Competency"; Quesada et al., "Structural Vulnerability and Health." On racialization, see, for example, Hansen, "Pharmaceutical Prosthesis and White Racial Rescue in the Prescription Opioid 'Epidemic'"; Hansen and Netherland, "Is the Prescription Opioid Epidemic a White Problem?"; Rouse, *Uncertain Suffering*.

12 | Adams, "Disasters and Capitalism . . . and COVID-19"; Biehl, "Pharmaceuticalization"; Biehl, "The Pharmaceuticalization and Judicialization of Health"; Caduff, "The Semiotics of Security"; Fassin, "Another Politics of Life Is Possible"; Mbembe, "Necropolitics"; Rose, "Biopolitics in the Twenty-First Century"; Stevenson, "The Psychic Life of Biopolitics"; Ticktin, "Where Ethics and Politics Meet"; Willse and Clough, *Beyond Biopolitics*. The pandemic is thus also a test case for the epistemes, institutions, and architectures of global health and particular strategies for security and financing, which have proliferated in recent decades and all emerge out their own particular histories, political economies, and ideologies, beckoning for critical analyses that provincialize singular narratives while also enabling granular insights into the contingencies that lead to particular institutional failings, even for seemingly universal and historic epidemics: see, for example, Farmer

et al., *Reimagining Global Health*; Adams, *Metrics*; Biehl and Petryna, *When People Come First*; Frankfurter, "Conjuring Biosecurity in the Post-Ebola Kissi Triangle"; Lakoff, *Unprepared*; Richardson, "On the Coloniality of Global Public Heath"; Richardson et al., "Ebola and the Nature of Mistrust."

13 | Biehl and Neiburg, "Oikography." See also Marcelin, "A linguagem da casa entre os negros no Recôncavo Baiano."

14 | Kleinman, "How Rituals and Focus Can Turn Isolation Into a Time for Growth."

15 | In his total corpus of seven single-author books, four multiauthor books, twenty-nine coedited volumes, and hundreds of journal articles and book chapters, Arthur Kleinman has devoted himself to exploring the social and structural predicaments of suffering, creating a whole genre of philosophical study aimed at grasping the nuances of psychic and social distress. His edited collections have covered the ground from global mental health, violence, and social suffering to global pharmaceuticals and subjectivity. For a complete list of his publications, see Kleinman's Harvard University faculty webpage at https://anthropology.fas.harvard.edu/people/arthur-kleinman.

16 | See, for example, Nichter, *Global Health*; Scheper-Hughes, "The Primacy of the Ethical"; Singer, "Critical Medical Anthropology"; Singer et al., "Syndemics and the Biosocial Conception of Health," and any number of the critical science studies inflected critiques of medical knowledge, including, among others, Kaufman, *The Ageless Self*; Kaufman, *Ordinary Medicine*; Latour and Woolgar, *Laboratory Life*; Lock, *Encounters with Aging*; Mol, *The Body Multiple*; Young, *The Harmony of Illusions*.

17 | Kleinman, "The Background and Development of Public Health in China"; Kleinman, "Medicine's Symbolic Reality"; Kleinman, "Some Issues for a Comparative Study of Medical Healing"; Kleinman, "Toward a Comparative Study of Medical Systems."

18 | Kleinman, *The Soul of Care*, 236.

19 | Winter, "Un-settling the Coloniality of Being/Power/Truth/Freedom," 264.

20 | Kleinman, *What Really Matters*.

21 | Lévi-Strauss, *The View from Afar*, 287.

22 | Butler, *Notes Toward a Performative Theory of Assembly*, 43.

23 | Baldwin, "The White Man's Guilt," 723.

24 | Kleinman, *Rethinking Psychiatry*, 14–15.

25 | Wilkinson and Kleinman, *A Passion for Society*, 163.

26 | Lévi-Strauss, *The Savage Mind*, 17.

27 | Benjamin, *The Arcades Project*, 591–92.

28 | Moten, *Black and Blur*, 33.

29 | Stainova, "Enchantment as Method."

PART I

Traversing Imperiled Worlds *and* Envisaging Human Futures

IN OUR CURRENT WORLDS ON EDGE, what prospects remain for the figure of the human as social?

Here, anthropologists consider the ways in which sociopolitical dynamisms and human futures might be eclipsed by forms of epistemological certainty. Exploring metrics and technological fixes, the authors theorize anthropological ways to deprivilege the centrality of human experience and politics under conditions of ecological threat. They suggest that the present moment calls for a renewed human science of the uncertain and unknown and that maintains an ethnographic focus resolutely on the diversity of human conditions, entangled as they are with myriad nonhuman forces.

Throughout his career, Arthur Kleinman has persistently returned to the primacy of the social in shaping experience and the possibilities for and nature of care. He developed the concept "local moral world" to underscore his perspectives on the human conditions, practical solidarities, and intersubjectivities that are situated in and emergent from networks of social relations, even amid structural forces that are global in scale. As he put it, "For almost all of us, everyday life experience in communities and networks—no matter how influenced we are by global forces of communication, commerce, and the flow of people—centers on what is locally at stake."[1] Kleinman went on to apply this critical perspective throughout his career to other types of knowledge that rest on notions of a bounded, autonomous patient: normative rationalities of care (bioethics); static social systems (epidemiology); and the promises of universal fixes for health problems (global health).

Our current predicament, in which ongoing environmental, social, and political upheaval color peoples' everyday existences the world over, beckons for more pliable analytics of "local," "structure," "the social" and "community." Political forces on all sides mobilize notions of moral certainty in ways that conflict, and technocratic regimes of social reform promise inclusion while also carrying with them the possibility of more deeply entrenched inequities. Toxicities and exhausted ecologies—the collateral byproducts of growing middle classes and excessive consumerism—threaten human suffering on a massive scale and prompt us to consider how practices of care might be extended to (and emerge from) nonhuman actors, as well. Anthropologists in part I thus probe, tweak, and swerve from Kleinman's trailblazing work on social suffering, structural violence, and local moral worlds for these troubled times while carrying with them the humanism and moral impetus that has always defined Kleinman's commitments to contemporary medical anthropology.

"The angel of history . . . is on fire," Vincanne Adams writes in her chapter, exploring the harrowing figure of the self-immolating Tibetan. How might the desire for moral certainty in a place where socialist, modernist, and Buddhist demands have become inextricably set against one another, Adams asks, have twisted into a predicament in which death by fire becomes thinkable and at times inescapable? Moral certainty, she writes, cannot be summoned from a common rhetoric of moral philosophy, or even from a coherent sense of what a local moral world look like in this place, when death is the effect of such certainty.

David Carrasco comes to a different conclusion, taking up the figure of the migrant who dies and disintegrates "into human dust" in the Mexican-American borderlands to explore the storytelling of devotional *retablos*. What might be learned from the violence of forced migration through barren and "killing" deserts, but also from the forms of meaning making and religious practice—the "redressive actions"—that also color migrants' experiences? Beyond abjection and "necroviolence," he asks how attending to moral formations of care in relation to the sacred, family ties, and aesthetics can fight erasure and enrich our concepts of human presence and responses to suffering.

Finally, Adriana Petryna's chapter considers how wildfire experts and ecologists are reckoning with "runaway climate change," yielding "intricate superstructures of surprise" and the sense that humanity has "run out of time" as it faces the real and devastating toll of unpreparedness—a predicament for which dominant scientific models and existential improvisation can neither provide adequate reassessment nor transformative potential. Rather than obliterate the human, Petryna argues that this "vast abrupt" necessitates "horizoning work"—a mode of thinking that considers disaster against "a horizon of expectation" that translates panic into tests of collective care and, in the process, shapes human futures in which people "can still act."

Note

1 | Kleinman, "Moral Experience and Ethical Reflection," 70.

Death by Fire

The Problem of Moral
Certainty in China's Tibet

TIBET IS ON FIRE.

The video footage is of a flaming person. His tortured face appears to suggest a posture of equipoise. And yet his flesh starts to melt as the winds pull the flames up and away from his body. Women in the crowd are screaming in panic. Policemen try to put out the flames with blankets and fire extinguishers. This self-immolator did not, but others have wrapped themselves in barbed wire, stymieing efforts to keep them alive. Who can blame them? Who would want to live after being burned alive? In truth, most of the Tibetan self-immolators have died, and only a few live on with grievous injury.

The problem of self-immolations in China's Tibet was, by the summer of 2018, catastrophic. Starting in 2009, roughly 154 Tibetans had self-immolated there, not including the ten or so among exile Tibetans who lived in India.[1] The most recent in China's Tibet, as of the writing of this chapter, was on March 7, 2018: a man in his forties named Tsekho Tugchak, from the Ngaba Prefecture of the eastern Tibetan Autonomous Region (TAR). Even though the number of self-immolations has slowed since that time, the persistence of their perceived rationale, and the ease with which they are called on to signal a life that has become intolerable, continues as if self-immolations were still happening in great numbers today. The maintenance of official security gates at high-traffic tourist sites in most TAR cities affirms the ongoing fear that persists regarding anyone carrying petrol (or smelling of it).

Just what are the perceived rationales of these self-immolators? Mostly, deaths like Tsekho's occurred in public places, often with self-immolators calling out praise for the Dalai Lama while setting aflame their petrol-drenched bodies. Some left behind notes about their motivations being directed at religious freedom and against political oppression. Still, even with these messages, and even with the need for these immolations to be meaningful in ways that seem obvious, there continues to be a great deal of debate and concern over what they mean and what to do about them. Just how to decipher self-immolations had become, by the time they reached more than a hundred, a source of great concern and a dilemma in regard to the moral contours of caring about them. In this chapter, I interrogate the problem of moral uncertainty that is both triggered by and, I would argue, *a cause of* this tragic set of enactments.

To make something morally certain, Arthur Kleinman argues, is to carve a path through worlds that are formed by social demands that, in fact, frequently make morality unclear. To find moral clarity is to achieve a form of care, and care, he writes and often reminds us, is "the invisible glue that holds society together."[2] Kleinman's work and approach (and particularly his 2006 book *What Really Matters*) have been pathbreaking in defining both morality and the ethical, and not simply as forms of culturally constituted reasoning about right versus wrong. Rather, he calls for an insistence on *an imperative toward relevance* in a world where being moral is sometimes conflicted and often tightly wrapped up in the ordinary acts of everyday life. His work clarifies that *to be ethical* means considering morality in our ethnographic engagements that are both intimate and social, as well as professional and discursive. He asks us to think about *what really matters* in our effort to make ourselves moral agents, especially at times of threats to our existence—in times of existential precarity—as a way of not just living but also doing ethnography *carefully*. What can be said, then, of how care-ful ethnography may also mean embracing the prospect that morality cannot be certain or that certainty is dangerous? In what follows, I interrogate the challenge of deciphering and relying on moral certainty among Tibetans whose morality drives them to death and of efforts to do care-ful ethnography in the face of such tragic deaths in China's Tibet.

Self-immolations in China's Tibet are events largely crafted by history and by the long-brewing and complicated problem of modern secularism that has entangled both Tibetans and their Buddhism in particular kinds of demands that, in a word, are morally confusing. These demands have made moral certainty—even about things such as self-immolation—a necessary burden. Following Kleinman, we might ask: What are the limits to moral certainty? And given this insight, what kind of anthropology is of use here?

Self-Immolation as Communication

Self-immolation could be seen as a form of suicide, as death in life before it has been fully lived by self-choice. In this sense, the self-immolator is never silent. In fact, the opposite is true: the self-immolator speaks too much, says too much, about both death and the limits of a life that can be lived. But what, exactly, is he or she saying in China's Tibet?

My Tibetan colleague and friend Phem Phuti, who talked with me about Tibetan self-immolations when there had been about 130 of them, said that this is not an easy question to answer. "Many explanations can be found," she said, "but not all of them agree." The obvious rationale gleaned from the evidence performed and left behind by self-immolators is that they are political, done in protest of the Chinese occupation of Tibet, and thus are acts of moral certainty through self-sacrifice.[3] But, not surprisingly, official Chinese press reports on self-immolations in Tibet characterize them as the opposite—as enactments by unstable people; by those who had been already deemed *mad* and thus were incapable of being logical, intentional, or (especially) political or moral. In this official view, the suicides do not and cannot speak for widespread discontent in Tibet because these people chose to kill themselves; they are acts of people who renounced their claims to moral certainty. In other words, the self-immolators are but a few irrational malcontents who have lost their moral compass. It would not be wrong to note that this official reasoning makes a certain kind of sense. Phem Phuti affirmed this partly when she asked me, rhetorically, "Does a suicide ever truly make sense?" The mere act of setting oneself on fire demands at least some recognition of a departure from rational and reasonable moral action.

The fact that many of the self-immolators have been monks (and a few nuns) only makes the claims about the morality and rationality of the acts more confusing, and it certainly disrupts official explanations. The exemplar for Tibetan self-immolations, Phem Phuti's husband Jangba told me, is Thích Quảng Đức, the Vietnamese monk whose self-immolation in 1963 at a crowded intersection in Saigon is widely recognized as a political and reli-gious protest against rising Catholicism and discrimination against Buddhists under conditions of the US-funded war in his country. That Tsekho (the lat-est self-immolator in Tibet), from Ngaba, lit himself on fire on March 7, 2018, echoes the embers of Thích Quảng Đức, since Tsekho chose to self-immolate during the same week that would commemorate the famous Tibetan Uprising Day (March 10, 1959) when many Tibetans came out into the streets of Lhasa to express opposition to the then nearly decade-long presence of Chinese forces and Communist Party governance. Thus, one might be led to think that these religious people are self-immolating as an act of moral certainty. Monks and nuns are the people most likely to be burdened by restrictions on religious freedom in China's Tibet, thus lending credence to the idea that self-immolations blur politics with moral action and moral certainty.

It is true that religious acts are often (and always have been) also *political* in Tibet. The historical theocracy held that seats of political power (at least since the rise of the Buddhist government in the thirteenth century) were monastic, and sectarian conflict (among other things) played a role in creat-ing the political vulnerabilities that led to the success of China's "Liberation" there in the 1950s.[4] Since that time, religious institutions ostensibly have been carved off from politics (under the demands of the Cultural Revolu-tion and the communist state), but this does not mean they are not also seen as political threats. Religious institutions in China's Tibet were stripped of autonomous political power, but under secular rule they were seen as hotbeds of political resistance in new ways. Because of this, monks and nuns were told what they could and could not study and who they could and could not worship, and these impositions were crafted in relation to Beijing's antipathy for the former Tibetan leader (the Dalai Lama) and his particular branch of Tibetan Buddhism (Gelukpa), which had been the base of national power for centuries. Although the region is called an "Autonomous Region," Tibet has been controlled by Communist Party directives emanating from Beijing since the "Liberation."

In sum, rather than political seats, as in historical Tibet, Tibetan religious institutions became a thorn in the side of government in China's modern-izing Tibet. The Chinese government has consequently had to maintain a persistent form of doublespeak about religion, patterned after their political position on all minorities in China: Tibetan Buddhism is to be preserved and admired as a treasure of the greater Chinese nation *and* it is a problem for modern secularist rule and thus persistently needs government interference and management. To make matters worse, the active and reactive political resistance from the Tibetan exile government in India has augmented the degree to which these religious institutions have been a source of political trouble for the Beijing-controlled government in China's Tibet. This history surely plays an important role in the predicament of moral certainty among self-immolators.

The Chinese government's explicit effort to drive a secular wedge into the institutions of religion, to divide church from state, enabled it to craft notions of civil morality that were and are disconnected from moral discourses of Buddhism and are based instead on notions of socialist ethicality. In this way, and not unlike in the rest of China, the pathway to Chinese modernity in Tibet created many rifts over moral certainty. Again, this history helps to make sense of how and why self-immolations *feel* and are scripted as political. To self-immolate as an act of religious devotion in Tibet is to perform an act of politics against the state, even if the official media portrayals of these suicides are that they are *not political*. Since voicing political opposition to the state in Tibet is officially illegal, self-immolation could be seen as a way of not just speaking but, rather, *shouting* political discontent as an act of moral (and religious) certainty. Still, many Tibetans are not so sure about this.

The ambiguity over the morality of self-immolation, even while many pronounce it decidedly morally virtuous, stems partly from the fact that Tibetan Buddhism considers suicide the ultimate *unvirtue*—an act that shouts not just moral uncertainty but a kind of *immorality*. So even though Tibetan Buddhism (like other forms of Buddhism) is based on the notion of preparing oneself for the inevitability of death, suicide is considered a very morally problematic form of death. It is, in a word, karmically burdensome in ways that make it hugely immoral—a karmic burden that cannot be rectified. That Tibetan self-immolators are seen by many Tibetans as moral heroes in relation to their sacrifice for a religious and political cause thus comes up against other Tibetan insights about how these deaths fail to accomplish the moral outcomes for which their politics hope, thus becoming both morally and politically bereft.

Phem Phuti's husband, Jangba, explained this to me when he said that self-immolations are a most violent instance of the failure of religion, morality, and politics. The idea that self-immolations suggest is that hope for a "free Tibet" is quite literally lost with the burning flesh of its once breathing citizens. If religious virtue must be shown in this way, he reasoned, then what is the point of fighting for religious freedom? What kind of Tibet would this achievement be hoping for? Worse still, he noted, it could be said that such heroism prompts even more deaths in copycat gestures, joining the cause of

Tibet's liberation through self-sacrifice ultimately destroys the very forms of virtue that Tibetans hope to preserve through political independence. Despite Jangba's view that Tibet was an occupied nation, he refused self-immolation as morally heroic. To valorize self-immolation as heroism would be to valorize the *death* of religion, to turn it into *no more* than a political battle. In other words, self-immolations could not be simultaneously politically and morally virtuous in China's Tibet.

The sea of conflicting rationales and explanations for self-immolations suggest a nightmare for moral virtue for many Tibetans. Moral certainty becomes itself an invitation to the death of not only the person but also of Buddhist morality, creating a series of nested confusions about the purpose of these deaths. Self-immolation as a moral act gets tangled in a politics that make deciphering these suicides impossible, full of messy confusion and silences, even while (again) speaking too loud. The ambiguity over how to read self-immolations will not likely be cleared up anytime soon in China's Tibet, even as the politics and moral demands that drive them continue to be enough to drive one mad—mad enough to light oneself on fire.

One might, from this account, be led to think that self-immolation in contemporary Tibet arises from discontent over the occupation by China and its political demands, but I would also argue that the moral ambiguities deriving from tensions between religion and political secularism were forged long before Chinese occupation in the 1950s. These earlier pressures point not to Chinese but to European and American investments in making Tibetan Buddhism itself a project of secularism. The predicament of moral uncertainty in relation to self-immolation in China's Tibet, in other words, may also arise from generations of entanglements between Tibetans and Westerners for whom Tibet has been seen as, ironically or tragically, a place where moral certainty is a given.

To trace this entangled history—a project that requires much more than can be done in this short essay—I offer a cursory tracing of several moments of historical encounters between Tibetans and others. First I look at the arrival of British and American scientific forms of reason in Buddhist Tibet in the late nineteenth and early twentieth centuries. I then look at the modern-day incarnations of these fascinations as they appear in the work of American scientists who are trying to translate Buddhist moral practices into secular knowledge. In these encounters, we can see how Tibetans have long been thought to be bearers of moral certainty—a projection that has become deeply troubling to the political movement to rid Tibet of Chinese occupation.

These historical threads point to what Talal Asad identified as forms of epistemic rupture in the meaning and routes to morality and to the impositions of notions of moral certainty on Tibetans in relation to their identity, knowledge, and truth.[5] While my explorations here cannot prevent self-immolation in China's Tibet or resolve their meaning definitively, my hope is that they can shed light on how demands for moral certainty may themselves become deadly. They also invite reflection on what it means to do morally informed, care-ful ethnography in a place such as China's Tibet.

European and American Science in Tibet:
Making Certain the Moral Basis of Truth

In the early twentieth century, British and Americans were fascinated with Tibet as a land of spiritually esoteric and mysterious beauty. Much of this fascination was created by traveling explorers who imagined themselves as translators of religious exoticism, having secretly and sometimes in disguise made their way into this remote and forbidden region.[6] It was, however, not until the early 1900s that Western colonial aspirations appeared at the edges of the Tibetan plateau, and they arrived in and through forms of technological violence. For instance, the British Younghusband expedition arrived in 1904 in Lhasa, where British soldiers killed hundreds of monks whose muzzle-loader rifles were no match for the Gatling gun the British managed to wheel all the way over the Himalayas.

This event, and the stationing of a British representative in Lhasa thereafter, created new kinds of encounters that put religious thinking in conversation with modern European science and created a love-hate relationship with secular forms of reason among the Tibetan elite. The impact of these guns, for example, was apparently so impressive that the then reigning Dalai Lama tried soon after to purchase more of them for his own government.[7] The Tibetan embrace of modern European scientific technologies and secular forms of reason eventually led to great rifts within the Tibetan aristocracy—rifts that (alongside sectarian disputes) weakened the government just as it was confronted with the rise of Communist China.[8] Debates over the utility of such technologies and modern scientific methods stirred the pot of moral certainty among educated literati who sought to weigh the moral value against the moral risk of things such as the Gatling gun and of secularity itself.

Sir Charles Bell, Britain's political officer for Bhutan, Sikkim, and Tibet described the fascination of the then Dalai Lama (the thirteenth) with the technologies of modern science that were finding their way to the Tibetan plateau.[9] The theocratic ruler was apparently enamored of watches and microscopes, revealing himself to be a curious and independent thinker even if distinctly unmodern in his commitment to religious claims about the world. Alex McKay has documented the embrace of modern biomedical technologies among Tibetans along the borderlands and edges of the theocracy's reach.[10]

One of the most robust renderings of the early Tibetan encounter with European science is offered by Donald S. Lopez Jr. in his book *The Madman's Middle Way* (2006), about the politically progressive and controversial monk Gendun Chopel, who lived at the turn of the twentieth century.[11] Chopel was a prolific writer, producing the monolithic text *The White Annals* (translated in 1978), as a cultural history of his country. Chopel's love for European science and technology put him in opposition to the educated literati of the Buddhist aristocracy of his time. He characterized his Buddhist peers' resistance to European science on grounds that it was *without morality* as shortsighted and wrongheaded. They believed European sciences were immoral because they often contradicted Buddhist scriptural claims. Chopel argued against this reasoning, noting that the challenge modern European science offered to scriptural knowledge was superior to Buddhist forms of knowledge because it was "an empirical knowledge derived from observation, and therefore superior to the knowledge gained from books."[12] For challenging the notion that all truth comes from the scriptural teachings of the Buddha, Chopel was considered a heretic, but, perhaps surprisingly, to defend his position he argued that accepting European science should be done on Buddhist moral grounds. To dismiss European science would be to hold stubbornly to prejudice and recalcitrance, which in its own way would be antithetical to Buddhist ethical positions. It would, in other words, be immoral in a Buddhist sense to reject European science outright.

Chopel's praise for European technologies was carefully constructed with the use of empirical and moral statements. He described scientific technologies as being able to make visible what could not previously be seen: the radio, the X-ray machine, slow-motion photography, and color spectography. "A spyglass constructed by new machines," he wrote, "sees across thousands of miles as if it were the palm of one's hand, and similarly, a glass that sees what is close by makes even the smallest atoms appear the size of a mountain; one can analyze the myriad parts, actually seeing everything."[13] To reject these technologies would be unvirtuous; to accept them as useful tools of knowledge would be taking the moral high road. But Chopel also used

Buddhist scriptural linguistic referents to make this argument. He described scientific reasoning as "holding sunshine in one's hands," an epithet used to describe the Buddha's teachings. Even more tactically, he refused to see science as antithetical to Buddhism and instead proposed the reverse: that "any essential point in Buddhism can serve as a foundation for science."[14] Although Chopel's argument was radical for his time, it presaged the work of later scholars and intellectuals who would embrace European modernity as an imperative of the Tibetan state, much as Chopel did.[15]

Chopel's views were probably inspired in part by epistemic murkiness around the acts of translation that were required to make sense of the engagement between Buddhism and science. He spent time in northern India and was influenced by Europeans there who, in their own ways, were enamored of Tibetan Buddhism. He met the theosophist Madame Helena Blavatsky and learned about her rationalist view of Buddhism, arguing that most of the so-called mystical aspects of Buddhism could be seen as rational in the same ways that science was rational.[16] Mysticism was not beyond the pale of reason; it was its own, competing form of reason.

As if prismatic alter egos, Blavatsky read Buddhism as a rational, even scientific, religion, while Chopel read secular science as capable of serving Buddhism by standing on equal moral footing to religious teachings. Neither of these was true. Buddhism is not a rational religion, and secular science does not offer a moral code. But these misreadings enabled an engagement in which both parties could assume parity and shared moral conviction. This was why, Chopel wrote, "Among the foreigners, some of the many scholars of science have acquired a faith in the Buddha, becoming Buddhists, and [some] have even become monks."[17] These early encounters presage many of the slippages between Buddhism and secular forms of reason that would follow.

At the same time, Chopel knew that his Tibetan compatriots might not share his optimism about these European converts and their ideas about the rationalism of Buddhism. Careful to use language that was familiar to his Tibetan audience, he wrote: "Like the light-rays of the sun and moon in the vastness of space, ... the two, this modern reasoning of science and the ancient teachings of the Buddha, may abide together for tens of thousands of years."[18] In other words, Chopel aimed to carve out space for secular forms of reason within the fold of Buddhism, making the embrace of science a moral certainty and making moral certainty a reason to become modern.[19]

As I said, huge misrepresentations and misunderstandings were going on here. That the theosophists (and modern translators) misrepresented

Buddhism is resoundingly underscored by other work by Lopez.[20] Still, the optimism of an easy marriage of Western science and Buddhism arises from an aspiration that was born in the colonial soup of encounters between practitioners and experts in both science and Buddhism. These encounters bent and blurred notions of religion and science in and around desires for a meeting of the minds, but these early encounters were orchestrated as moral practices under conditions that were challenging, at best. What is interesting about them, however, is how important questions of moral certainty were in the encounters. The idea I am getting at here, following Asad, is that moral certainty was used to establish secular forms of reason in the theocratic state.[21] But these secular forms of reason created ruptures of knowledge and ethics that resonate to this day. Buddhist versions of morality, in fact, have very little in common with the forms of reason that underpin modern technologies such as the Gatling gun, the spectrograph, and the X-ray machine, which, in and of themselves, as noted, have no inherent moral index.

The embrace of European science in Buddhist Tibet required a willingness to believe that moral certainty could exist across both kinds of reason—indeed, despite their different versions of reality—that often contradicted each other. What science offered (but neither Chopel nor the Theosophists accounted for) is the proposition that secular forms of knowledge and reason could provide a basis for moral certainty, but this also meant rejecting Buddhist reasoning about morality. Rather than creating a seamless conjugation of Western modern science to Buddhist ideas of morality, these encounters created huge rifts that, I argue, trickled down to Tibetans trying to live a moral life in an increasingly secular (especially post-Liberation) state. Chopel suffered a sad demise during the reign of the thirteenth Dalai Lama because of his heretical views, but, not surprisingly, he was resurrected as an early modern hero by the Chinese secular state in the early twenty-first century.

Debates over how to be modern in Tibet today point to ruptures around notions of moral certainty that emerged in the early twentieth century and that still inform politics in Tibet. Efforts to modernize in secular ways were ushered in forcefully after Chinese Liberation in the early 1950s, and they were supported by the installed government of Tibet. The secular push, coupled with Communist Party tactics of purging ideological resistance, hit full stride in the Cultural Revolution with various state-sanctioned regimes of political surveillance, incarceration and a persistent suspicion of Buddhist religion. Of course, national policies that variously valorized and demonized traditional religions of the minorities were hard to navigate, and while some religious figures were supported by the government, others were denounced mostly along sectarian lines.

Various programs of social reform (at different times, with differing degrees of force) in education, politics, religion, and social life made it very clear to most Tibetans that secular ideals of morality as propounded in Communist Party socialist ethics were frequently at odds with Buddhist ideals of morality. These ideals created ambiguous medical, social, and political predicaments for Tibetans in regard to their ability to be moral people. I have documented many of these predicaments as instances of ethical rupture and uncertainty in different locations: reproductive health for women and the politicization of suffering, in scientific research and modernizing efforts in Tibetan medicine, and in problems of truth-telling under conditions of state-mandated lying. Certainty about how to be a moral person in Tibet, over the twentieth century, became a complex mess that tangles truth and virtue into a hornet's nest of danger, in which it becomes imperative to steer clear of the secular state's fears of political dissent but, in doing so, requires one sometimes to do immoral things.

My point in walking briskly through this history is to suggest that it is, at least in part, the demand for moral certainty in a place where such certainty is always up for grabs and contested that has spawned self-immolations in China's Tibet. What self-immolations make clear is that moral certainty is itself almost impossible to decipher. To make the case more strongly, I turn now to the other encounters where Tibetans—who, after all, are not self-immolating in a geographic void but, rather, pronouncing their complaint to the world writ large—are possibly provoked by the stirrings of confusion over how to be morally certain.

Tibet in Science: Compassion Laboratories

In 1904, the same year that the Younghusband expedition was mowing down Tibetan monks with a prototype machine gun, the Theravada monk Anagarika Dharmapala was brought to Cambridge, Massachusetts, to give a lecture at Harvard on the Buddhist conception of mind. Evan Thompson reminds us that it was probably this lecture that convinced William James of the rich empirical ground for cross-cultural research and the development of a psychology committed to exploring the subjective seat of perception. According to Thompson, James stood at the end of the lecture on Buddhism and proclaimed that "this is the psychology everybody will be studying twenty-five years from now."[22]

He was largely correct. The path is long and winding that traces the Buddhist religion in the early and mid-twentieth century (including the work of the theosophists) to a contemporary psychology of *mindfulness*. A thread of continuity on that path, however, is the desire to treat Buddhism as a rational, science-like form of knowledge. The effort to bring Buddhist principles of mind training to Westerners begins with a variety of Western Buddhist scholars (trained in Zen, Tibetan, and Theravada traditions) and, especially, the work of Jon Kabat Zin, who invented Mindfulness Based Stress Reduction. Even more secularized iterations of this training are found in therapeutic protocols of cognitive behavioral therapy.

Although there are many overlaps and divergences in the histories of Buddhism in Europe and the United States, one of the more interesting end points of this conversation has been the birth of something called the contemplative sciences—the Western scientific study of Tibetan Buddhism. Starting with a series of conversations with the Dalai Lama, this field has exploded over the past two decades and returns us to questions about how questions about morality are navigated between secular and Buddhist forms of reason.

One of the chief proponents of the contemplative sciences is Richard Davidson, a neuroscientist from the University of Wisconsin, Madison, who wrote about his motivations and inspirations for this work. As a graduate student at Harvard in the early 1970s he became fascinated by both the neurosciences and meditation. He took a retreat in Asia, and his meditation studies enabled him to learn about "generating compassion toward those with whom we may have had conflicts and those who are less fortunate." Through that, he became convinced "that the contemplative traditions of the East had something meaningful to offer us in the West and that this dialogue and synthesis could occur without sacrificing the scientific method that [he] held to and continue[d] to believe in so strongly."[23]

Research (by Davidson's predecessors) that, I believe, is a precursor to work in the contemplative sciences was carried out by Herbert Benson, a Cambridge medical doctor. His work entailed hauling devices up to Himalayan meditation caves to record blood pressure and heart rate, vasodilation and vasoconstriction, among monks who were in the midst of multiyear meditation retreats. By the time of Davidson's research several decades later, Tibetan monks were being brought to the United States, where functional MRIs and CAT scans would be used to ascertain the anatomical and neurochemical pathways of minds in advanced states of meditation. Today, contemplative science researchers hope their findings will translate into clinical therapeutics in work with people on the autism spectrum, trauma victims, and those with high-stress jobs (e.g., security guards). They also study the benefits of meditation for posttraumatic stress disorder, depression, and the reduction of symptoms in autoimmune disorders.[24]

Just as with the theosophists and Chopel, there are many obstacles and misreadings in this translational work that involve assumptions about moral certainty. The surprising death of one Tibetan monk soon after his return from the United States, where he had participated in this research, led other Tibetans to worry about the potential effects of the electrode sensors on the body's subtle energy, especially on what Tibetans call the *srog rlung,* or life force that flows through the inner channels.[25] "Subtle energy" didn't even exist in the scientific episteme, but here it was getting in the way as if it were a real thing, raising questions about how ethical the technologies may or may not be from a Buddhist perspective. This work has thus required the invention of new languages that could and can accommodate invisible things, turning subtle energies into "biofields" that may operate through signaling at chemical/ molecular and physical/atomic levels. The possibilities of *techno-enlightenment* are here being offered through randomized clinical trials, a methodology that is perceived as morally neutral for those who use them but can be seen by those subjected to them as modes of knowing that are harmful.[26]

It would be tempting to talk about how the moral becomes mapped as a technological and measurable end point in these studies or how ethicality is repackaged in the form of *fidelity of research design* and *robustness of the data.* But the attempt to offer neurological mappings of religious behavior can also violate moralities because the religious underpinnings of those moralities are effaced. As the benefits of meditation are primarily based on moral apprehension of the world, the remaking of meditation as an object of scientific inquiry must also reject the prospect that there is no world (no action, no condition) without a moral underpinning. This problem becomes visible in large and in the most minute and subtle ways.

For instance, one of the goals of contemplative science research is to *measure* what Buddhists deliberately and thoughtfully refer to as the *immeasurables* of Buddhist ethical comportment (love, compassion, joy, equanimity).[27] One might ask: What kinds of morality are being crafted here? The terminology of immeasurability is itself a translation, of course, but one that is intentional, signifying the unfathomability of karmic cause and effect. The notion, as I understand it, is meant to incur a sense of insight about wisdom (an experiential state). It is immeasurable in the sense that it cannot be counted both because it is endless and because it is based on experience. The irony of trying to measure the immeasurables is that to do so, one may have to ignore the moral purpose of calling these qualities immeasurable.[28]

If the efforts to translate Buddhism into science in the United States, just as they have been in Tibet, are undergirded by a fundamental assumption—that all of this work is in service to moral virtue—then we should also recognize that these compassion laboratories also produce certain kinds of morality and efface others.[29] For instance, the scholars in this field tend to remain conspicuously silent about the hideous necropolitics of Tibetan self-immolations. I am not suggesting that these scientists should take up the political cause (or be more vocal about their politics than, say, their working with the Dalai Lama already is). But I do think it is worth noting that the framework these studies offer to deal with these ethical fragilities sometimes undermine the very moral indices associated with the Buddhism from which they derive. The proposition that Buddhist training in compassion labs is being studied as an antidote to serious mental health problems becomes an ironic solipsism in view of the fact that highly skilled Buddhist monks in Tibet are sometimes propelled by this training to suicide by self-immolation.

As Tibetan engagements with science have continued to make religious underpinnings of morality speak in and through secular idioms of science and technologies, they continue to make demands on moral sensibilities at the most vulnerable and fragile sites in Tibetan culture and everyday life. Tibetans are not unaware of the role they play as moral arbiters (or as holders of a kind of moral certainty) in the US and European contexts.

Moral Certainty: The Ongoing Life of Death

The motivations of Tibetan self-immolators are ultimately unfathomable, even if they are often wrapped in political verbiage about the independence of Tibet and the return of the Dalai Lama, and even if they are imbued with a type of moral certainty that awkwardly calls on both secular claims to political freedom and religious claims to moral obligation. In proclaiming moral certainty, self-immolators and those who have jumped in to decipher their acts are hoping that these actions will be read as unquestionably virtuous, especially in the eyes of an international community that looks lovingly at Tibetans as purveyors of spiritual and moral insight. I suspect, and what I have tried to trace historically in this essay, is that what is going on with these immolators has less to do with the specifics of political subjugation than with the ongoing effects of living in a place where moral certainty is so needed and so confusing. In this sense, performing certainty through self-immolation might seem like a way to stabilizing morality or to create moral certainty where there is little opportunity to do so, but it ultimately fails.

Tibetans disagree with one another about these things. As I have said, for every Tibetan who feels the need to make a political statement about independence through self-immolation, there are other Tibetans who find these actions of monks deplorable, immoral, and useless. The figure of the Tibetan on fire is one that circulates far and wide even now, many years after the epidemic of them. They call on viewers to both witness and offer some kind of response. In this sense, the participation of those who want Buddhism to provide moral certainty are asked to read the Tibetan who has set himself or herself on fire with a particular lens. But these images and stories don't resolve death as a call to arms to liberate Tibet; rather, they simply make death live on, and on.

Taking this seriously, I turn to the notion that Tibetans might be thought of as "suffering experts," like those described by in Kafka's *A Hunger Artist* (also called *A Starvation Artist*): "Back then the starvation artist captured the attention of the entire city. From day to day while the fasting lasted, participation increased. Everyone wanted to see the starvation artist at least once a day. During the later days there were people with subscription tickets who sat all day in front of the small barred cage. And there were even viewing hours at night, their impact heightened by torchlight."[30]

A subjugation expert is a human subject who is so good at being a political subject, who bears a subjugation so vast and oppressive, who can articulate personal and collective oppression and his people's social suffering in such clear and stunning terms that he or she becomes the subject of anthropological inquiry and writings, time and again, as well as of political interrogations, time and again—with all of this destined for "reports to the academy."

The motivations and aspirations for leading an ethical life in times of ongoing conflict and existential threat in Tibet create all kinds of ambiguities and conceal all kinds of potential violence. Anthropologists like me get caught up in efforts to sidestep one sort of danger, only to reproduce another, even while the self-immolating Tibetan compels us to think in new ways about history, occupation, and moral uncertainty that are specific to the history of this place, and even while asking for a shared sense of obligation to do something. Perhaps moral certainty, in the end, is not one of these things that we need, always, to be pursuing.

Care-ful Ethnography

A painting by Paul Klee titled *Angelus Novus* shows an angel looking as though he is about to move away from something he is fixedly contemplating. His eyes are staring; his mouth is open; his wings are spread. This is how one pictures the angel of history. His face is turned toward the past. Where we perceive a chain of events, he sees one single catastrophe that keeps piling wreckage upon wreckage and hurls it in front of his feet. The angel would like to stay, awaken the dead, and make whole what has been smashed. But a storm is blowing from Paradise; it has got caught in his wings with such violence that the angel can no longer close them. This storm irresistibly propels him into the future to which his back is turned, while the pile of debris before him grows skyward. This storm is what we call progress.[31]

Anthropology frequently runs the risk of two kinds of danger that Walter Benjamin understood. One is reading history as solely a product of structural conditions—the kind Karl Marx wrote about and that changed whole nations forever, but not necessarily all for the better from where Benjamin was sitting. The other danger is in overly sentimentalizing the particular, the irreducible moments of specificity of encounters, affects, and contingencies—fragments of memory that are aesthetically beautiful but ineffectual at preventing such horrors as the forms of postsocialist fascism he witnessed. Benjamin tried to walk the line between the tactics of structure and aesthetics, as his angel of history does, in his overly quoted passage about Klee's painting. Taking only fragments of the real, he lends credibility to the ominous danger that exceeds what could be told as a linear progression of causes and effects. This angel who is thrust into the future with his back turned, able to see only what is already past, attends to the monstrous problem I see in Tibet as a problem of moral rupture.

The angel of history in Tibet is on fire. By reading the crisis of self-immolation in Tibet through this lens, I hope to have shed light on how problems of everyday morality are products not just of everyday living, but also of histories and epistemic formations that make things like truth and moral certainty deeply conflicted. Moral rupture and attempts to promote moral certainty remain open wounds of a past that is full of ignited conflicts and a present that remains unquenchable. Leaving open the question of what self-immolation truly signifies, then, I want to end with the image of the burning angel whose silence and incomprehensibility nevertheless, as I have said, speaks—or, perhaps, shouts—in anguish.

Notes

1 | "Self-immolations by Tibetans," International Campaign for Tibet, accessed May 30, 2019, https://www.savetibet.org/resources/fact-sheets/self-immolations-by-tibetans.

2 | Kleinman, *The Soul of Care*, 236.

3 | See the *Hot Spot* collection in *Cultural Anthropology*, especially the introduction by McGranahan and Litzinger, "Self-Immolation as Protest in Tibet."

4 | Goldstein, *A History of Modern Tibet*.

5 | See Asad, "The Concept of Cultural Translation in British Social Anthropology."

6 | The most sensational of these was Alexandra David-Neel, who wrote such popular books as *My Journey to Lhasa* (1927) and *Magic and Mystery in Tibet* (1932), among more philosophical treatises on Tibetan Buddhism.

7 | Venturi, "The Thirteenth Dalai Lama on Warfare, Weapons and the Right to Self-Defense."

8 | Goldstein, *A History of Modern Tibet*.

9 | Bell, *Tibet*.

10 | Bell, *Tibet*; McKay, *Their Footprints Remain*.

11 | Translated by Lopez, *The Madman's Middle Way*. His journey began in the company of the Indian Sanskrit scholar Rahul Sankrityayan. Perhaps ironically, Pandit Rahul was traveling in Tibet to study an earlier ideological revolution—that of Buddhism's arrival and root taking in the Kingdom of Tibet some 1,300 years earlier. Chopel's assistance to Rahul in his study of Buddhism's history would bring him face-to-face with another ideological revolution as a kind of history in the making. Over his twelve-year residence in India, Chopel became enthralled with science and politics— notably, the communist movement in China and the Independence movement in India.

12 | Lopez, *The Madman's Middle Way*, 18. Janet Gyatso, working through historical medical texts, points out that Tibetan scholars during the seventeenth century had carved out space for an empiricism beyond Buddhist scriptural claims, long before European science arrived on the plateau: Gyatso, "The Authority of Empiricism and the Empiricism of Authority"; Gyatso, *Being Human in a Buddhist World*. Observations of corpses and knowledge of geography and history, for instance, were used to contest medical accounts of the body in Buddhist scriptures. These scholar physicians, however, argued that such empirical realities could reinforce, or accord with, a Buddhist theocratic state. Chopel's goals ultimately were somewhat different.

13 | Lopez, *The Madman's Middle Way*, 19. Lopez offers a short discussion of all of this: see Lopez, *The Madman's Middle Way*, chap. 1.

14 | Lopez, *The Madman's Middle Way*, 19–20.

15 | Goldstein, *A History of Modern Tibet*.

16 | In Europe, science had fully established itself as the authoritative source of knowledge separate from, and often in conflict with, the Christian Church, but Christian missions in Asia were busy undermining Buddhism by calling it idolatry and superstition.

17 | Lopez, *The Madman's Middle Way*, 19.

18 | Chopel, in Lopez, *The Madman's Middle Way*, 21.

19 | Lopez offers several examples that Chopel used to make his case for enter-
taining and accepting European reason, all of which made use of Buddhist
framings even while exceeding them. One of these cases was the scientific
notion that the world is spherical rather than flat. Buddhist depictions of
the world with Mount Meru at the center and four continents spread one to
each side could not be easily reconciled with European notions of the world
as spherical. Chopel calls on the Buddha's notion of *provisional*, rather than
definitive, truth to make the case that they can both be true. Thus, the Buddhist depiction of the universe as flat was "provisional," while the notion of
a spherical world could be seen as definitive. Using another tactic, he argues
that even scriptural forms of reasoning can lead to false truths, such as the
Jaina position that plants have consciousness, which all Buddhists know is
not true. Again, his provocation is to enable European forms of reason and
knowledge to find a home within a Buddhist episteme, or to create space in
Buddhism for the acceptance of scientific claims that would, on their own
terms, efface (if not erode) Buddhist foundations of knowledge. He was a
clever rhetorician and tactician.

20 | See Lopez, *The Scientific Buddha*.

21 | Asad, "The Concept of Cultural Translation in British Social Anthropology."

22 | Thompson, "Neurophenomenology and Francisco Varela," 21.

23 | Davidson and Harrington, *Visions of Compassion*, 108.

24 | See Dahl et al., "Cognitive Processes Are Central in Compassion
Meditation"; Davidson, "Mindfulness-Based Cognitive Therapy and the Pre-
vention of Depressive Relapse"; Davidson, "Well-Being and Affective Style";
Davidson and Harrington, *Visions of Compassion*; Davidson et al., "Alterations
in Brain and Immune Function Produced by Mindfulness Meditation"; Da-
vidson and Kaszniak, "Conceptual and Methodological Issues in Research on
Mindfulness and Meditation"; Lazar et al., "Functional Brain Mapping of the
Relaxation Response and Meditation"; Light et al., "Electromyographically
Assessed Empathic Concern and Empathic Happiness Predict Increased Pro-
social Behavior in Adults"; Lutz et al., "Regulation of the Neural Circuitry of
Emotion by Compassion Meditation"; Maclean et al., "Intensive Meditation
Training Improves Perceptual Discrimination and Sustained Attention";
Rosenkranz et al., "Reduced Stress and Inflammatory Responsiveness in
Experienced Meditators Compared to a Matched Healthy Control Group";
Wallace, *Contemplative Science*.

25 | Davidson and Harrington, *Visions of Compassion*.

26 | Adams, *Metrics*.

27 | See the Shamatha Project, run by Clifford Saron, a neuroscientist at the Uni-
versity of California, Davis: Saron Lab website, https://saronlab.ucdavis.edu.

28 | In other contexts, Evan Thompson explores critical questions about the
contemplative sciences and how they forge certain translations by finding
epistemic overlaps and points of similarity: see Thompson, "Is the Brain a
Decomposable or Nondecomposable System?" What might a neurological
notion of plasticity mean in relation to impermanence, he asks.

29 | Davidson sees science as the arbiter of virtue here, but he also refuses to make decisions without first obtaining approval from the Dalai Lama (including making themselves available for interviews with outsiders such as anthropologists).

30 | I thank Robert Desjarlais for these insights and suggestions offered as personal communication. Earlier translations gave the title as "A Hunger Artist," but more recent translations have gone with the more accurate "starvation."

31 | Benjamin, *Illuminations*, 257–58.

Bringing Up the Bodies

Erasing and Caring for Mexicans
in the Mexico-US Borderlands

Preface

This essay begins with sadness and travels into an earthly inferno where medical anthropology confronts an extreme challenge: how to care for dead bodies disintegrating into human dust in the Mexican American borderlands. This radical form of human erasure takes place in "the land of open graves," where human violence extends its career to anonymous, deceased bodies in a practice Jason De León calls "necroviolence."[1] We now know that, for decades, the US government has employed the Sonoran Desert as a vast killing machine in its policy of PTD, or Prevention through Deterrence. I use terms such as *inferno* and *erasure* to alert the reader to the purposeful obliteration of Mexican bodies, families, and histories that this essay reveals. Given the intensity and depth of the social and psychological aggression against Mexicans in the examples that follow, it is appropriate to be blunt about the challenges we face as anthropologists, historians of religion, and others in the academy.

The term *erasure* has often meant the collective social aggression that makes certain people and groups invisible though they are living among us. It now means dismissing and deporting problematic people from our historical and bureaucratic records and lands. To confront this radical kind of erasure, I present six tableaus to *bring up the bodies* of Mexicans who appear and disappear in multiple locations in the Mexico-US borderlands.[2] The locations are the city morgue in El Paso; a train boxcar in the Arizona desert; a watermelon field in Colorado, the Greater Southwest of Sadness; and the land of open graves where human remains and the precious objects they left behind are identified as *basura* (trash) by some and sacred bundles by others; finally to a hospital in Los Angeles. I use the language of *tableau*, or dramatic historical scene, and *retablo*, or ritual re-creation of miracles in the desert, to write about the religious dimensions of caring for Mexican bodies. Each tableau, or scene, begins with human life, dignity, energy, and action and is reduced by the killing machine to a tableau of death, indignity, stillness, decay. Each *retablo* is a ritual storytelling (through words and images) of human and divine caregiving.

My claim is that religious experience is an indispensable part of many Mexican peoples' experiences, beliefs, and family ties. As William B. Taylor has shown us in his writings on the history of religion in Mexico, many people in contemporary Mexico experience and value their world in part through their awareness of the presence of the sacred in their daily lives. God, the saints, and experiences of the sacred are more than complex ideas. They are living forces that exist nearby and within the daily lives of many Mexicans. Factoring religiosity into our research, policy building, and writing is crucial for those who wish to care for and interpret the bodies on the border. The point is not that scholars should claim an (impossible) certainty about others' worldviews and phenomenologies of migration, suffering, living, or dying. Still, to discount or efface the centrality of religious experiences, beliefs, and practices of migrants in scholarly efforts to evoke migrants' suffering, structural violence, and death is also a kind of erasure—that is, a *denying* of the points of view of others that we seek to understand.

This essay adds these necessary dimensions of caregiving and survival to the existing scholarship on the US-Mexico border through a dialogue with the position of anthropological advocacy taken in the work of Arthur Kleinman. In his work and in the religious art of many surviving migrants, we see "redressive actions": ritual, aesthetic, intellectual, and political actions designed to bring relief, expose the malice of the killing machine, and help mend the suffering.[3] What remains to be seen in innovative strategies for new knowledge is whether the worldviews and religiosity of these ritual, aesthetic, and family ties will be included in the repertoire of anthropologists working and living in the local worlds of the borderlands in truly meaningful and effective ways.

My Father in the El Paso City Morgue

A few months before he took his own life in El Paso, Texas, my father told me a story of horror about Mexican bodies that was a doorway into his crushing depression. He was the founder and director of the El Paso Job Corps Center, where he dedicated the last two decades of his life to helping thousands of teenagers, mainly Mexican Americans who had dropped out or been pushed out of school, to receive education in the vocational trades as a basis for future employment. He was carrying on the tradition of his father, Miguel Carrasco, who had founded the Smelter Vocational School in the 1920s, where hundreds of Mexicans, documented and undocumented, received vocational training and moved out of poverty.[4] My father was born in the Segundo Barrio of El Paso, notorious as one of the poorest and toughest neighborhoods along the nearly two thousand-mile border. He had become widely respected in El Paso for his effective and relentless caring for El Paso youth, but as he approached his seventieth birthday, his Anglo supervisor—a close colleague of Texas governor John Connelly, who was known for his arrogance and bias against Mexicans— began to take psychological and bureaucratic steps to force him out of his job. It was during this painful struggle to survive professionally that he witnessed a deeply troubling scene in the El Paso city morgue. He told me:

> After midnight a few weeks ago, I received a phone call that several of the Job Corps students had been killed in a horrendous car wreck. The students, all Mexican-Americans, had gotten weekend passes from the Job Corps Center where they lived and went joy riding. On I-10, the driver lost control and crashed into a median column, and all five were killed. I knew these young people personally from working with them at the center and had met their mothers when we were considering them for admission. I'd been to the morgue before to identify a few other students over the years, but the neglect of the bodies I saw that night rattled me down inside. To tell you the truth, I haven't been able to go to sleep one night, lying in the darkness, without seeing the bodies piled up in the morgue.
>
> An attendant met me at the door of the morgue, took me down the hall to identify the bodies who were dressed in their Job Corps uniforms.

In the cold room with bright lights there they were—the five black-haired Mexican kids just thrown into a big pile, bodies on top of one another on the table, arms and legs sticking out at odd angles, blood on their heads and clothes, broken and bashed in. A heap of death. A wave of nausea rushed over me, and I had to turn my head and cover my eyes. After a moment's silence an anger rose in me, and I said to the attendant in a harsh voice, "Yes, these are my Job Corps Students. Can't you show some *dignity* to these kids even in death? They deserve *respeto*, hombre." He looked at me as though bored. "We can't move them until the coroner arrives in a few hours," [he said] and walked out of the room. I stood alone with the bodies of the youngsters for a few minutes and looked them over and a flood of heat rose up in my shoulders and neck and I wondered if it was the beginning of a heart attack. Back in the car I sat there for a while and a bitter thought came to me. "All that I've worked for, and it comes to this tonight. These Mexican kids are insulted even in death." You know, son, this is the border; this is El Paso, and maybe I can't take it anymore.

Arthur Kleinman's Caregiving and *Retablo* Practice

My father's tale speaks to my title, "Bringing Up the Bodies," and I choose to bring up and interpret Mexican bodies located in various extreme situations— morgues, boxcars, wars, deserts, and watermelon fields in what Carlos Vélez Ibañez calls "Greater Mexico" and the "Greater Southwest": the "greater" meaning parts of northern Mexico, as well.[5] It is remarkable that these situations of extreme suffering, erasure, and sadness also result in practices of caregiving by scholars who seek to find and, perhaps, change the causes of what put the Mexican bodies down in the first place. My concern with the potency of caregiving in the extreme borderlands is inspired by Kleinman's views:

> I wished to see my own subjectivity—self, sensibility, commitments, will—experienced not as moral theory, but as authorizing feelings and values that could sustain my engagement in the world and connect me to others who mattered to me. Hence my deep subject was not experience as a philosophical problem; it was experience as practice that I was after. And such practice is always about action among others, upon others, best of all, for others. It is through mentoring and caregiving—as doctor and teacher—that I have come closest to finding the object of my quest for wisdom . . . that redeems our humanness amid inevitable disappointment and defeat.[6]

I choose this passage because Kleinman's commitment to the practice of caregiving "among others, upon others, best of all, for others" allows me to test this practice against the extraordinary suffering that Mexicans face in the borderlands. For instance, how can anthropological work qualify as effectively caring for immigrants in maximum travail, in death and decay, and far from their homes and family? In a different essay, "Caregiving as Moral Experience," Kleinman gives us an assist in approaching this pragmatic question. He writes about caregiving as "a different kind of reciprocity . . . a gift exchange and receiving among people whose relationships really matter."[7] It is relationship between the caregiver and the person receiving care that rises to the level of moral caregiving for Kleinman. But again, how does reciprocity work when the anthropologist is faced with caregiving for the dead and disappearing in the fields and deserts of the killing machine in the Greater Southwest? We are forced to ask questions such as: What can become of a relationship of exchange, a gift exchange between the living researchers and the physical remains of Mexicans found and examined in the Sonoran Desert? How can my father's cry about dignity for the dead in the morgue be addressed?

Let's go into the territory where, in the past fifteen years, more than six thousand lost and abandoned bodies have been found, often in barely identifiable conditions, and see how a painter, a filmmaker, a cultural anthropologist, and a new anthropological practice try, against many and sometimes all odds, to be bring dignity to the dead through art and science. I insist that for Kleinman's method to be effective in the killing fields of the borderlands, we must attend more seriously to the point of view of the Mexican families themselves for real moral caregiving to take place. We will see that for many of these Mexicans, one of the most potent, hopeful, and sometimes desperate fight backs to the structural violence of border crossings is religion, taking the form of material memories of divine aid in what I call the "*retablo* pattern." Each *retablo*, a word that comes from two others—*retro* and *tabula*, meaning behind the table (the sacred table in front of the altar of the church)—is a "sacred thank-you note" addressed to God or the saint who cared for and sometimes saved an individual in life-threatening travail. This *retablo* pattern, in its many examples, demonstrates a variety of the "local moral worlds" (to use a Kleinman phrase) that together reveal a sense that the most crucial examples of social solidarity include the presence of divine or spiritual helpers. They live not only behind the table, but also in front of the migrants moving in the borderlands.

Borderlands as a "Boxcar" and Caring as Filmmaking

We begin to come face to face with the dangers of borderlands suffering *and* an attempt at redressive action by looking at *Box Car*, a painting by the Chicano artist George Yepes that was the playbill cover for a production by the same name (figure 2.1). *Box Car* depicts a single Mexican migrant in three phases of descent from life into death, into a skeletal condition in a slow-burning inferno. On the right, the Mexican migrant appears young, strong, determined. With a gaze of human purpose, his eyes are crossed by what appears to be the narrow winding river of the Rio Grande. His face is filled with bright reds, living whites, and firm facial lines that say life is at its full. The man's face and gaze shift in the middle into a look of shock. The reds are replaced by creeping blues and purples, and his frightened eyes are now looking not at the river but through one of the slats of a boxcar abandoned in the Arizona desert. We see this desert and the night sky painted on his forehead. Finally, on the left the man's head is shriveled and losing its living form. Deathly yellow whites spread across his forehead and cheeks; he is now a death mask, his eyes sunken into the skull and his teeth protruding as a result of baking to death. Yepes has depicted a Mexican's erasure from life.

This painting reflects actual, repeated events of migrant deaths in train cars and trucks and torturous desert landscapes. My coeditor, Nick Cull, and I wrote about one such scene in the introduction to our book *Alambrista and the US-Mexico Border*. A 911 call from a cellular phone alerted an emergency dispatcher that people were asphyxiating in a trailer somewhere:

> Before the dispatcher could summon a bilingual assistant to help, the call ended. . . . At around 2:30 a.m. on the morning of May 14th sheriff's deputies from Victoria, Texas, about 175 miles north of the border, found an abandoned trailer at the truck stop on US route 77. In and around the truck lay seventeen dead bodies. . . . The dead included a five-year-old boy, later identified as Marco Antonio Villaseñor Acuna, and his father, José Antonio Villaseñor Leon, aged thirty-one, from Mexico City. . . . Around eighty-five would-be immigrants from Mexico, Honduras, and Guatemala had been packed into the insulated trailer to cross the border into the United States. Trapped for hours without fresh air and in record heat for the time of year, they had begun to die. In despair some had clawed holes into the side of the trailer for air and to attract attention. The driver— Tyrone Williams of Schenectady, New York—had panicked when he realized that his human cargo had begun to die. . . . He told investigators that

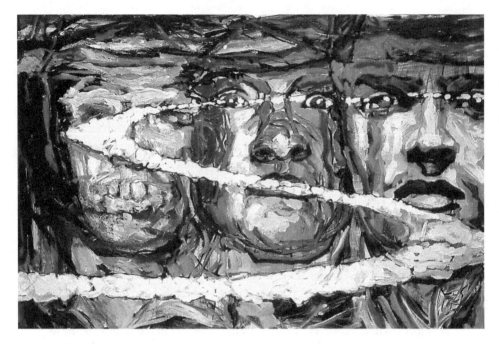

FIGURE 2.1 | George Yepes, *Boxcar*. Painting. ©1991 George Yepes.

he had been paid the sum of $5,000 to haul the migrants from Harlingen, Texas (near the border town of Brownsville) to Houston. Although other arrests followed, the masterminds behind the smuggling operation remained at large.[8]

Fifteen years ago, when disturbed by these and other scenes of Mexican farmworkers' suffering, I turned to the filmmaker Robert M. Young, who had put a human face on these migrant deaths. Young calls his films *dramas of the commonplace*, saying: "All my stories are the same. They're about people to whom life gave a raw deal. But they're not losers. They have dignity."[9] It was his attraction to the physical and emotional suffering of Mexican farmworkers that launched his breakthrough film project, *Alambrista* (The Wire Jumper), and that brought us together years after its release.[10]

After hearing Cesar Chavez speak at a rally for striking farmworkers in the Coachella Valley in California, Young followed farmworker families to learn about their lives and became friends with the Paolo Galindo family, who were traveling on the migrant trail in the Southwest. He learned about the *underground* existence of undocumented farmworkers recruited by growers and picking by day and even by lantern light at night. Young also heard a story about a Mexican woman who had crossed illegally into the United States while pregnant and gave birth clinging to a pole at a border crossing to ensure that her baby was born in the United States and wouldn't need papers to find work.

In the subsequent film, *Alambrista*, which won the Camera d'Or at Cannes and first prize at the San Sebastian Film Festival, the hopes and travails of Mexican bodies are symbolized when the protagonist Roberto finds his long-lost father dying in the baking sun of a Colorado watermelon field, where each is working without knowledge of the other. An early scene showing Roberto about to leave his family in Michoacán sets up this later, heartbreaking reunion. It also signals the power of religious symbols and humble places for Roberto's family. When Roberto is just about to leave his family and travel north, he meets his mother at a roughshod family chapel, and they pray in front of a statue of the Virgin of Guadalupe. Leaning against Guadalupe is a photograph of Roberto's father, who went north years ago along the migrant farmworker trail and never returned. His mother says, "No te vayas, hijo. . . . Tu Papa nunca volvío" (Don't go, son. . . . Your father never returned). But just like his father before him, Robert leaves his young wife and new baby and heads for *el Norte* to earn a living wage he can send back to them.

Following harrowing and humiliating experiences working in the United States as an undocumented farmworker, Roberto is deported to Mexico and then clandestinely recruited by a labor boss working for watermelon farmers in Colorado who desperately need laborers. On his first morning in Colorado, Roberto and his cohorts are picking watermelons and heaving them toward the supply truck when he hears a commotion among nearby workers in which the name "Alberto Ramirez" is yelled out. Roberto runs to the spot where an older man is dying of a heart attack. When he looks more closely, Roberto realizes that the man is his long-lost father; after not seeing him for twenty years, the man is dying right before his eyes.

In a state of shock and sadness Roberto is taken to an abandoned school bus, where a kind coworker of his father shows him Alberto's bunk and his worn suitcase and its contents, which include a book in English, a toothbrush, a $50 money order for a woman (not his mother), pictures, and some letters. As a fly lands and crawls on his face, Roberto realizes that the life of his lost father is *exactly* the kind of life he has now entered—a dead end.

Reminiscent of *Box Car*, Roberto has just witnessed his father and himself turning into the third face, the death mask of the painting. In defeat and disgust he hitchhikes on the highway, knowing he'll be picked up by the Border Patrol and deported to Mexico—which is his goal. The film ends as

Roberto sees a Mexican mother clinging to the flagpole at the border crossing in front of border agents and two Mexican women assisting her in childbirth. Roberto, in ironic disgust, walks with other undocumented workers back into Mexico.

Young tells us, "This film is about people who pick the fruits and vegetables we eat, but because they are moving they don't have time to ripen themselves. Moving like that gives you the illusion of freedom. You think you are making choices but you're not."[11]

Short Historical Context for the Land of Open Graves

As the Chicano historian Albert Camarillo writes, "Immigration from Mexico to the United States in the twentieth century is not only the most prolonged movement of people in American immigration history, it is also the largest sustained international labor migration in the world."[12]

The twentieth century saw four periods of intensive immigration of Mexican people northward to the United States, making the century one long period of Mexican migration into US territory: "the first 'Great Migration' (1910–1920s), the 'Bracero Era' (1942–1964), the so-called 'Los Mojados' period (1950s which coincided with the bracero programs), and the 'Second Great Migration' (1970s–2000)."[13] During these migration waves, Mexicans and Americans worked alongside each other in fields, factories, and railroad yards. Some attended schools together and intermarried. Mexicans who came and went in seasonal labor periods laid down personal and social tracks, formed friendships, and became part of Mexican American social networks in towns across the Southwest and North, in cities such as Chicago, Grand Rapids, and Milwaukee. Several generations of Mexicans had gained direct and indirect social knowledge about working in the United States and the act of migrating "al Norte" as wage laborers had become a common practice for several million Mexicans. This Second Great Migration (1970–2000) was triggered by weakening economic conditions in Mexico and wage labor opportunities and demands in the United States. It was also the period of huge financial investments by the US government to detain and deport undocumented Mexicans, which led to the shadowed lives of many Mexican migrants portrayed in Young's film.

In the past two decades, the killing machine of the hostile PTD policy has turned the borderlands into something akin to Dante's vestibule of hell, and the Río Bravo/Rio Grande has become a kind of Acheron, or river of woe, a landscape of immense and sometimes unimaginable suffering and debasement of individuals, families, and, especially, human bodies. This politically created inferno on Earth raises the challenging question for medical anthropologists of how the teaming up of science, arts, and humanities can respond with pragmatic caring for the peoples who have been systematically stripped of human dignity—as my father witnessed that night in the El Paso morgue.

The Distribution of Sadness of the Greater Southwest

These scenes of migrant workers roasting to death in the boxcars and dying in a watermelon field recall the insightful anthropological work of Carlos G. Vélez-Ibáñez in his book *Border Visions: Mexican Cultures of the Southwest United States*. Velez-Ibáñez shows a long history of social and cultural "bumping" in the borderlands, whereby successive waves of peoples—Native Americans, Spaniards, Anglos, and Mexicans—migrate and "bump" their predecessors to marginal conditions. This bumping has had an impact on Mexicans in specifically negative ways so that they suffer a greater "distribution of sadness . . . the overrepresentation of Mexicans in statistics on poverty, crime, illness, and war."[14] Central to this extraordinary distribution of sadness among many Mexicans is their formation as tools, as bodies to be worked, and as undervalued commodities rather than as full human beings.

As the Yepes image of the boxcar victims showed us, Mexicans and now other Latin American migrants have become a "type of price-associated group to be used and discarded not unlike disposable materials or any used manufactured goods."[15] The best example of the rise in Mexican workers' value (but that in its name shows the reduction of Mexican value to body work) was the Bracero program. Labor needs in the United States between World War II and the Korean War resulted in a binational agreement that brought nearly five million Mexican farmworkers and railroad workers into the United States. It was the US growers who lobbied for a robust guest-worker program to solve their labor shortages that threatened the productivity and profits of agricultural products during the war years. An agreement with Mexico resulted in a recruitment program that brought temporary, seasonal workers into the United States. The deal required American employers to provide housing and transportation for the workers, but in many cases the housing, health services, and pay they provided was subnormal. By 1956, when more than 450,000 braceros had arrived in the United States, growers in Texas and California had grown dependent on these laborers for crop production. It is ironic, as Velez-Ibáñez shows, that during the early years of the Bracero program, thousands of Mexican immigrants and Mexican American farmworkers were inducted into the Armed Forces or became urban dwellers in the United States, filling job opportunities as part of the war economy. The irony of the commodity Mexican is that, while the Mexican migrants helped save the US agribusinesses at home during the war years, the children of Mexican Americans who had been here for generations were off fighting in the wars and getting wounded and killed.

These hyperphysical contributions and sacrifices led many Mexicans to see themselves, psychologically and physically, as *braceros* (working arms)— that is, valuable as bodies but not as full human beings in the United States. Add to this sense of stigma the overrepresentation, in terms of percentages, of Mexicans serving and killed in the wars fought by the United States and we gain a better grasp on the overdistribution of sadness in Mexican American families. Consider these facts about how Mexican bodies were brought up to Marine, Army, and Navy units to fight wars. In some cases, many members of Mexican households in war included most male and some female members for several generations. "In one family of fifteen, for example, ten had joined the armed services between 1941 and 1965, five served in World War II and one returned, wounded, scared, and scarred for life. The sixth and seventh sons served in Korea, and later a marine was killed two weeks after celebrating his eighteenth birthday."[16] In one street of a Mexican community in Illinois during a period between World War II and the Vietnam war, eighty-four men and women served in the wars. Eight were killed, and many returned maimed and traumatized. While only 11 percent of the US population was Mexican (in the Southwest in the years 1961–67), almost 20 percent of those killed in Vietnam were from Mexican families.[17]

Vélez-Ibáñez's book is an outstanding example of anthropological caring in that he struggles with the limitations and untapped resources of the social sciences to generate hybrid crossover knowledge. He models how research, writing, reporting, and teaching about Mexican American sadness can be linked to the redressive spirit of Mexican American creativity—that is, the aesthetic creations of Chicanos striving to reveal the historical presence and human dignity of Mexicans in Mexican American life. He presents Chicano writings and paintings of Mexicans and their mixed-race bodies as potent expressions of political protest *and self-caring*. Authors, painters, dancers, and muralists since the Chicano civil rights movement of the 1960s have sought strategies to diagnose the causes of Mexican suffering, reveal the spirits of resistance to sadness, and embrace the dignity of Chicano families."[18]

And yet we are forced to ask again, amid this celebration of Chicano art, "Where is the acknowledgement of religious sensibilities among the very people anthropologists and artists strive to care for?" This question becomes even more pressing as we now travel into the "land of open graves" of the landscapes of the Sonoran Desert.

Jason De León and the Killing Machine

Jason De León's *The Land of Open Graves: Living and Dying on the Migrant Trail* is at once a political revelation about what he terms *necroviolence*, an effective application of four-field anthropology, and a devastating critique of the US policy of PTD. However, what is largely absent from De León's achievement, closely attending to the bodies of the dead through the innovative archeological and forensic methods he draws on, are the religious imagination and practices of the living migrants whose remains he cares about. What alternative survivals are indexed by the profound religiosity of these families and their feelings, their sacred grief about the bodies of the lost?

De León's work of caring through the application of his anthropological training teaches us that US policies have turned the Sonoran Desert into a "killing machine that simultaneously uses and hides behind the viciousness of the Sonoran Desert."[19]

The motto of the killing machine is Prevention through Deterrence, and its origins take us back to El Paso, where this essay began. The PTD policy began in 1993 just months before the North American Free Trade Agreement (NAFTA) induced a near-flood of laborers who were unofficially invited into cheap labor positions along the border. The basic premise of PTD was to build human barriers in the form of more and more Border Patrol agents and fencing to stop the many would-be laborers from flowing through El Paso and to force them, instead, into much rougher terrain in the desert. There, they would die or at least be deterred by the punishing terrain. More deaths followed; more deterrence did not. The structural violence of the El Paso experiment was considered a success and became the model for a border-length security policy that is being bolstered in gargantuan rhetoric today.

De León powerfully reveals that the US policy has taken the form of *necroviolence*, violence toward the migrant bodies that continues even after death. He emphasizes what my father experienced briefly in the El Paso morgue—namely, that the bodies of migrants and Mexican Americans have a political afterlife whose main theme is war and hostility toward the dead.[20]

De León gives the reader a pathos-filled example of this hostility when he and his students attempt to show some care for the dead body of a migrant woman whom they come upon in the Sonoran Desert just as vultures are circling overhead. They cover her with a blanket; stay with her to ward off the vultures; and take pictures to record her last resting place while some students weep and grow nauseated. De León, like my father in the El Paso morgue, is confronted with the problem of how some human *dignity* can be saved for this isolated, dead body. He tells us: "Some months later someone will corner me after a talk and complain that the photo I showed of this woman's body robbed her of her dignity. I will point out that the deaths that migrants experience in the Sonoran Desert are anything but dignified. That is the point. This is what 'Prevention Through Deterrence' looks like. These photographs should disturb us, because the disturbing reality is that right now corpses lie rotting on the desert floor and there aren't enough witnesses."[21]

De León strove to wrest a bit of dignity for the woman who, they later learn, is a forty-one-year-old mother of three named Marisol. He called the family and told them he had come upon Marisol already dead: "I was with her at the end, and we put a blanket over her to bring some dignity to her there in the desert. I told them that my students and I stayed with her for seven hours waiting for law enforcement to come and take her away."

Forensic Humanitarianism and Religiosity

The travails of De León and the lost migrants resonates with work done by other researchers in the borderlands, as illuminated by Claire Moon's writing on forensic humanitarianism in "Human Rights, Human Remains: Forensic Humanitarianism and the Human Rights of the Dead."[22] Moon and others show that forensic anthropologists are often motivated by humanitarian impulses, and more humanists are joining forensic scientists in their investigations. At the heart of forensic humanitarianism, which "entails the exhumation of mass graves in the effort to establish, forensically, the individual and collective identities of the dead victims of mass atrocity and the causes of their deaths," beats a profound relationship between the scientist and the corpse.[23]

Moon's work is aimed not at a general or global conception of the dead but toward the extremely marginalized dead bodies of the tortured and disappeared in Argentina and the disappeared in the Spanish Civil War, in the former Yugoslavia, in Rwanda, and in Mexico. What also stands out from her work is that forensic humanitarians often seek an ameliorative approach to this suffering that strives to protect the dignity of the dead and address the needs of the bereaved. This approach draws directly on humanitarian values that configure "not only the living but also the dead as the subject of humanitarian concern and object of intervention."[24] This configuration of the dead as worthy of dignity depends on a partnership between the living and the dead—and, especially, the abandoned dead who continue to suffer indignities. We can ask, "Do the dead have rights to dignity?" In Moon's views, these rights are not abstract but relational. She writes, "I would argue, they [the dead] can be seen to be rights holders insofar as the living behave as if they have obligations towards the dead, treat them as if they have rights, and confer rights upon them in practice."[25]

Moon and the forensic humanitarians draw on a long Western discourse on rights and dignity, arguing that all humans have an innate right to be valued and respected and to receive ethical treatment. I applaud this caring approach and the multidisciplinary strategies to alleviate the erasure of the dead and disappeared. Yet I wonder whether this language of innate rights may also be pushed in the realm of religious worldviews and practices by Mexicans who often connect the "innate" to a creator.

I return to my earlier question to Kleinman about how a meaningful and effective relationship of exchange can take place between the living anthropologists and the physical remains of Mexicans found and examined in the desert. The question carries deeper meaning especially when, in the hearts and minds of many Mexicans, one's dignity while alive or deceased is tied to another kind of gift: the gift of life given by ancestors, God, and the spirits of saints. When we put the claim of innate human rights to dignity in contact with the local cultures of the dead, we may find ourselves in the presence of peoples raised with experiences of and beliefs in divine presences through their whole lives. The Mexican bodies, peoples, and families who populate this essay may have internalized, to one degree or another, a religious worldview (Protestant, Catholic, indigenous, evangelical) that locates the origins of innate dignity in a nonhuman entity and source. For the Mexicans in these stories, the innate right to dignity almost always comes from a reality prior to and beyond the human, a Creator. Some migrants who survive the journey say they were accompanied by Jesús Amigo (Friend Jesus), with whom they formed a profound friendship that will serve them for the rest of their lives. Therefore, the exchange between anthropologists and medical professionals that can evoke dignity must involve a third being—beyond the filmmaker or the anthropologist and the Mexican dead. That third being is a divine being. It is a being created *in the likeness of God* combined with the caring actions of others toward this likeness, the human being, that is the source of dignity. While Moon as humanitarian does not attend in her work to this particular dimension, it is often attested to by the migrants themselves in some of the objects they carry and leave behind (crosses, images of the Virgin of Guadalupe, pictures of saints, prayer papers), by the many prayers they speak, and even by the shrines they create along the miserable migrant trail. Likewise, though De León makes little of the religious dimension in his work, listen to the words of Vanessa when he shows her a photo of Maricela's dead body covered by a blanket in the desert: "In case this is her buried here, thank God we have the body. It is a miracle of God that she came back to us."[26]

My point is that God or the saints, in the Mexican and Latin families, is the third presence who guarantees dignity in the reciprocal world that Kleinman imagines. In this view, there is a dual caregiver: the anthropologist/filmmaker/artist *and* the religious force or divine presence longed for and experienced by the migrants. *Retablos* are storytelling devices ritually used to help visualize how a divine presence intervened to save a life or protect and cure a person.

One of the most vivid and profound Mexican practices for assigning rights of dignity and respect to the dead are the Día de los Muertos celebrations, which are ancient, contemporary, and growing among Mexicans and other peoples in the United States. Every year, family altars and shrines are set up and celebrations are carried out in graveyards. In part, it is because these religious beliefs and practices are so vital to many Mexicans that the loss of a family member forever in the desert or along the migrant trail throws them into states of extreme grieving. Research disciplines such as medical anthropology and forensic humanitarianism that seek both to draw attention to the egregious structural and interpersonal violence of the borderlands *and* to bring up the Mexican bodies to be understood with respect and dignity must maintain a space, in the morgue, in the watermelon fields, in the classroom, in the lab, and in the book for the saints to appear and claim their places.

Tableau to *Retablo*

"Naturally, most *retablos* commemorate successful crossings and good fortune," Jorge Durand and Douglas Massey write in *Miracles on the Border: Retablos of Mexican Migrants to the United States.* "But sometimes they acknowledge sadder outcomes in which luck ran out. One such *retablo*, reported to us by another colleague who saw it in San Juan de los Lagos in 1982, offered a mother's thanks to the Virgin for the recovery of the bodies of her two sons, who drowned while trying to cross the Rio Grande into the United States."[27]

This chapter has surveyed five tableaus, or dramatic historical scenes, filled with Mexican bodies, dead and alive. Each scene—the El Paso morgue, the detached boxcar, the dying father in a watermelon field, the workers and soldiers of sadness, the open graves in the Sonoran Desert—begins with human life and action that is reduced to a tableau of death, stillness, decay. Each has raised the question of human identity and human dignity among Mexicans. In the passage from Durand and Massey, we see how the "recovery of the bodies of her two sons" provided a mother with direct access to the identity and dignity of her children's remains. We also see that her response is a religious one: in her mind it is the Virgin of San Juan who is responsible for this gift of the return. This gesture of making a *retablo*, a sacred thank-you note, brings into clearer focus the religious dimensions of identity and dignity in the Mexican worldview.[28] *Retablos* are usually kept at home or deposited at a shrine; in either case, they function as images of divine presence in the life of the individual or family.

A central tenet of much contemporary, reflexive anthropology is that an other's phenomenology or worldview may never be wholly captured, understood, or ethnographically rendered. Attending to the worldview of others is a matter of careful discernment, relational inquiry, observation, and care; it is never something that can be presumed. Still, my point in centering the work and reflections of these *retablos* is that many Mexican migrants and their families—themselves from heterogeneous backgrounds—readily emphasize the centrality of religious experience alongside the presence and care offered by religious forces throughout their journeys north. Without more attention to the religiosity of the Mexican bodies I have brought up, and that many Mexican Americans and migrants consistently articulate, scholars may continue to skirt—or even evacuate—knowledge of how the subjects of inquiry understand their own bodies in key ways and the moral orderings and spiritual allies that color their lives and deaths. Religious experience and the knowledge that God, the saints, and the sacred are close at hand in the Mexican environment are indispensable spheres for these people. Factoring this sphere into our research, policy building, and writing—in addition to continuing to account for the structural and political violence that metes out such suffering and death on the borderlands—is crucial for those who wish to care for and interpret the bodies on the border. How can Kleinman's insistence that medical anthropology give much more weight to the practices of caregiving and reciprocity be realized if a full encounter with this potent dimension of Mexican worldviews is not part of the medical approach?

One modest way to show the religiosity of Mexicans is by switching our focus from the tableau of graves and sadness to the Mexicans' *retablos*. I think of *retablos* as redoing the tableaus of danger and death in the borderlands by showing the presence of a divine ally. *Retablos* show us that God, saints, ancestors, crosses, and their miracle-making capacities travel with the undocumented migrants and appear in the tableaus of death and rescue. To get a sense of the abundance of religiosity and its bodily orientation in Mexico, consider this scene in the "Virgin's Chamber" inside the Church of the Virgin of San Juan de los Lagos, Mexico, when the faithful and the desperate come to worship, ask for miracles, and make vows: "Each day hundreds of thankful supplicants transform the walls of the sanctuary with new votive offerings: drawings, photographs, letters, crutches, bouquets, locks of hair, plaster casts, orthopedic devices, diplomas, driver's licenses, examination results, and dozens of metal charms in the shape of [arms, legs, feet, and hands.] In some places, ten or more layers are superimposed on one another."[29] What stands out in the church among this near-pandemonium of material pleadings and thanksgivings about vulnerable bodies, families, and careers are the *retablos*, colorful paintings on sheets of tin usually ten by fourteen inches in size. These paintings, ever present in Mexican churches and often present in homes and some art museums, tell the story of threatening, dangerous events in which someone is protected or rescued by a miracle brought by the presence of a sacred image of Jesus, the Virgin Mary, or one of the saints. The imagery is always accompanied by a text that describes the miracle. Numerous *retablos* tell of border crossings and depict the suffering and salvation of Mexicans in the desert or the river. The content and emotion reflected in the combination of imagery and text speak directly to the themes of caregiving, reciprocity, and healing within the Mexican imagination and sphere of religion.

According to Durand and Massey, the origin and spread of the practice of *retablos* "arose from a spontaneous desire on the part of the people to placate supernatural forces they believed controlled their fate."[30] But placation misses the more fundamental attitude in Mexican religious history of the role and power of shrines and miraculous images, as revealed in abundant detail in William B. Taylor's historical analysis: the long historical record shows that Mexicans developed "deep rivers of devotion" to places and images that were experienced as filled with "bursts of divine presence," signaling that "extraordinary consolation and favors for the faithful were available to the faithful there."[31] Placation, yes, but also, and more so, joyful embrace, gratitude, and rituals of moral and emotional identification with the divine presences that can and do appear throughout landscape and social places. What the description provided earlier of the abundance of offerings at the Virgin's Chamber shows is that as these Mexicans live their lives—they travel through urban, rural, and desert landscapes—seeking constant connections with divine beings. Their lives and deaths are linked to the presence of God, saints, and Jesus through vows and offerings they make, not only after they survive an ordeal, but all along the pathways they travel. Let us consider just two border-crossing *retablos* to bring religious experience in touch with the key conceptions of identity and dignity.

RETABLO OF BRAULIO BARRIENTOS

Retablo of Braulio Barrientos (figure 2.2) shows how a group of desert crossers on the edge of death portray themselves in a relationship of dependence and gift exchange with the Virgin of San Juan. It shows four men stranded, having run out of water, under a blazing desert sun that dominates the upper half of the painting. The four men are trying to make their way up a high desert hillside,

FIGURE 2.2 | Anonymous, *Retablo of Braulio Barrientos*, 1986. Church of San Juan de los Lagos, Mexico. Oil on metal. Photograph by Douglas S. Massey.

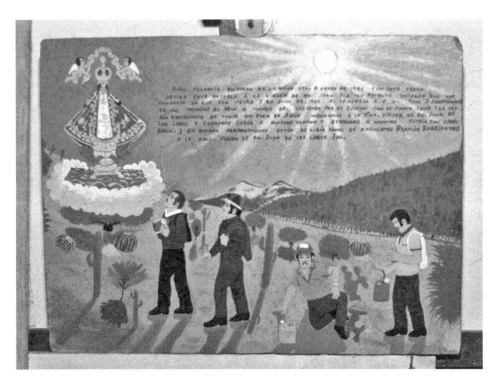

as indicated by the snowcapped mountain in the background. One of the men has collapsed to one knee, exhausted and with an empty water bottle. A man next to him seems stunned as he gazes at the sunbaked sand. But the other two men look skyward at an apparition of the Virgin of San Juan dressed in her blue, gold, and white costume, with two angels above all, floating on a cloud on top of a desert shrub.

The accompanying text tells us that one of the men, Braulio Barrientos (who probably hired a *retablo* artist to produce this scene), dedicates the *retablo* to the Virgin of San Juan "for the clear miracle she granted on the date of June 5, 1986." The text says that Barrientos was returning to the United States with three friends, who ran out of water in the desert: "And without hope of drinking even a little water, we invoked the Virgin of San Juan and were able to arrive at our destination and return to our homeland in health." For this miracle of life and health Barrientos has reciprocated by having this *ex-voto* painting produced and placed in the Sanctuary of the Virgin in San Juan de los Lagos, Mexico. The implication is that he will forever be devoted to this Virgin, who showed herself to his companions and him when their bodies could no longer survive.

RETABLO OF MARÍA DE LA LUZ CASILLAS AND CHILDREN

A final tableau turned into a *retablo* has more to say about another Mexican family's attitude toward medical treatment and the need for modern medicine to be linked with a religious practice and the role of miracles. In *Retablo of María de la Luz Casillas and Children* (figure 2.3) we see a scene of surgery being performed on a woman joined to a vision of a miracle to save her life. We can imagine that the woman and family depicted in this *retablo* are poor migrants, most likely with limited English skills, and have had equally limited exposure to the kind of technology and medical practices common in surgery.

The picture shows a woman, who had migrated to the Los Angeles area, undergoing an operation in 1960. On one side of the painting, all of the action is in white, while on the other side, the action is in color. We see María de la Luz Casillas lying face-up on an operating table, arms immobilized at her side and two surgeons dressed in white gowns and surgical masks. One may be holding her shoulders down while the other, with a pair of scissors held above her chest, is perhaps ready to make incisions into her body. A nurse dressed in white stands at the foot of the bed with her hands reaching for María's feet. A nearby table contains medical instruments. On the left side of the painting we see postoperative María dressed in a red skirt and blue

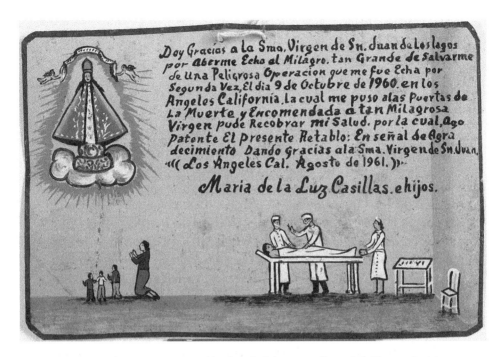

FIGURE 2.3 | Anonymous, *Retablo of María de la Luz Casillas and Children*, 1961. Oil on metal; 17.3 × 26 cm. Princeton University Art Museum. Gift of Jorge Durand and Patricia Arias (2020–21).

blouse kneeling behind her three standing children, who are also dressed in colorful clothes. The four family members are all looking up to the largest figure in the entire *retablo*: a colorful image of the "Holiest Virgin of San Juan de los Lagos." The Virgin's blue-and-white costume, her golden crown, and the two angels above are surrounded by a golden corona and are floating on a cloud. The revealing text shows how modern medical treatment and Catholic miracles are united in this Mexican's imagination:

> I give thanks to the Holiest Virgin of San Juan de los Lagos for having made me so great a miracle of saving me in a dangerous operation that was performed on me for the second time on the 9th of October 1960, in Los Angeles, California. Which put me at the door of death but entrusted to be so miraculous a Virgin I could recover my health, for which I made apparent the present retablo: in sign of thanksgiving, I give thanks to the Holiest Virgin of San Juan. Los Angeles, California. August 1961. María de la Luz Casillas and children.[32]

The message is that the surgery was successful—that is, María's life was saved *not just* by the surgeons, but mainly because of a miracle by "so miraculous a Virgin," who is the cause for the recovery of her health.

Conclusion

The trauma and necroviolence suffered by Mexicans as summarized in this chapter leave open the question of whether the work of De León, forensic humanitarians, medical anthropologists, and other scholars attuned to the political forces creating such death on the borderlands can rise to the level of Kleinman's search for moral reciprocity or my own concern for attention to religious experience in the practice of caregiving for abandoned bodies and for the disappeared, even if they are someday recovered. Recall what Kleinman teaches us: caregiving is "a different kind of reciprocity . . . , a gift exchange and receiving among people whose relationships really matter." But where is the real gift exchange when the bodies are brought up in the wake of the killing machine? Is it only the living, the medical anthropologist, who benefits by being a moral agent in interacting with the deceased body? Is Moon correct when she argues that if the living behave as if we have obligations toward the dead, then we confer the right of dignity on them, even if they are sometimes anonymous to us?

What these tableaus and *retablos* show is that the recovery of dignity for the Mexican bodies and families may come most readily when a sacred object, divine presence, or sense of miracle is also present or, at, least acknowledged. The *retablo* is a memory device. It enables the family to be caregivers for their memories of the deceased, which keeps them alive in an alternative way. Those memories and the divine presence may be materialized through an image of Jesus or the saints or in some other object or ritual action. Most of all, what is necessary is the *presence* of all three: the caregiver, the person in some form, and a miraculous image. Or, to put it another way, the caregiver for these Mexicans is, more often than not, a dual caregiver that includes a human being and a divine ally working together.

Perhaps the real gift exchange of dignity in the work of anthropologists who work with these remains is to the families, to the surviving members of families, and to the wider Mexican population who learn of, remember, and memorialize these brought-up bodies in their works and days.

Notes

1 | This phrase is from De León, *The Land of Open Graves*.
2 | I borrow this phrase from Hilary Mantel, whose historical novel *Bring Up the Bodies* is part of her trilogy about the rise and fall of Thomas Cromwell; Mantel, *Bring Up the Bodies*.
3 | The anthropologist Victor Turner developed the notion of the "social drama," in which a social group suffering a profound crisis undergoes a dynamic four-stage process that includes the practice of "redressive actions"— actions that include political, social, and, especially, theatrical, artistic productions. These productions aim at both diagnosing the causes of the collective injuries and working toward some healing: Turner, *Dramas, Fields and Metaphors*.
4 | Perales, *Smeltertown*.
5 | Vélez-Ibáñez, *Border Visions*.
6 | Kleinman, "A Search for Wisdom."
7 | Kleinman, "A Search for Wisdom."
8 | Cull and Carrasco, *Alambrista and the US-Mexico Border*.
9 | Cull and Carrasco, *Alambrista and the US-Mexico Border*, 151.
10 | Robert Young's *Alambrista* won the Camera d' Or at the Venice Film Festival in 1977. I worked with him to produce the award-winning *Alambrista: The Director's Cut* in 2003.
11 | Cull and Carrasco, *Alambrista and the US-Mexico Border*, 160.
12 | Camarillo, "Alambrista and the Historical Context of Mexican Immigration to the United States in the Twentieth Century," 27.
13 | Camarillo, "Alambrista and the Historical Context of Mexican Immigration to the United States in the Twentieth Century," 15.
14 | Vélez-Ibáñez, *Border Visions*, 7.
15 | Vélez-Ibáñez, *Border Visions*, 7.
16 | Vélez-Ibáñez, *Border Visions*, 201.
17 | Vélez-Ibáñez, *Border Visions*, 205.
18 | Vélez-Ibáñez, *Border Visions*, 263.
19 | De León, *The Land of Open Graves*, 16.
20 | Here is De León's definition of *necroviolence* and statement of his purpose in studying and changing it. Necroviolence is "violence performed and produced through the specific treatment of corpses that is perceived to be offensive, sacrilegious, or inhumane by the perpetrator, the victim (and her or his cultural group, or both). . . . By labeling this phenomenon, I seek both to connect it to modern forms of political power and to provide a framework for facilitating a conversation about this postmortem violence across sub-disciplines of anthropology. Much can be learned about ideologies of conflict and social inequality by interrogating necroviolence across time, space and fields of study": De León, *The Land of Open Graves*, 69–70.
21 | De León, *The Land of Open Graves*, 213.

22 | Moon, "Human Rights, Human Remains."

23 | Moon, "Human Rights, Human Remains," 49.

24 | Moon, "Human Rights, Human Remains," 57.

25 | Moon, "Human Rights, Human Remains," 58.

26 | De León, *The Land of Open Graves*, 258.

27 | Durand and Massey, *Miracles on the Border*, 92.

28 | The phrase "sacred thank you note" comes from María Luisa Parra.

29 | Durand and Massey, *Miracles on the Border*, 2.

30 | Durand and Massey, *Miracles on the Border*, 9.

31 | Taylor, *Theater of a Thousand Wonders*, 1.

32 | Durand and Massey, *Miracles on the Border*, 47.

In the Vast Abrupt

Horizon Work in an Age
of Runaway Climate Change

Runaway States

Epic storms from warming oceans, wildfires burning with unprecedented intensity, rising sea levels, massive crop failures, extreme heat, prolonged droughts: models of risk are insufficient for grasping what might come next. As one structural engineer who is working to improve infrastructures to withstand hurricanes on the US North Atlantic coast notes, "There is a 'switch' beyond which we cannot plan."[1] Relatively stable environments—coasts, landforms, wetlands, habitats, and soils—once afforded engineers the opportunity to build the stable infrastructures of modern life. Today, the very thing we look to experts for is compromised; expectations are routinely undermined as ecological behaviors morph into intricate superstructures of risk. In the words of a former director of the US Geological Survey, who spoke in the wake of Hurricane Sandy: "We have already crossed a threshold."[2] The "crossing" points to a basic insight. Climate change is breaking a fundamental aspect of our relationship with the environment: that we tend to have a sense of how it acts over time and that we can make models and predictions based on it. Risk is a problem not of modeling but of navigating superimposing events that set the stage for further surprises.

In recent years, certain heuristics have dominated how we think about surprise—specifically, the role of expert intuition in averting disaster. In what is now a standard anecdote, a firefighting commander leads a crew into a burning house. The crew points a water hose at a fire in the back of the house. The commander expects the temperature inside to cool, but instead it gets hotter, and he orders the crew members to leave. Within a minute of evacuation, the floor they had been standing on collapses (from a fire that, unknown to the crew, is burning in the basement). The commander could "think fast" (or make that split-second evacuation call) because his knowledge of fire patterns allowed him to sense the anomaly. He wasted no time—or, rather, he made the gap between what he thought was happening and what did happen as small as possible. He also used pattern recognition that allowed for rapid decision making, which, in turn, afforded intuitive leaps (fast thinking) that meant he could project relatively accurately.

The scholars of "fast thinking" acknowledge that intuitive expertise can evolve only in stable environments, not in environments that switch or are highly unstable.[3] The idea of runaway climate change, defined as a rapid departure from long-established baselines or historical trends, speaks to such instability: projections whose accuracy is continually undermined by the chaotic potentials of "crossed thresholds." I documented such chaos in the aftermath of the 1986 Chernobyl nuclear disaster in Ukraine. A runaway chain reaction contributed to a powerful explosion and the meltdown of a nuclear reactor core. A radioactive plume, crossing the globe and depositing radioactive material in waterways, soils, and rocks, likely condemned far more people than the United Nations' projected long-term death toll of 4,000. Those who survived found themselves suspended in a terrible gulf in which links between knowledge and the scope of suffering were constantly unmoored. Amid the official pronouncements that the disaster had been contained, sickness and symptoms had a way of outpacing predictions, as well as people's own ability to keep up with them. In the "switch" into exponential uncertainty, there were no experts to tell someone like Maria Ivanivna, a collective farmer who had achieved a secondary education, what symptom might materialize next ("No one tells me what is happening with me," in her words). She was resettled once, then again, only to return to the area from which she was initially resettled. She could no longer work, she said, because "my strength has left me, and I do not know from what." She drew the "wrong" conclusions from her symptoms—for example, she said she had a disease called "leukemia of the knee joint." I took her diagnostic misnomer to represent her effort at calling out a vacuum of expertise. I saw how Chernobyl acquired a language that concealed within itself the logic of its own progressively more destructive force. This runaway state seemingly "switched on" Ivanivna's ailments and made it impossible for her to know what to do next. There was no fast thinking there; she engaged the personal stakes of environmental and political instability as she desperately clung to her own capacity to be its knowledgeable agent.

Elements of this runaway state of being, as well as of a Chernobyl survivor's search for actionable time and of finding a foothold within it, have migrated into our own lives. People affected by the Camp Fire in Paradise, California in 2018 and record-breaking wildfires in subsequent years have asked themselves whether they can return home, whether it is environmentally safe, whether there is support for them, and how they can rebuild their lives—and whether it makes sense to do so in fire-prone areas. Their sense of the future must somehow be shored up and articulated within the failures of expertise (e.g., in the case of Paradise, in which a poorly conceived urban plan turned the town into a firetrap). Short-term horizons have been the rule as various political and financial actors have framed wildfires as merely episodic, allowing them to avoid serious action on a predictable, long-term, and chronic hazard. The ability to collect taxes and limit exposure to bad credit ratings is at stake. Yet this mode of quick "recovery" denies vulnerable publics a foothold in changing realities that are themselves contributing to a rapid degeneration of knowledge about the realities of new and unstable states.

What is at stake is change that is extensive enough to make projection seemingly impossible. The geoscientist James White underscored this point in a public briefing about anticipation in a time of abrupt climate change: that scientists must address "areas of observation where we are largely blind.... As a scientist, my hope is that we can study the planet well enough, monitor it well enough, understand it well enough, that we're not going to be blindsided. As a realist, I'm pretty sure we're going to be blindsided."[4] At a time when some psychologists continue to claim that the human brain just isn't "wired" to grasp the urgency of the climate crisis, I point to a different problem: How do we learn to be blind—or tolerate becoming blindsided by forces we cannot grasp? We can be certain that survivors of large-scale fires aren't thinking about fantasies of poor wiring but of how lives and immediate futures are being caught up in the miscalculations of larger institutions.

How should we think about this thing called expertise in the rapidly evolving realities of climate change? How should it be recalibrated for worlds that no longer exist, and how do we capture our own senses of threat as sources of knowledge and expertise? Looking at the extent of wildfires from year to year, a wildfire researcher framed the problem of runaway change in these terms: "So there's not a ton of horizon." His pithy phrase suggested that previous modus operandi for quantifying risk—risk assessment based on probability, the maximization of expected utility, cost-benefit calculation, or scenario forecasting—have not given him him the tools that are required for planning and intervening amid repetitive disasters. Neither have the conventional modes of stabilizing the situation—that is, of fighting wildfire, a practice that dates to the early 20th century, when practices of fire suppression evolved, and that can involve anything from hand crews digging out fire barriers (or fire lines) to the use of chemical flame retardants to slow wildfire spread. The efficacy of these efforts has proved to be poor in many instances, even contributing to long-term wildfire risk.[5]

As I would learn, something had to replace the old practices; "acquiring" a horizon was a challenge in itself—as if a horizon were some finely calibrated instrument that was missing in calculations of how to navigate rapid change. If these firefighters had one, they could address this time of exponential uncertainty—or, as one researcher put it to me, what "we actually are going to do over the next week, not, like, the next hour"—and maybe their roles could be different, helping to restore forests to reduce fires and absorb carbon, rather than release it. But mainly, they—along with the constituents they serve—could be *horizoning*, confronting vested interests and harmful policies, turning the void where practices to hold back climate chaos fail into forms of collective action for securing desired future conditions.

Marking Horizons

In everyday language use, a horizon denotes an object at a distance, out of our immediate grasp. But the wildfire scientist quoted above thought it was salient: a quantifiable material thing that is also politically and ethically charged. The word *horizon* derives from the ancient Greek ὁρίζω (horizō), meaning, "I mark out a boundary," and from ὅρος (oros), meaning "boundary" or "landmark." Renaissance architects used the contrivance of horizon lines to properly orient objects in three-dimensional space. Early modern surveyors devised mercury-filled "artificial horizons" to create an image of a level surface against which the "inconstancy of the terrestrial horizon" could be judged.[6] Today, extraterrestrial rovers are equipped with so-called predictive horizons, which calculate optimal routes for autonomously navigating the rugged terrains of Mars.[7] In the last example, the fate of a machine agent (a remotely operated Mars exploration rover) would be at the mercy of a "dearth" of horizon. Conversely, each horizon points to a possibility of maintaining a response—a space of reflexive intervention into an unknown that sets up an interaction between the faculty of perception and previously imperceptible events. This process can create movement, prevent a crash, or forestall the disappearance of a whole system (a rover, an ecosystem).

To emphasize this act of risk mediation, I turn the noun *horizon* into a verb—*horizoning*—and use it as a device to concretize some very abstract processes amid life on borrowed time. I think of horizoning as a conceptual device of "interference" at multiple levels—epistemological, moral, and political—and one that relates to thinking and intervening in climate-related and other runaway phenomena. Using words in new ways can make room for unexpected meaning within settled grammars of crisis. For instance, Shakespeare, employing a poetic technique (*anthimeria*), called on the greater energies of the verb form, as in "And I come *coffin'd* home."[8] To heighten a foreboding feeling, the poet John Milton, in his epic poem *Paradise Lost*, turned nouns into verbs ("sea-monsters *tempest* the ocean"). Or to amplify a sense of the unknown, he turned adjectives into nouns, as in "the palpable obscure" and "the vast abrupt." Wildfire survivors, firefighters, and emergency workers are caught in a vast abrupt and a degree of unsettlement in which not only is the physical environment changing, but expectations for how the environment should act are being constantly violated. When environmental changes "run away" from received explanations or models, validating the climate crisis as a race against time, one can ask, what is horizon acquisition as a basic human capacity and, by the same token, what is horizon deprivation?

In my book, *Horizon Work: At the Edges of Knowledge in an Age of Runaway Climate Change*, I consider this question in terms of local and highly practical forms of research that attempt to bring a runaway future into the present and to turn it into an object of knowledge and intervention. Such horizoning work is an imaginative exercise first and foremost, one that is not limited to experts alone. It entails grappling with present and near-future shifts, but also retrieving the possibility of desired future conditions. This work also brings us full circle to anthropology, and particularly to medical anthropology, a field that has shifted biomedicine's focus from an exclusive clinical domain of positivistic expertise to health as a value, a societal construction, and a multitudinous way of being in the world. The sea of meaning attributed to the word *health* includes various efforts of navigating physical forces we cannot always grasp—that is, to see ourselves (and others we care for) within a horizon of expectation in which such efforts matter. How that ground is gained or lost or subjective judgments about where one stands in relation to disease processes does not invalidate the effort, or the meanings derived therein. The process itself can become a vital source of expertise, furthering a sense of how to pursue or direct health-care efforts or identify needs and information gaps. What would otherwise be called uncertainty is a difficult problem of acquiring or losing a horizon of intervention, especially in the case of a loved one whose life hangs in the balance.

Nowhere is this medical anthropological imaginary of struggle in a vast abrupt more applicable than in caregiving. Along such lines, Arthur Kleinman frames caregiving as a type of understudied expertise, especially for complex medical conditions for which there is treatment uncertainty around often inexplicable symptoms, such as dementia. As he shows, the toll of unpreparedness is both real and devastating.[9] Where biomedical thinking is often limited or too time-constrained to dwell in complexity, patients and caregivers themselves have to pick up the pieces of a fragmented care system and reimagine "arcs of interference" on their own terms.

Today, medical anthropology must tap this expertise as a form of horizoning work and enter into dialogue with processes that stand to threaten species, whole communities, and ways of life; overtax medical systems; and ravage global food supplies. For many, runaway climate change means both unpreparedness and catastrophe as foregone conclusions for the foreseeable future. As one famous broadcaster and natural historian put it, "If we don't take action, the collapse of our civilizations and the extinction of much of the natural world is on the horizon."[10] Or, as an American journalist stated, we are on course toward an "uninhabitable earth."[11] Along the way, one must ask about the nature of that trajectory: if runaway climate change signifies an inability to avert worst-case scenarios, what could tell us that we have broken free of this horizon? What, if anything, would be a theory and indicator of progress in holding back a tide of incalculable losses? Such questions bridge environmental science and medical anthropology, inasmuch as the concerns of both fields delimit the conditions of knowable, and thus livable, worlds.

My ethnographic work in the "vast abrupt" of the climate crisis has taken me into two disparate but related fields.[12] The first concerns ecological theorists who are not focused on wildfire specifically but are, on a planetary scale, attempting to define varieties of critical thresholds that, if crossed, may entail irreversible ecological change, and who are characterizing early warning signals for such changes. The second concerns ground-level actors who are directly caught up in abrupt environmental change while being tasked with trying to contain wildfire proliferation in the United States. In this second field, fire behavior analysts are going back to basics in wildfire science to understand a phenomenon they thought they already knew. My research among these scientists, training and technical specialists, and engineers has led me to explore at length how fire's new qualities and dynamics can eclipse human and technical competencies. In other words, the "runaway" forms of wildfire have orphaned the practices meant to control them. They drive an ever bigger wedge between wildfire threat and its institutional frames of response. As disasters rush in, horizoning turns the voids where projections fail into opportunities to rethink collective response. It cannot be left to one set of experts, but must be undertaken by interdependent knowledge holders who, in their partial comprehension of ecological shifts and how they occur, can expand a breadth of resources with which these shifts can be responded to. Such coordination also requires a reckoning: in the United States, with the settler colonial legacies that have excluded fire as part of a genocidal erasure of Indigenous peoples; these legacies haunt the very same landscapes that are now ready to ignite. Futurity is at stake, but not the dystopic kind from which others must be "saved," as Indigenous philosopher and environmental justice scholar Kyle Whyte writes.[13] Normalized societal divisions around who is the rescuer and who is the saved should be rethought, and this in itself points to other theoretical and ethnographic potentials of horizoning work to interfere in public domains of climate discourse and future anthropology.

In the Vast Abrupt

By the time it had ended, 2015 was seen as the worst wildfire year on record in the United States. Wildfires consumed ten million acres, and the war on wildfire cost taxpayers $2.6 billion. In California alone, about 3,400 wildfires were fought, one thousand more than the average over the previous five years. Fire seasons are lasting, on average, eighty-six days longer than they have in four decades. For two weeks in 2015, recruiters in the national dispatch and coordination system hit a resource limit: there was simply nobody left to recruit to fight the fires. Military personnel, volunteers, and even prisoners were conscripted into emergency response efforts. These numbers (of acres burned or costs accrued for any given year) become distant benchmarks of runaway change. In 2017, new records were set, and dispatch services once again hit novel breaking points with exhausted fire crews and widespread pollution and destruction. California, with more than nine thousand fires, saw the first ever wintertime mega-fires in December of that year, during "what should be the peak of the state's rainy season."[14] As one observer of these fires noted: "I was expecting to see snow on that mountain, and now the thing is on fire." There is no shortage of broken records.[15]

In the past decade, scientists have engaged in a peculiar exercise of time reckoning with certain aspects of a changing global climate system. Concepts that aim to ascertain sudden or far-reaching modifications in ecosystem dynamics, such as critical thresholds and regime shifts, have proliferated in ecological science. Critical thresholds are theorized moments at which characteristic behavior deviates from known patterns or trends. Regime shifts manifest as breakaway processes—for example, in the structures and functions of ecosystems. As these breaks occur, they can make certain ecological niches in which species thrive no longer suitable. Different, unforeseeable constraints on survival or possible extinction arise. The suddenness of the shifts also causes hardships. Changes can register as anomalous at first ("That fire season was long") but stabilize into a new state of ecosystem organization ("Fire seasons are getting longer"). Their impact can be observed at a regional or more context-specific scale ("That mountain is burning"). But by this time, the realization that the new conditions may not be survivable comes too late.

Bill Armstrong is a forest fuels specialist for the US Forest Service (USFS) and veteran of a select group of wildland firefighters in the Southwest with whom I first spoke in 2014. He was of thin frame; his worn grey USFS-issued coveralls looked oversize; his blue eyes, with crinkles seemingly formed from years of watching, staring at, and fighting fires, seemed oceanic. Armstrong had described to me what the community of wildland firefighters considers the decades of the regime shift, a time of an "exponential rise in area burned." One particular fire stands out for this community: the 1996 Dome Fire in northern New Mexico, whose physics was unlike anything they had ever seen. Armstrong told me, "In the '80s, when I started, intense fires were anomalies. What we thought was a freak incident became a wakeup call that nobody woke up to. It was a plume-dominated fire—more like a firestorm, so much energy is released in such a small period of time. We just weren't expecting that kind of fire behavior."

Huge updrafts of burning embers and material that get sucked high into clouds characterize a plume-dominated fire. "As material moves up through the clouds, it cools off, and when it cools off, the weight of the clouds can no longer sustain themselves," he said. "Then the clouds collapse, and when they collapse, they throw stuff everywhere." In fact, they can do this many times.

Critically, plume-dominated fires have become more likely over the past few decades because the fuel substrate for forest fires has become progressively drier, creating a higher intensity and greater coupling between fire and atmospheric conditions.

By the mid-2000s, what had been a freak incident became the norm. Armstrong was a first responder in the Las Conchas fire of 2011, which, like the Dome Fire, defied the behavioral assessments coming from the USFS's fire modelers in Missoula, Montana. Fires usually move with winds, but a plume-dominated fire such as Los Conchas "burned with greatest intensities and greatest rates of spread against the wind," according to Armstrong. "It actually managed to push its way up against the wind." This meant that "with the power of the fire and what it was generating, with its own internal winds and its own weather system . . . , it was feeding itself." Such fires actually move around based on areas of highest fuel availability or driest fuels and do not follow any particular logic.

Also, unlike previous fires, the Las Conchas fire eerily and aggressively "burned into areas where we thought there was absolutely nothing left to burn. It burned through the Cerro Grande wildfire scar of 2000. It burned through the old Dome Fire scar of 1996. We could not have predicted that kind of fire behavior." What Armstrong described to me is a fatal mismatch between what modelers can model and what emergency workers face. In the absence of knowledge of superstorm or mega-fire dynamics, what accumulates is an intricate superstructure of surprise, consisting of overlaid events whose net physical interactions and intensities are unpredictable. The gap between what is expected and what is encountered, in his mind, is growing too wide to bridge. According to Armstrong, "We should be treating these fires the same way we do hurricanes. Get the hell out of the goddamn way."

With Armstrong's emphatic words in mind, let's recall the fast thinking expert: the fire commander who knew enough about patterns to sense anomalies and to tell his crew to evacuate the burning home. Now imagine a fire commander standing before a large wildfire; it is burning out of control—hotter and faster than it would in previous years because of prolonged drought conditions. What if she doesn't have the tools or experience to exercise similar intuitive powers—to make the right split-second call to protect her crew? Indeed, there are plenty of things that can't be seen or anticipated here: the random gust of wind carrying a burning ember across a highway and into a nearby suburb, sparking a new fire, or the gust that takes the ember into a neighboring mountain range, igniting parched vegetation in one of its canyons.

While the fire commander of fast thinking derived expertise from a mental model of fire that allowed him to sense patterns and deviations, the opposite seems to be happening here: mental models don't work as much, and there is little to draw on to build intuitive expertise (about disaster or about when and where the next one will be). There was a time, wildland firefighters tell me, when there *was* enough constancy in wildfires' shapes and behavior to afford some pattern recognition. They told me about how they carried "slides" of previous fires in their heads; they instinctively called on these mental slides to predict the behavior of fires. Today, relying on these mental slides can obscure the new realities they face.

Trust in patterns has become an occupational hazard, and wildland fire researchers at the USFS Research Station in Missoula are going back to the basics of learning about the properties of fire ignition and the dynamics of wildfire spread. The Rocky Mountain Fire Station and its Fire Lab are at the center of an interdisciplinary research endeavor. There, basic scientists and engineers study the changing dynamics of physical phenomena such as fire, making experimental sense of exponential change (e.g., how a fire becomes a mega-fire). Here the reality of "the switch" confounds not only coastal planning but also wildfire management. "Instead of being, instead of just this gradual buildup, it's like a switch," says Matt Jolly, Fire Lab research ecologist. "And that switch is thrown, and it changes; and once you're in that situation, you better have a way to get out."[16] Jolly's work on fire growth and dynamics feeds directly into reformulations of risk and response in the field, where wildland firefighters are confronting the switch to an alternative ecological stable state.

Now imagine a firefighter who happens to be in a parched canyon where a switch is about to occur, scouting out structures and properties that may be at risk. The public is expecting action; retreat isn't an option. But the canyon fire professional is standing in is more like a wind tunnel. A creeping little fire is just one wind event away from turning into a fireball. He will not see it coming; he might hear a sudden roar and not know where the sound is coming from. As he struggles to gain his footing, the fire overwhelms him, raising the question: should he have been in a situation that does not lend itself to expertise anymore?

Unlike their counterparts in many other wildfire-prone countries, US wildland firefighters often work in immediate proximity to fire. They are trained to remain aware at all times of available escape routes, nearby clearings, and safe spots that have already burned over (called "the black" by firefighters). To minimize the risk of entrapment, they are trained to "keep one foot in the black"—that is, to maintain access to a designated safety zone. They deduce the size and location of a safety zone from flame geometries and on the basis of (continually updated) guidelines for how to make these deductions. As changing conditions are more readily felt, these practices of enhanced, situated awareness become less reliable. Sometimes there is no black, and with unburned fuel, drought conditions, and rising temperatures, even the black somehow burns. Crewmen can lose their way in the shifting smoke and flame, particularly as they depend on others (squad leaders, lookouts, superintendents, and so on) to radio them about what is going on or what to expect next. When information is limited or communication breaks down, they must focus on getting to a safety zone or else, in a worst-case scenario, prepare for imminent entrapment and deploy their emergency fire shelters—four-pound devices of last resort used by US wildland firefighters when they run the risk of wildfire entrapment.

A fire behavior analyst referred me to his colleague, Tony Petrilli, a former smoke jumper who now works at the Forest Service's Missoula Technology and Development Center. In this onrush of disaster, he told me, sometimes survival comes down to a coin flip. Yet when a fast-moving wildfire swept through Yarnell, Arizona, in 2013, killing nineteen highly skilled firefighters who had deployed their fire shelters, Petrilli told me that there was "no flipping of nothing." A postaccident investigation of the Yarnell Hill Fire cited surrounding temperatures higher than 2,000 degrees Fahrenheit. The fire surprised the firefighters, who were in a narrow box canyon. Its vertical walls blocked their ability to gauge the spread and speed of the flames. As Petrilli told me, "Fifteen-mile-per-hour winds were pushing flames pretty much parallel to the ground in a ton of red-flame contact." The deployment site was "not survivable."

Petrilli himself survived a disastrous blaze (the 1994 South Canyon Fire) by deploying a fire shelter; fourteen of his fellow firefighters did not survive. Conducting numerous postaccident forensic reviews, he has also trained people in the complex art of deploying these shelters. He showed me a video (used in wildland fire-safety training courses) of firefighters who found themselves in a situation of imminent fire entrapment, pointing to the challenges of securing borrowed time. As he suggests in the following exchange, some firefighters on the verge of entrapment might even hesitate to deploy their shelters:

TP: One of the guys had his cell phone video going, and it's, like, "The fire's coming. They're talking about it. They have their fire shelter in their arm. And it's like—as I'm sitting there watching it—it's like, 'OK, how about now? How about now?'" [...].

AP: OK.

TP: You're starting to get the burning embers. They're just trying to make [the safety zone] as big as they can.

AP: Thinking that's going to work.

TP: The bigger, the better. I don't blame them for that, but it's time to call it.

As this work continues, it becomes apparent that the firefighters will soon be entrapped. Petrilli points out how the fire "is starting to suck in all the oxygen." He is eager for them to "get in their shelter, *right now*." Just before that moment arrives, and in spite of all the shelter deployment training, they are still working on their safety zone (and one crewmember continues to film away). They think they're following protocol, or they're in denial or underestimating the speed of the fire or relying too heavily on mental slides from previous fires. Regardless of their motives, their time is up; they deploy their fire shelters in the nick of time (I don't see that part because they have dropped their camera). As such scenarios suggest, making self-preservation a common value out of divergent intuitions about correct courses of action is hard to do. They also provide powerful lessons; they remind viewers that these firefighters are just like "anybody and everybody," in Petrilli's words, and that "it can be you" who thinks that it isn't going to be all that bad. He brings the viewer (me) to a precipice at which certain projections fall (or must fall) apart and make way for new intuitions and responses. The philosopher of science Gaston Bachelard once wrote that fire is a scene of emotive states, of "rigid mental habits," of "phobias" and "philias" that cripple the objectivity of a science of fire.[17] What is the threshold in which perceptions of fire become *too* variable?

"There is an expression that everyone says," the fire behavior scientist Mark Finney told me. "'Spreads like wildfire.' Yet we don't even know how wildfires spread." I am sitting with Finney in his office near the entryway of a two-story building on US Highway 10 in Missoula. From here, a quiet hallway leads to a multistory burn chamber, where a palimpsest of experiments have tested or simulated fire ignition, buoyancy, and vorticity (fire-spinning motion). There are used, abandoned, and ready-for-reuse apparatuses everywhere—wind tunnels and a combustion laboratory; one-of-a-kind air torches and a fire whirl simulator—all built over five decades and surrounded by heaps of ignition sources such as cut cardboard and shredded wood. Highway 10 runs northwest from Missoula past the airport and merges onto an interstate that soon narrows into winding stretches of valley and high-mountain roads. We are right in the middle of the northern Rockies, where fires consumed more than a million acres in 2017. At the nearby Aerial Fire Depot, visitors can sometimes spot smokejumpers parachuting from aircraft into the Missoula Valley, training for upcoming fire seasons.

The situation of potential fire entrapment suggests that dominant models of fire behavior are losing some of their power of foresight (figure 3.1). Wildfire's rogue nature erases comfortable distinctions between dead fuels (that burn) and live fuels (whose burning differs from that of dead woody fuels and is less well understood). It also erases distinctions between rural wildland fires and urban conflagrations. In the words of the noted wildfire research scientist Jack Cohen, such geographic distinctions are "not relevant to the physics of what is actually happening."[18] Or, as the wildfire historian Stephen Pyne observed after the firestorm in Santa Rosa, California, in 2017, the fires "seem to be going where the houses are."[19] Given fundamental changes, researchers are going back to the basics of fire, researching mechanisms of wildfire spread and even the properties of ignition. These phenomena seem elementary— stunningly so—especially if one considers that more than half of the USFS's budget is now focused on fighting fires. But the long-standing fixation with suppression, especially after World War II, meant that the science of wildfire had limited itself to an image of *controllable* wildfire. Cold War ballistics experts, who once dominated the relatively small field of US wildfire science, created "hypothetical universes in which fires burn only small, uniform, dead fuels on the forest floor," Finney told me. But fire does not spread according to averages: "It's actually the excursions, or the nonsteadiness, that allows fire to spread." By "averaging out nonsteady physics" and creating patterns that don't exist, these models conjure images that could prompt misjudgments in the field.

Expertise in this tricky context means confronting not only gaps in expertise but also faulty intuitions about physical patterns; it means making perceptions and "mental slides" of fire spread align with the physical trajectories of fuels. Where fire's combustibility confronts fire's "hypothetical universes," well-intentioned but misinformed suppression responses can create new paths for wildfires to travel, worsening conditions for the next fire (a condition known as the "wildfire paradox").[20] Scenes of the things wildfire is not supposed to do—spreading *against* the wind and even pushing its way up against it; burning into old fire scars and into places fire should

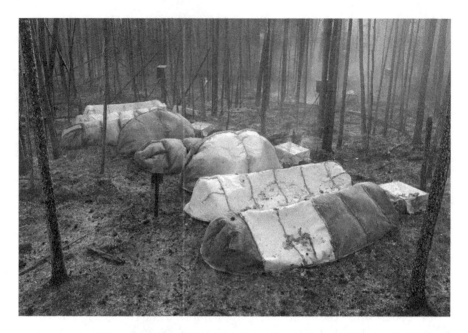

FIGURE 3.1 | New-generation fire shelter test in Alberta, Canada: high temperatures melted the aluminum covering, exposing heat-resistant silica cloth (2015). Photograph courtesy of Ian Grob/US Forest Service.

not be able to burn—are harrowing. In the gap between the expected and what actually occurs, that intuitions and projections will be undermined is axiomatic. Trainers tell firefighters to throw away their old mental slides; fire researchers tell their colleagues in the field that they have been looking at fire in the wrong ways; and engineers seek otherworldly materials to thermally enhance emergency fire shelters. They recently tested materials from the National Aeronautics and Space Agency (NASA) designed to thermally protect spacecraft upon atmospheric reentry, but these materials did not hold up well against fire temperatures on Earth.

Acquiring a Horizon

The concept of runaway change suggests not only shifting ecological patterns. It points to conditions that oblige emergency responders to revise knowledge calibrated to a world that no longer exists, as well as to an apparent futility of certain expertise. Fire experts are using their insights into changes in fire behavior to avoid what one called "diligent insanity" (i.e., the day-to-day and ineffective tactics of fire suppression). They also work toward "acquiring a horizon" in which time might be leveraged or borrowed. What is at stake in all of this? A concerned wildfire researcher said it best: "What I really mean is that we need to act in a way that we are not cutting off options for future generations."

The ability to horizon implies an ability to learn, act, or, at least, reconstruct the terms of understanding of ecological phenomena like fire. Moreover, the fire experts and others I interviewed are attempting to gain an empirical foothold in new fire dynamics while avoiding being cut off from the prospect of knowing them. They are cultivating what feminist scholar and historian of science Donna Haraway calls "response-ability," which precludes a "surrender [of] the capacity to think."[21] Haraway cautions against any such surrenders in a time of "onrushing disasters, whose unpredictable specificities are foolishly taken as unknowability itself."[22] These fire scientists agree. Yet declarations of new epochs—as if we know their beginnings and can contemplate their ends—reinforce an anthropocentric knowing that anthropologists have countered. By the same token, the conceptual grounds of projecting forward in time should not be ceded to scientists alone. They too are uncertain about the new conditions, or of how near, far away from, or over we are with respect to tipping points for particular biomes. Putting any label on that kind of uncertainty is, at best, premature.

What we can say is that temporal horizons of any sort are political; they can demarcate or dissolve spaces of political action or justify inaction or "quitting thinking."[23] In the meantime, forms of planetary rescue, including geoengineering, promising to stabilize the warming effects of greenhouse-gas emissions, are being promulgated. Largely untested, they can include injecting billions of sulfur dioxide particles into the upper atmosphere, producing chemical clouds that reflect sunlight. But geoengineering approaches can never reverse what has already happened to Earth's fuels. Halting the fossil fuel combustion that drives the climate crisis is the best path of stabilization. So are the efforts that create worlds that are compatible with life. The Brazilian Indigenous leader Davi Kopenawa—whose community has endured massacres, land theft, and violent resource extraction, speaks of an obligation to safeguard whole systems when he states, "protect the [Amazon] forest. Prevent the river waters from flooding it and the rains from mercilessly drenching it. Repel the cloudy weather and darkness. Hold up the sky so it does not fall apart."[24]

The anthropological analysis of runaway change, when attuned to the visions and pragmatics of stabilization, returns some kind of possibility or temporality that is graspable as it reaffirms a possibility of maintaining futures that are recoverable and not denied.[25] Actionability of this sort hinges on lessons learned from the past, as well as ethnographic analyses of improbable fights and how they are won by people under siege.

―――――――――――

It was ten years after the Chernobyl disaster when the Ukrainian health physicist Vadim Chumak posed this question to me: How did they survive? He was referring to the workers who had been conscripted to do Chernobyl cleanup and exposed to six to eight times the textbook definition of a lethal radiation dose, and he didn't know the answer. Their collected tooth samples, providing an indicator of absorbed dose, evidenced the unthinkable: improbable lives for whom the textbook of survival was not yet written or imagined.

I had the opportunity to revisit what has been learned from the unnatural experiment/catastrophe of Chernobyl and how it has evolved scientifically: what is known now that wasn't known before about the human effects of chronic, high, and low-dose radiation and how such knowledge should figure into revised epidemiological understandings of the health effects of accidental and massive releases of radiation. Over thirty years later, the textbook does not exist. The research networks required to translate Chernobyl survivors' reconstructed doses into an internationally recognized gold standard of clinical data have all but disintegrated. Populations affected by Chernobyl have by and large become vestiges of larger—and mostly unsystematized—bodies of fragmented studies.[26] Ukraine, and the world, still face a legacy of incomplete knowledge about Chernobyl's public-health consequences.[27] Accounting for these is not a closed matter; it hinges on what kinds of research and funds are applied, and over what timescale. The scientific establishment's short-term purview made contending with complex health outcomes almost impossible. It is no surprise that Chernobyl continues to be framed as a unique, one-off event with no lessons for bettering response for future disasters.[28] All this amounts to a narrowing of Chernobyl into a "quasi-event," minimizing the potential for informed action in the future. The painful lesson here is that some horizons are really fleeting.

The question, "How did they survive?" suggests at least two distinct (temporal) dimensions. One is linked to the lives of individual citizens and immediately assessable damages to ecologies and species. The other is linked to longer timescales and to other events—for example, of Chernobyl and the nuclear disasters at Fukushima, as well as refusals to deal with them on comparable terms. Such events, examined within a broader stretch of historical time, register notions of failure, resourcefulness, and recovery. Along this second dimension, one would hope for lessons and opportunities taken for scientific research to build and crystallize into a social science of survival: disasters become touchstones, rather than flukes, and arcs of knowledge inform a capacity to prevent or face future disasters. This social science would, however tentatively, articulate a learning curve that could stretch from one catastrophic and routinely data-scarce environment to the next. It would also engage the public about what information is available or missing, but required, to obtain a fuller picture of devastating tolls. It would also be about improving templates of data collection and using them to predict and, one hopes, to better respond the next time disaster comes. In the barrage of tipping points, anthropologists are tasked with building heuristic and material responses that become more fortified and just.[29] As new baselines of knowledge are built where old ones disappear, such anticipatory anthropological work interrogates the conditions that can prevent vulnerability and expand resources with which chances for "success" can be preserved, not forever lost.

Such social sciences of survival, shorn amid constant exposure to jeopardy, can set the ground for revolutionary acts of resistance in the future, as is the case in Ukraine. When, in February 2022, Putin's army invaded the country, it chose the Chernobyl zone as its initial staging ground in an attempt to impose the rule of a petro-state. Among the many war crimes that have been committed, its troops destroyed and looted sensitive radiological equipment in an area in which radiological information is vital. Ukrainian technical experts had painstakingly labored to achieve nuclear security at the site over decades. As nuclear instability becomes weaponized, so too does the terror of a disaster that could force the country's population back into dangerous decontamination work.

Insofar as horizoning carves out futurity as an expansive rather than a collapsing resource, it is very much at work as other tipping points loom. Indeed, the universe of risk with respect to the climate crisis now includes an unwieldy range of such tipping points. If this is true, our image is not really of an isolated point but, rather, of a messy, frayed vastness of causally intertwined risks that make up a broad, undulating border of tipping points that is more like a cliff. Depending on various factors (such as wind), some things on its jagged edge will fall sooner rather than later, while other things will be able to withstand greater erosive forces, at least for a while. This undulating edge represents countless threshold conditions and a huge range of events in waiting: states of "climate chaos, global militarization, and the mass displacement of people and other species" in which so many now live.[30]

To paint such states with images—whether it is an isolated point or an undulating cliff—is to call out shifts that are taking place along boundary lines that are neither stable nor predictive. Such instability necessitates conversations about what it means to look into a future and to say that we cannot project into it. Rather than running toward fear, how can we circumnavigate this vast abrupt with our forests, oceans, biospheres, and lives still intact?[31] If we think this circumnavigation is possible, then we will have to have new mental models to prepare ourselves for this collective maneuver.

Saving forests, lives, and rivers and "holding up the sky" is about more than just borrowing time, but plumbing the lines of a durable world.[32] Such lines run through violent histories, misguided policies, and ongoing structural inequalities. They run through the extractive fossil fuel regimes that generate massive transfers of risk that overdetermine who is protected and who is sacrificed in environmental regime shifts, placing Indigenous communities on the frontlines of climate change and unjust forms of disaster response. Only in contending with these concerns can benchmarks for concerted action be effective, and further damage on a planetary level be stopped. Along the way, it won't just be target-setting for limiting greenhouse gas emissions, as imperative as that is, but coordinated acts of stabilization that can stop the drift toward an inhospitable planet.

Coda

In his haunting series of seascape photographs, the Japanese photographer Hiroshi Sugimoto captures a struggle to enable the act of seeing in conditions of opacity: to grapple with a loss of how to imagine the dimension of loss. The viewer's sense of distance and time are lost in an image of "nothing" that also opens into an unknown magnitude. With closer scrutiny, Sugimoto's images give, and the viewer takes in, clues: tidal patterns, for example, gesture toward yet unseen paths that also beckon the viewer to undertake an arduous process of reckoning with an unseen object. Without a stable horizon line, the viewer finds signs as clues to a pathway.

Horizons suggest a conceptual interiority and a space for deliberation with whatever critical detail can be coaxed out of the scene. They are also age-old instruments that create effective perceptual range in "invisible presents."[33] The physicist John Huth writes in his book *The Lost Art of Finding Our Way* that seafarers, finding themselves trapped in dense fog or storms, have a special ability to grasp the kinetics of uncertain situations.[34] They demarcate increments using known parameters—the smell of a certain forest, certain patterns in tidal waters—and deduce their positioning vis-à-vis a previously estimated location or "fix." Their so-called dead reckoning (from deductive reckoning), like those of the fire and ecological scientists I spoke with, makes good on faulty or fleeting information, forestalling the prospect of exponential uncertainty or preventing a crash (or disappearance) of an entire system. In other words, such horizoning allows for a constant reentry into a navigable present and a still recognizable future. In and beyond the immediacies of the climate crisis, horizoning turns panic into a test of collective care. There is no preconceived protocol for this work of translation, only to say that it has to be done.

Notes

1 | Nordenson, "Probabilistic Coastal Hazards Mapping for the United States."
2 | Marcia McNutt, Public lecture, National Council for Science and the Environment, Disasters and Environment Conference, Washington, DC, January 2013.
3 | Kahneman and Klein, "Conditions for Intuitive Expertise."
4 | James White, Public briefing on National Research Council report, "Abrupt Impacts of Climate Change: Anticipating Surprises." Washington, DC, January 10, 2014, https://www.youtube.com/watch?v=uh3auNaQbhc.
5 | Today, 1 in 6 Americans are exposed to significant wildfire risk, with communities of color experiencing the highest risk. See Muyskens et al., "1 in 6 Americans"; Davies et al., "Unequal Vulnerability of Communities of Color."
6 | Thomas, *The Artificial Horizon*, 21.
7 | Binet, "Model Predictive Control Applications for Planetary Rovers."
8 | From Coriolanus 2.1.193: see Brogan, *Anthimeria*.
9 | Kleinman, *The Soul of Care*.
10 | Attenborough, cited in Wallace-Wells, "Time to Panic."
11 | Wallace-Wells, *The Uninhabitable Earth*.
12 | Petryna, *Horizon Work*.
13 | Whyte, "Our Ancestors' Dystopia Now"; and Gilpin, "Urgency in Climate Change Advocacy"; also see Callison, "The Twelve-Year Warning."
14 | Holthaus, "The First Wintertime Megafire in California History Is Here."
15 | Downey, "Why Are California's Wildfires So Out of Control?" By mid-September of 2020, entire towns went up in flames in California, Oregon, and Washington in the worst fire season on record. In early 2022, both Colorado and New Mexico saw the most destructive wildfires in their states' histories.
16 | Matt Jolly, interview by the author, Missoula, 2017.
17 | Bachelard, *The Psychoanalysis of Fire*, 6.
18 | Curwen, "California's Deadliest Wildfires Were Decades in the Making."
19 | Curwen, "California's Deadliest Wildfires Were Decades in the Making."

20 | The wildfire community refers to this sociotechnical aporia as the wildfire paradox, such that, as one fire behavioral analyst told me (reflecting a generally accepted fact), that the harder you try to suppress wildfires, the worse they get when they happen.

21 | Haraway, *Staying with the Trouble*, 35.

22 | Haraway, *Staying with the Trouble*, 35.

23 | On inactivism as a pernicious form of climate denial, see Mann, *New Climate War*. Jack Cohen, interview by the author, Missoula, 2017.

24 | Kopenawa, *The Falling Sky*, 32.

25 | For an analytic of temporal framing as it remakes experimental methods and frameworks within unstable social systems, see Fischer, *Anthropology in the Meantime*.

26 | Petryna, *Life Exposed*. Also see Brown, *Manual for Survival*.

27 | Arguably, researchers have more knowledge about the genetic and reproductive vulnerabilities of voles, mice, and birds in the abandoned Chernobyl dead zone than they do about human recoverability.

28 | Petryna, "How Did They Survive?," in *Life Exposed*.

29 | Bonilla and LeBrón, *Aftershocks of Disaster*.

30 | McClintock, "Monster: A Fugue in Fire and Ice."

31 | Wallace-Wells, *The Uninhabitable Earth*.

32 | Kopenawa, *The Falling Sky*.

33 | Magnuson, "Long-Term Ecological Research and the Invisible Present."

34 | Huth, *The Lost Art of Finding Our Way*.

The Category Fallacy *and* Care amid the Experts

HOW CAN MEDICAL ANTHROPOLOGY SPEAK to multiple audiences to break open hegemonic forms of expertise and technocratic certainty and, in so doing, propel broader movements for health equity and justice in our imperiled times?

The chapters in part II force us to reckon with the technocratic valuations that produce and reify unequal burdens of disease and patients' access to care. The anthropologists Salmaan Keshavjee and Janis H. Jenkins and the historian David S. Jones draw on their experiences speaking to different "publics" (clinicians, global health technocrats, policy makers, social scientists) to critique and decolonize commonsense practices in medical care. Their essays highlight interdependent dynamism between critical interference and social change making; in doing so, they nod toward the epistemological and moral commitments central to clinical medicine that might cross-pollinate anthropological work that has consistently critiqued the "thinness" of biomedical care without necessarily examining its own analytic abstractions, dispassionate tendencies, and paralyzing obfuscations.[1]

The analytical orientations of these chapters are all in line with Arthur Kleinman's sweeping critiques of the dominant epistemological and empirical methodologies of transcultural psychiatry. "Much of [this] work has involved a breathless search through large amounts of data from different societies looking for 'universals,'" such as depressive illness or other psychiatric diagnoses, he wrote.[2] While such studies were motivated by a desire to parse out the culturally specific from the universal, in merely searching for the presence of Western psychiatric categories within other patient populations, researchers a priori precluded the possibility of producing nuanced knowledge on the role of culture in shaping mental illness.

Kleinman termed this trap "the category fallacy." His main point at the time was that cross-cultural health researchers must always keep in mind that culture does more than merely color the experience of illness; it also informs the very categories by which it is lived, understood, and cared for. Kleinman's insights have been taken up and pushed forward by medical anthropologists concerned with the social construction of illness categories and what are deemed "possible" treatments. This perspective has also deeply informed the work of many of Kleinman's physician-anthropologist trainees (including Keshavjee and Jones), who have used notions of the category fallacy to critique the social construction of assumed scarcity in health-care resources. Anthropologists here do their own analyses of the social construction of diagnostic categories and treatment possibilities across diverse settings and demonstrate how this form of critical medical anthropology can have profound practical implications for decolonizing and making more just health policy and practice.

Salmaan Keshavjee, an infectious disease physician and anthropologist who has devoted his research career to implementing more effective programs to treat and prevent multidrug-resistant tuberculosis, shows how logics of tuberculosis (TB) treatment in global health have been shaped by colonialism and neoliberalism, creating a presumed sense of scarcity that structures TB treatment guidelines sustained through racialized logics of scarcity and privilege. This clinical "common sense" (codified in TB treatment protocols and standardized interventions) is actually rooted in economic and colonizing ideologies. It not only reifies vulnerabilities to the infection among poor populations but also serves as a foundation for the global institutions that now constrain the public health and broader societal responses to TB epidemics, actually increasing the number of cases of drug-resistant tuberculosis. This, in turn, converts a treatable disease into an often fatal outcome for poor patients. Keshavjee argues for an ambitious overhaul of the transnational TB treatment infrastructure that consists of both decolonizing the epistemological certainties that have put cost-effectiveness above all else and drawing on the histories of other social movements in efforts to increase access to safe, effective, and modern TB treatment for all.

David S. Jones takes on the case of heart disease and its erasure under the burden of infectious disease-focused models of international and global health in India and the Asian subcontinent. He explains how the very designation of what is deemed an epidemic is embedded in political, economic, and cultural assumptions, such that public-health epidemiologists assumed that a disease common to "rich societies" could not exist in India. Here, regimes of care embedded in political economies are legitimated and scaled up to meet categorical assumptions held by global health experts, and these assumptions, in turn, lead to the obfuscation of an entire burden of disease.

In her chapter, Janis H. Jenkins reviews the at times fraught relationship between anthropological and clinical/epidemiological studies of mental disorders. Jenkins's attention to the primacy of experience of the mentally ill reveals that public-health studies continue to fall prey to the category fallacy—that is, to ignoring the roles of culture in shaping mental illness. But such omissions also can be found in anthropological work, where critiques and efforts to situate mental illness as purely a social construction may deny the legitimacy of patients' suffering. Reimagining mental health disorders as "extraordinary conditions" may thus humanize the afflicted by attending to the interplay of broader social conditions and the phenomenological experience of psychiatric symptoms, and peoples' struggles to sustain an ordinary rhythm of life amid disruptive experiences of mental illness. Mental illness, in other words, remains an indeterminate form of suffering that must be understood in relation to a patient's own agency and existential efforts to make sense of and make do through their condition.

Notes

1 | Franklin and Munyikwa, "The Thinness of Care."
2 | Kleinman, "Depression, Somatization and the 'New Cross-Cultural Psychiatry,'" 3.

Justifying a Lower Standard of Health Care for the World's Poor

A Call for Decolonizing Global Health

TUBERCULOSIS (TB), an airborne bacterial disease that has been treatable since 1948, causes the death of more than one-and-a-half million people annually—more than four thousand people every day. With the exception of the COVID-19 outbreak, it is the leading infectious killer of adults globally and the leading killer of people coinfected with the human immunodeficiency virus (HIV). Out of the estimated ten million people who become sick with TB each year, one million are children. Almost one third of TB patients go undiagnosed and continue to spread the disease in their families, communities, and places of work. The majority of those affected live in some of the world's most impoverished settings.

Over the past almost thirty years working in global health, and more than twenty years working in the area of TB treatment, research, and policy, I have noticed that, despite the dedicated efforts of many people and programs, the best word to describe the pace of progress in ending the global TB pandemic is *glacial*. While a cure for the disease is available—and well-understood strategies to stop the epidemic have been used in high-income countries with great success since the early 1960s—global rates of new cases of TB drop only 1.5 percent per year.[1] In this chapter, I explore one of the reasons tuberculosis treatment delivery is the global health poster child for what we might call "failure to deliver."

To be sure, the simple biomedical answer is that we have not properly deployed in poor and middle-income settings tried and tested strategies for stopping the epidemic.[2] But this does not fully explain the problem. Rather, we need to look at the double standard of care between high-income settings and low- and middle-income settings—a double standard that has become naturalized, or taken as a natural order of things, by experts who are in a place to determine people's access to lifesaving care, rather than as a man-made and reversible situation—what the physician-anthropologist Paul Farmer has referred to as the result of "the fixing of protocols and policies based on a lower standard of care."[3] To understand how this naturalization occurs, we need to explore how the "subject" of global health—or, rather, the subject who is worthy of care—exists today in part as a legacy of prior eras, both colonial and postcolonial.

Tuberculosis as a disease came to the forefront as an epidemic—or, more accurately, pandemic—at a historical moment shaped by colonialism and the imperatives of empire. The logics of colonialism contributed to an enduring legacy of substandard health policies in the postcolonial and global health eras. Indeed, the foundational assumptions about who TB affected and how it mattered in these places shaped colonial health interventions, and these assumptions were rekindled in the postwar, postcolonial era under similar rubrics of implicit racial superiority. The era of global health has also inherited these assumptions, though they appear in different forms today, as perceived conditions of scarcity are used to rationalize limited health aid, and the logics of a naturalized and inferior subject who may or may not be worthy of aid persists. My point is not that static hierarchies of worthiness and care were simply transmitted across colonial, postcolonial, and now neoliberal public health but that, to understand global health failures around TB today, it is important to think about how the subjects of colonialism have been constructed through histories of imperialism and statecraft and how expert notions surrounding their health end up justifying the brutality of empire. By exploring these logics and the epistemological systems that have persisted and reemerged over many different eras of clinical interventions, we can better understand the processes that perpetuate various forms of inequality and ineffectiveness in relation to stemming the spread and mortalities of TB.

This exploration builds on and interrogates critical insights offered by Arthur Kleinman in some of his earliest work: the problem of the category fallacy. In his work on the cultural construction of disease and illness, he described how care could be derailed by mistaken assumptions about shared understandings of diagnosis and therapy. In my work, I take the category fallacy to mean the mistaken assumption that difference in health status and resource acquisition were and are natural, fixed, and unable to be altered, and, indeed, come to be built into the medical and scientific rubrics for clinical care as driven by biological givens rather than as social constructs and political choices. To this day, few have explored how assumptions surrounding the European or "white" body as dominant both justified the extractive capitalism of colonial eras *and* continue to be woven through postcolonial and global health programs.[4] In this chapter, I trace these threads of racialized category fallacies that can be seen in a variety of historical accounts of the colonial and postcolonial health encounter.

Colonial Health Priorities and the Dominance of the "White" Body

Historians have offered a clear picture of how the health of indigenous populations in the colonies was a low priority for colonial governments that devoted considerable energy to keeping the colonizers healthy but reserved health care for the natives only when it affected their ability to work or there was a perception that lack of care was putting the health of the colonizers at risk.[5] In this way, health during the colonial era became an instrument of extraction and protection for the colonizers and the colonial metropole rather than caregiving toward the colonized. This shaped the dominant discourse about the etiology of disease among the colonized. For instance, in his very detailed work on the US colonization of the Philippines (1898–1930s), the historian Warwick Anderson describes the colonial encounter "as a process and category in the history of medicine and public health more generally" in which ideas around disease and the treatment of illness among the colonized was transformed.[6]

According to Anderson, the result was that disease was divorced from the social conditions of the Filipinos and became naturalized as part and parcel of being Filipino. Similarly, in his work on tuberculosis in South Africa, the historian Randall Packard shows how the "evolution of medical ideas concerning the history of TB among Africans did not occur in an intellectual vacuum but was shaped by wider currents in the political and economic history of South

Africa."[7] And although it is problematic to compare colonialism in different places as if they entailed the same operations, Anderson's and Packard's accounts show how drivers of sickness among the colonized populations—and the risks they posed for the settlers and soldiers—were constructed. Examples such as these offer a particularly useful insight about how assumptions about deserving subjects of health care, though certainly driven in part by political and economic considerations, were fashioned around racial categories that naturalized health worthiness along lines of racial difference. Packard, who compares TB in South Africa to TB in nineteenth-century England, goes as far as to say that "the South African experience with TB has not been produced by a unique set of social and biological phenomenon (either the racist state or the racially susceptible African)." Rather, he argues, it "must be seen . . . as a product of a particularly pathological intersection of political, economic, and biological processes that have a much wider distribution."[8]

In Anderson's work, one can clearly see the movements over time in the explanations of disease. In the early part of the United States' colonial encounter in the Philippines, Anderson argues, there was a feeling that the "white soldier" needed protection from a climate that was "unnatural" to him, one that produced a deterioration of the "white" physique and mentality. As a result, much was done to protect the population of soldiers and prevent their physical and emotional deterioration. Under this rubric, the spread of diarrhea and disease was viewed as due to the "alternate heat and rains of the tropical climate and by the lowering of vital powers consequent on heat exhaustion."[9] As the US occupation continued, new technologies such as bacteriology emerged as an important factor in defining disease locally. Local resistance to occupation was also increasing. Previous concerns about terrain and climate became increasingly displaced by understandings of natives as "natural" hosts and carriers of microbes—as dangerous. "Filipinos were thus armed . . . with a weapon more insidious than any rifle," Anderson notes, capturing the insights of one colonial official who stated, "The Filipinos are never free from contagious disease of one form or another, . . . and we can never be sure that they are not bringing infection into our midst."[10] The discovery that Filipinos, including children, were carrying germs "secretly" and were a source of fatal infection to Americans of European descent sealed their fate. Medical officers forbade contact with natives, suggesting that no matter how clean local Filipinos "might look or smell," they were to be distrusted. Thus, as Anderson tells us, "Together, the Bureau of Science and the Army Board for the Study of Tropical Diseases produced a white male body that was more or less indifferent to tropical relocation and . . . with apparently natural, though not naturally fixed, differences in disease carriage and susceptibility. That is, science helped to reframe the boundaries of whiteness in the Philippines, neutralizing or overcoming containment and making racial contact even more salient and medically significant."[11]

Local "immunity" to malarial parasites—that is, the possibility that Filipinos may have, in the context of endemic malaria, lived with chronically fluctuating levels of malaria parasites in their blood that could, in turn, be transmitted to American or Europeans there—was viewed as proof that the "Malay race" or "Oceanic Mongols," as the Filipinos were called, were "no amigos." This sealed the fate of sick Filipinos, who were viewed as inherently sick and infectious—not only unworthy of the same care but also warranting physical separation.

Similarly, in South Africa race and disease were used as one of the bases of the system of apartheid—segregation. Packard points out that in the late nineteenth century, massive urbanization resulted in the growth of TB in the African population. He links this to the arrival in South Africa of individuals with TB, primarily from England, who hoped that the climate would help them heal, and Polish and Russian Jews who had come to South Africa to escape poverty and persecution. The "consumptives," as the TB-afflicted Europeans were known, included Cecil Rhodes, who came to South Africa from England because of fears that he had TB. After being cured, he went on to make a fortune in the diamond trade and to lead the charge for European imperialism and white supremacy. Many of the European settlers sick with TB were not that lucky. According to Packard: "Some who arrived too ill to work and without resources died soon after their arrival. Others who were able to work but lacked resources were forced to seek employment in low-paying, physically demanding jobs that further weakened their condition. In addition they frequently lived in cheap tenements and overcrowded boarding houses, and there they became sources of infection to other residents who shared their economic condition and eventually their disease."[12]

Similarly, the European Jews, who were called "Peruvians," came from countries with high rates of TB. According to Packard, "Prevented from making a reasonable living, forced to live on the margins of white society, and unable to properly care for and feed themselves or their families, these less fortunate settlers often suffered reactivation of their disease and became open sources of infection within the community."[13] Poor Blacks and poor whites ended up in interracial tenements and somewhat mixed neighborhoods, and the result was almost predictable: tuberculosis rates among the Africans also began to rise rapidly.

The *explanation* for the rise in TB among Africans varied, but Packard points out that "the weight of both medical and lay opinion on the subject favored an explanation that stressed the 'natives' incomplete and inadequate adjustment to the conditions of urban life, their ignorance of sanitary conditions, and their adoption of European patterns of dress and behavior."[14] The mixing with Europeans, especially wearing European clothing, was seen as a particular *risk to the indigenous population*. While there was recognition that urban poverty played a part, TB was linked to particular behavior of the indigenous population: "Other reports pointed to the unsanitary conditions in which urban Africans lived, their habit of living in overcrowded houses, of spitting indiscriminately, of sleeping with blankets pulled over their heads, and 'habits of inebriety and depravity'" as other indications of their maladjustment to civilization and reasons for their susceptibility to TB."[15]

The view of the African as prone to disease and a carrier of disease pushed the drive for public-health laws that would move and isolate Black and Brown populations; limit the movement of labor and the interaction between races; and, de facto, limit access to health care. This had been done before. During the epidemic of plague in Cape Town in 1901, the government used the Public Health Act of 1897 to create "native locations" on the outskirts of the city, even though the plague was not limited to the Black African population.[16] The medical administrator at the time, Barnard Fuller, argued that the interventions were necessary: "Rest the blame where it may. These uncontrolled Kafir hordes were at the root of the aggravation of Cape Town slumdom brought to light when the plague broke out. Because of them, it was absolutely impossible to keep the slums of the city in satisfactory condition."[17] This is what the historian Maynard Swanson referred to as "sanitation syndrome": using health regulations and rules in the name of "sanitation" to segregate populations. In the case of the plague, the Prime Minister William Philip Schreiner is said to have exclaimed about the Black population: "They lived all over the place.... We could not get rid of them. They were necessary for work. What we wanted was to get them practically in the position of being compounded."[18] The feeling was that segregation would not only protect the European settler population; it would also allow more control over the African population.

And thus, much like the situation in the Philippines, "sanitary conditions" were used as an excuse for racial segregation. According to Packard, "Physical segregation heightened racial consciousness and moved conceptions of the causes of African susceptibility to disease toward a more explicit racial conceptualization of the problem. . . . Africans were, in effect, biologically ill-adapted to civilization and its diseases."[19] This, Packard argues, "increased the social distance between Africans and whites, creating for whites a definition of 'the other' which facilitated and justified the physical removal of Africans from 'civilized society.'"[20]

The view of the local population as dirty and a risk to the "white" population—a focus on the bodies and space occupied by the colonized themselves that is not, of course, unique to the Philippines or South Africa—is of great significance to global health in the twentieth century. This is because the focus on the race of the colonized—a system of logic that naturalizes difference or "otherness"—allowed for a demarcation of rights and access to medicine and public health.[21] The racialization of illness and the subjugation of colonial subjects on the basis of their being biologically inferior was seen throughout the colonial era. As Anderson suggests, this racialization provided the basis for naturalized assumptions about the social order that bled into the postcolonial era.

Postcolonial Reworking of the Category Fallacy

Many casual observers of history, including policy makers and global health experts, see the end of World War II and the creation of the United Nations as the birth of a new epoch of internationalism and equality. Moving beyond colonialism offered the promise of this hope for equality to many a newly independent nation. But the naturalized hierarchies that justified unequal treatment for the colonized were sustained in international health programs, leaving many of the underlying structural inequalities in place even though now presented under the rubrics of international health aid. Here, too, hierarchies were built on ongoing concerns with racial hierarchies and, specifically, white supremacy.

In his study of the United Nations, the historian Mark Mazower argues that "a great deal is assumed about the UN's past by both supporters and critics on the basis of cursory readings of foundational texts, with little acknowledgement of the mixed motives that accompanied their drafting."[22] Commentators and critics of the UN at the time of its founding saw the "rhetoric of freedom and rights as all too partial," and as "a veil masking the consolidation of a great power directorate" with an "imperious attitude to how the world's weak and poor should have been governed."[23] Mazower contends that the "new" system—really not that new but, rather, a modified version of the older League of Nations—was meant to maintain US and British power in the postcolonial period. Noting that the architect of the UN's stirring preamble, Jan Smuts, South Africa's former prime minister and elder statesman, was an ardent advocate of white racial superiority, Mazower points out that, for many, the UN was seen as a means for maintaining "a democratic imperial order" and for "civilizing inferior races."[24]

Smuts saw the British Empire as "the only successful experiment in international government" and wanted it to be extended on a world scale. Although he spoke of the importance of internationalism and blending nationalities, he was referring to European nations and "white racial unity."[25] Especially with respect to Southern Africa, Smuts felt that "the white race" should "act as trustees for the colored races."[26] Such an arrangement, Smuts contended, left Blacks and whites better off, with each having "their proper place" and both having "their human rights."[27] In his 1929 Rhodes lecture at Oxford University, Smuts argued that "Africans may have 'wonderful characteristics' such as a 'happy-go-lucky disposition,' but they nonetheless 'remained a child-type, with a child psychology and outlook.'"[28]

After the collapse of the League of Nations and the toll of World War II, Smuts and others advocated for the formation of a League of Nations–like institution that included all the "great powers"—the soon-to-be victors of World War II—which in their minds were the United States, the British, and the Soviet Union. On August 14, 1941, US President Franklin Roosevelt and British Prime Minister Winston Churchill signed the Atlantic Charter on the USS *Augusta* off the coast of Newfoundland. The document, which was a declaration rather than a treaty, defined American and British goals for the postwar period, calling for the improvement of economic and social conditions for all, the restoration of self-government to those deprived of it, and reduced trade barriers—the latter two clauses being a direct attack on European colonial control of global markets and a nod to the rising influence of neoliberal thinking. The document's importance was enhanced by the signing of the "Declaration by United Nations" in Washington, DC, on January 1, 1942, by twenty-six allied governments, including the United States, the United Kingdom, the Soviet Union, and China, which pledged to follow the Atlantic Charter's principles.

While many in the United States and the European colonies viewed the charter as a way of dismantling the European empires—in fact, some US businessmen who had been against Roosevelt's New Deal economics became supporters of the Atlantic Charter because of its business potential—Churchill and the British did not see it that way. In fact, Churchill reported to the

British Parliament that the charter's self-determination clause did not apply to India or any other country within the British Empire.[29] When African countries used the charter to demand freedom, Smuts and other defenders of European colonial rule viewed that interpretation as a false reading of the document and "called for international collaboration in the development of 'backward countries' and recast colonialism as a kind of depoliticized guidance toward higher standards of living."[30]

Smuts, whose racial and segregationist policies had raised the ire of Mahatma Gandhi in the early part of the twentieth century, saw human rights as pertaining to basic minimal needs, part of the "sacred trust" imposed on "the more advanced people to look after the more backward."[31] He was not alone in his view. By the time the Great Powers met at Harvard University's Dumbarton Oaks estate outside Washington, DC, in late 1944 to set the framework for an institution of global governance, there was no mention of freedom for the colonies. China, which attended the meeting and had proposed "that the principle of equality of all states and races be upheld," was convinced by the United States to drop the proposal.[32] Not wanting to upset its close British ally during a time of war—and not wanting to disrupt plans to set up a network of US bases in the South Pacific—the US delegation was convinced by the US Army Chiefs of Staff to drop any discussion of self-determination. Most notably, no mention of self-determination or racial equality was made in any of the proposals submitted at Dumbarton Oaks. The African American intellectual W. E. B. Du Bois described this as "intolerable, dangerous" and incompatible "with any philosophy of democracy.... The only way to human equality is through the philanthropy of masters."[33]

At the United Nations' founding conference, held in the spring of 1945 in San Francisco, suggestions from the Philippines to get a commitment for the independence of colonies written into the UN Charter were crushed, as was an Ecuadoran proposal for the UN General Assembly to vote a country into independence. Du Bois was so scandalized by the lack of willingness to change the status quo that he commented, "We have conquered Germany but not their ideas. We still believe in white supremacy, keeping Negroes in their place and lying about democracy, when we mean imperial control of 750 millions of human beings in colonies."[34] Speaking in January 1948, British Prime Minister Ernest Bevin ironically echoed Du Bois's position by stating that he saw the United Nations as an opportunity for Europe to recover in the postwar period by drawing on the resources of colonial Africa.[35]

Not only was the United Nations in many ways a continuation of the status quo.[36] Its technical agencies themselves maintained a significant continuity with the past, with a focus on preventing disease in Europe's colonies from reaching the colonial metropole. The idea of international cooperation around health had been around for a while. The International Sanitary Conference was initiated in Paris on July 23, 1851. This was the first of eleven meetings that took place over half a century, mostly linked to stopping the international spread of cholera. According to the historian Javed Siddiqi, "The national motives for participation were primarily political and commercial, with public health being merely an incidental issue. The primacy of concerns about shipping over those about public health were no secret, as this had been explicitly laid out at the start of the conference by its President."[37] This series of conferences gave rise in 1907 to a permanent international health office to centralize epidemiological information and oversee international quarantine arrangements called the Office International d'Hygiène Publique (OIHP). Other organizations with similar mandates were also created: in 1902, the Pan American Sanitary Bureau (PASB) had been created in the Americas. and in 1919 the League of Red Cross Societies had also established itself as an international health organization.[38] After the Treaty of Versailles came into force in 1920, the League of Nations formed its own health organization, the League Health Organization. The merging of the OIHP or PASB and the League Health Organization was vetoed by the United States. The OIHP—whose main mandate had been focused on quarantine as a means of stopping diseases from moving between nations—later became part of the World Health Organization (WHO), which moved into the OIHP offices in Geneva and inherited its staff.

Although the newly formed WHO was conceived by its first director-general, the Canadian psychiatrist Brock Chisholm, as an organization that would transcend the nation-state and focus on the health of the entire world, post–World War II and Cold War politics soon stopped that.[39] In contrast to its position with the League of Nations, of which it was not a member, the United States was a vigorous supporter of the technical health agencies, seeing the provision of foreign technical assistance as a critical component of preventing the spread of communism. In fact, in his State of the Union message to the US Congress in 1952, President Dwight Eisenhower stressed that the promotion of "world health" was "essential in the fight on reds."[40]

I digress into this tumultuous history of the founding of the postcolonial institutions of international health to point out that the health goals of these organizations have always been compromised and shaped by other political agendas—including direct linkages with the waning colonial agenda; the view of the colonial metropole as central; and, much as we saw in the examples from the Philippines and South Africa, the colonized as a source of disease that needs to be contained rather than cared for or cured. In this way, the postcolonial period had a continuity with the past that relied on social hierarchies that labeled some kinds of people capable of self-governance and others incapable of it, as hopelessly in need of foreign aid and the forms of governance—and domination—that came with it. These hidden agendas became coupled with new cartographies of neoliberalism as the fear of communism became intertwined with various logics of health aid as a bulwark against its spread.[41] These agendas also became another way for implicit agendas of racial and economic supremacy—in the form of Euro-American domination—to infiltrate and mix with assumptions about worthiness for receiving health care. In the postcolonial era, the idea that some countries were destined to be resource-scarce and in need of health governance by agencies such as the WHO and various bilateral aid agencies became a new kind of racialized domination dressed up in the language of neoliberal progress.

Old Wine in New Bottles: Sacrificing Treatment
Complexity on the Altar of "Scarcity"

The global response to tuberculosis is paradigmatic of the divergence in international health, writ large, between the standards of care provided to the sick poor in low- and middle-income countries—mostly the former colonies—and those for the rich. To be sure, this is partly a vestige of a logic that gave rise to colonial medicine and the construction of the colonial/postcolonial other as a naturalized racial inferior. Colonialism engendered a moral orientation toward the colonized—moral values that guide behavior—that justified substandard care and a lack of urgency in addressing health problems even while extracting resources from the local population and leaving in its wake widespread poverty. But as colonialism waned, a new force arose: neoliberal political and economic philosophies.[42] There are important differences between the political logics of colonialism and those that underlie neoliberalism. However, the logics of both political regimes deprioritized the provision of social services via weakened states and promoted markets as optimal distribution mechanisms for social goods, as well as the extraction of labor and wealth as conduits to "development." And most critically, colonial and neoliberal political regimes alike treated resource-rich but wealth-depleted (or wealth-extracted/impoverished) countries and communities as fundamentally and naturally different from wealthy nations and communities in ways that justified unequal systems for and expectations of medical treatment. While the particular justifications for naturalized inequities in access to care may be slightly different, the consequences—codified health disparities—were the same; the history of TB treatment policies for poor countries is reflective of this noxious synergy.

The first antituberculosis antibiotic, streptomycin, was isolated by Selman Waksman and his graduate student, Albert Schatz, at Rutgers University in 1943, as World War II was coming to an end.[43] In 1948, the British Medical Research Council (BMRC) conducted the first large-scale clinical trial of streptomycin, after which it became the standard of care for treatment.[44] The use of streptomycin immediately revealed the complexity inherent in treating tuberculosis with the available armamentarium. The BMRC found that, beyond its toxicity in some patients, a large proportion of patients relapsed after treatment, and most did so with streptomycin-resistant strains of tuberculosis.[45] This was no surprise. As early as 1942, the microbiologist René Dubos had hypothesized that, with the selection that can result from the use of antibiotics, strains of bacteria would emerge that were resistant to killing by those antibiotics.[46] From the earliest days, in other words, treatment failure and drug resistance became linked in the minds of tuberculosis clinicians, resulting in decades of painstaking studies to understand how to prevent this dreaded outcome.[47]

Part of the solution for preventing the development of resistance was to use drugs in combination. In 1948, two new antituberculosis medicines, thioacetazone and para-aminosalicylic acid (PAS), became available. When they were given with streptomycin, antibiotic resistance was less frequent.[48] In 1951, isonicotinic hydrazide (isoniazid) was tested by Irving Selikoff, Edward Robitzek, and George Ornstein at Sea View Hospital in New York. This old, off-patent drug provided dramatic results for patients with tuberculosis.[49] A number of other drugs were developed soon afterward: isoniazid (1952), pyrazinamide (1952), cycloserine (1952), ethionamide (1956), rifampin (1957), and ethambutol (1962).[50] Because of its high efficacy, rifampin was a particular game changer for tuberculosis treatment. In 1971, rifampin was approved for use in tuberculosis treatment by the US Food and Drug Administration; however, almost as soon as it was used—even under extremely controlled conditions—resistance to the drug was observed.[51]

As far as treatment was concerned, the scientific evidence was clear: multidrug regimens were essential to prevent the rapid development of drug-resistant strains.[52] Given the overwhelming scientific evidence that the use of multidrug regimens not only improved the probability of cure but prevented the generation or selection of resistant mutants, the main question facing scientists was: Which combination, and for how long? In a series of carefully conducted clinical trials led by the BMRC over a number of decades in several countries, it was ultimately demonstrated that a four-drug regimen based on a backbone of isoniazid and rifampin was highly effective, curing almost all patients who adhered to treatment when given for a period of six to eight months. Added to this were studies demonstrating that home-based tuberculosis treatment was safe and highly effective when appropriately supervised.[53] Thus, "short-course chemotherapy" became an option for treating tuberculosis even in settings with limited health infrastructure.[54]

From the very outset, however, policy recommendations around tuberculosis therapy in poor countries were clouded by nonmedical considerations, and this is where resonances and legacies of colonial othering and its naturalizing of social hierarchies become visible again. Despite all the data coming in from the various studies, in the 1950s the newly formed WHO advocated treating tuberculosis patients in poor member states with isoniazid monotherapy because it would cost less.[55] Despite much validated clinical trial data already available that revealed the critical importance of multiple drugs in tuberculosis therapy, a "study group" convened by the WHO argued that, since isoniazid-resistant strains of tuberculosis seemed to have lower virulence in guinea pigs, the use of isoniazid alone would be "acceptable practice" if the alternative was having no program at all (as was the case in many poor countries).[56] Not only was the claim about "attenuated strains" among guinea pigs incorrect, but in a series of four clinical trials conducted between 1957 and 1961, the BMRC showed that this "scientific" recommendation to some of the world's poorest and most at-risk countries resulted in unfavorable treatment outcomes (relapse, failure, and death) and higher rates of isoniazid resistance.[57] According to the historian Christian McMillen, some British physicians in Kenya, which at the time was still a colony of Britain, were so aghast at the recommendations from the WHO that they refused to provide this type of substandard treatment to their patients.[58]

Yet the idea that poor countries warranted different programs of care than those offered in wealthy countries endured. The racialized rubrics of difference seen under colonial regimes were maintained, having morphed into rubrics of scarcity. In both cases, the codified and explicit disparities in access to and expectations of care were based on a notion that such disparities were natural, immutable, and thus common sense. Indeed, the idea that health aid programs *had* to operate in an environment of scarcity—that no new money could be found to treat more tuberculosis patients in former colonies—was so pervasive that even Wallace Fox, one of the fathers of the BMRC program, wrote in an article in the *British Medical Journal* in 1964, "In this difficult situation, where the practical choice may be to give no chemotherapy at all to the great majority of patients or prescribe isoniazid alone, the clinician can hardly be censured for giving isoniazid alone even though he is departing from the practice of countries with abundant drug supplies."[59] Here we see the use of a sliding scale of deservingness based on locale: although fewer than 70 percent of the patients would be cured (the other 30-plus percent transmitting what would likely be drug-resistant strains of tuberculosis to their families and communities), the discourse was neither about demanding increased funding (from states and donors—often the current or former colonial masters) nor about lower-priced drugs, both of which would allow for the scientifically proved and medically sound standard of care. Rather, people were offered the care they could directly pay for based on where they lived and funds in their countries' treasuries (rather than the value of resources being extracted from them). This is all a far cry from claims about the universality of rights to health, care, and life based merely on being human.

A similar situation occurred with the use of preventive therapy for those infected with the tuberculosis bacilli but who had not yet progressed to active disease. Overwhelming data from a randomized controlled trial conducted by George Comstock and his colleagues in Alaska in the 1950s showed that preventive therapy for contacts, when given in conjunction with treatment of individuals suffering from TB disease, could not only markedly lower rates of TB but also mortality; this approach, however, was rejected *for* low- and middle-income countries.[60] In 1964, the WHO's Expert Committee on Tuberculosis argued against the use of prophylaxis therapy in resource-depleted countries because "cost, logistical difficulties, the likelihood of defaulting, and other concerns all made it unfeasible."[61] In 1974, despite the highly successful use of prophylaxis therapy as part of a comprehensive epidemic control strategy that had essentially stopped the tuberculosis epidemic in rich countries, another WHO expert committee called the use of the approach in low- and middle-income countries "irrational." In 1982, this was reaffirmed by the WHO and its partner, the Paris-based nongovernmental organization the International Union against Tuberculosis and Lung Disease (IUATLD), who said that "in practice [prophylaxis therapy] has virtually no role in developing countries."[62] Of note, the WHO changed its policy to recommend prophylaxis therapy for low- and middle-income countries—a mainstay of tuberculosis epidemic control in high-income countries since the 1960s—only in March 2018.

The late 1970s were notable for a watershed event in global health: the Alma Ata Declaration. This declaration, signed in what was then the Soviet city of Alma Ata (present-day Almaty, Kazakhstan), called on nations to make primary health care "universally accessible to individual and families in the community . . . *at a cost that the community and country can afford.*"[63] Although heralded as a breakthrough that could offer health care to people who had little or no access to care, the declaration called for health care that was "simple" and "inexpensive" and essentially maintained the status quo between rich and poor globally.[64] Sadly, and minimalist though it was, even the primary health-care movement had begun to falter by the end of the 1970s. Concern about cost led to the idea of *selective* PHCC (SPHCC): discrete, targeted, and inexpensive vertical interventions.[65] This approach, which focused on childhood interventions, immediately won the support of the United Nations Children's Fund (UNICEF) and, more significantly, the World Bank.[66]

Despite extensive criticism for being too vertical and for not contributing to the strengthening of health systems, the SPHCC approach offered a sense of simplicity that appealed to donors.[67] However, while SPHCC and arguments about cost-effectiveness outlined a framework that might have been suitable for one-off interventions, they were not suited for diseases of any complexity. For patients with TB, the framework imposed by SPHCC meant limited access to treatment and likely death: the disease was specifically labeled as too costly and complex an intervention to be a high SPHCC priority.[68] Thus, TB treatment in poor countries was deemed an intervention unworthy of global support.

In the early 1990s, a new measure of cost-effectiveness emerged: the disability-adjusted life year (DALY).[69] Through this lens, interventions were considered cost-effective in a country if the cost per DALY saved was lower than three times the per capita gross national product. Linking this measure, which placed a premium on individuals deemed to be in their most productive years of life, to short-course TB treatment provided on an ambulatory basis, changed the place of TB in the global policy hierarchy. In 1993, the World Bank's *World Development Report: Investing in Health* came out in support of TB treatment as an extremely "cost-effective" strategy that should have a place in the SPHCC.[70] Seizing the momentum, the WHO branded and began to successfully promote its DOTS (directly observed therapy short course) program.[71] The program consisted of five key areas: government commitment, case detection based on sputum smear microscopy, short-course chemotherapy, a steady drug supply, and standardized recording and reporting systems. The DOTS program was packaged in a manner that fit well with selective primary health care: simple to treat, algorithmic, no expensive inputs (such as laboratories or X-ray machines), and no complications (such as drug resistance). As a selling point for adopting DOTS in its 1997 TB guidelines, the WHO openly recognized the policy lineage of the program by stating, "The World Bank recognizes the DOTS strategy as one of the most cost-effective of all health interventions and recommends that effective TB treatment should be a part of the essential clinical services package available in Primary Health Care (PHCC)."[72]

All of this would have been a public health victory had there not been one major problem: in simplifying tuberculosis to fit within the SPHCC paradigm—health care tailored to provide minimal care for the world's poor—the fundamental complexity of treating the disease had to be disregarded. In its first decades, those driving the DOTS approach, mostly the WHO and its close partner organizations, advocated the use of sputum smear microscopy—invented by the German scientist Robert Koch in 1882 and well known to have a sensitivity for finding the disease of 50 percent or less—instead of cellular culture technology as the best or most appropriate tool for tuberculosis diagnosis. The stated reason: building basic laboratory infrastructure to diagnose TB and other diseases would be too expensive for poor countries, and they did not have enough trained human resources to sustain such an effort. This type of thinking was flawed on many levels. For TB, it not only ignored people with disease that was outside their lungs (extrapulmonary TB) but also children and people living with HIV, groups of individuals who often did not excrete measurable bacteria. Also, the use of smear microscopy alone was incapable of diagnosing patients with drug-resistant strains of tuberculosis—a phenomenon known and documented since the first antituberculosis drug was used—thereby resulting in their continued transmission of difficult-to-treat disease in families and communities. The DOTS program was built on a legacy of doing the minimum for low-income countries and a sense that nothing beyond the minimum *could* be done for them; thus, it served both to link the logics of colonialism and neoliberalism and to naturalize a global burden of tuberculosis heavily based on geography and race.

Arguments to alter DOTS were met with counterarguments about scarcity of resources and—similar to Fox's argument from the 1960s—the firm belief that in the setting of resource scarcity there was value in doing something, however substandard, rather than nothing. In many ways, this set the foundation for a codified program of essentially *bad biomedicine* for the sick in some of the world's most vulnerable settings.[73] The poor—many of whom lived in the former colonies—were naturalized as poor and unhealthy by public health experts, just as disparities in health and care had been naturalized by racial hierarchies during the colonial era. These were the very categories on which expedient health policy decisions could be made. And people's poverty—their inability to pay for care—continued to justify forms of care that were substandard compared with the care offered to TB patients in rich nations.

Our present failure to stem the tide of tuberculosis globally can be directly linked the divergence in health policy represented by more than two decades of the WHO's DOTS strategy and more than half a century of advocating substandard treatment for the poor. Although successful for some patients, this approach has left many nations ill-equipped to address the complexity of tuberculosis.[74] The fact that highly drug-resistant tuberculosis strains are on the rise and the disease continues to be the biggest infectious killer of adults has unmasked these failings in dramatic fashion. Not surprisingly, the majority of the world's nations that labor under high TB mortality are the poorest and often racialized as other.

Conclusion: Transforming International Health into a Truly Global Health

This very brief history of the colonial encounter and its noxious synergy with neoliberal doctrine, albeit in broad strokes, is aimed at helping us better understand *why* anyone would think it is acceptable that people in poor countries (former colonies) should receive health care different from that received by people in rich countries (the former colonial masters). By tracing the legacies of European supremacy—often based on the social construction of a "white" race—from the colonial area through the postcolonial health development era and to the era of global health, I have argued that there is continuity in the way the naturalizing of difference as a biological or God-given fact has been sustained: what was once a problem inherent to the racialized other is now a problem of the poverty-stricken (and often racialized) other living in a nation that is too poor to warrant the most effective medical care. These, too, might be seen as ongoing problems of social and economic domination and call on us to think about how efforts to decolonize global health might also require tracing these legacies of naturalizing difference.

The "right to health" often requires addressing structural barriers to care, and they are often historically deep and socially complex. It also requires untangling the hidden assumptions and category fallacies that have sustained rationales for health intervention that continue to be unequal and unfair. Exploring these histories and legacies requires a methodological approach that attaches anthropology and history to the pragmatic work of medicine and global health policy.[75] By recognizing that the constructs that have clouded health-care delivery for the past few centuries can change, we have, as the anthropologist and physician Paul Farmer describes it, "the privilege of reasserting our humanity. Against a tide of utilitarian opinion and worse, we are offered the chance to insist, *This is not how it should be done*."[76]

Notes

An earlier version of this chapter was first presented at the conference Distinct Histories, Entangled Futures: Towards an Epistemology of Coinfection, organized by the Institute of History of Medicine at the University of Zurich at the Brocher Foundation in Geneva, Switzerland, February 27–28, 2014. I am grateful for feedback from the participants in this workshop, especially from the organizers, Lukas Engelmann and Janina Kehr. I am also grateful for feedback from Vincanne Adams and João Biehl, the editors of this volume. Special thanks to Sue Kulkarni, Elizabeth Noyes, and Tim Nichols for their assistance in the preparation of the manuscript.

1 | Kyu et al., "Global, Regional, and National Burden of Tuberculosis."
2 | Keshavjee et al., "Stopping the Body Count."
3 | Paul Farmer, personal communication, 2016.
4 | While this applies to some extent to European colonialization of other European countries (e.g., English control and colonization of Ireland; Prussian control and colonization of Silesia), much direct extraction and control of European colonies ended after World War I and does not pertain to the discussion of the post–World War II period. It is also clear that while race is a salient category, it also lines up with what the French philosopher Michel Foucault refers to as "labor force medicine." Foucault, *The Birth of Social Medicine*, 152.
5 | Anderson, *Colonial Pathologies*; Brown, *Rockefeller Medicine Men*; Fanon, *The Wretched of the Earth*; Hunt, "Rewriting the Soul in a Colonial Congo"; Packard, *White Plague, Black Labor*; Vaughan, *Curing Their Ills*.
6 | Anderson, *Colonial Pathologies*, 4.
7 | Packard, *White Plague, Black Labor*, 31.
8 | Packard, *White Plague, Black Labor*, 19.
9 | Anderson, *Colonial Pathologies*, 39.
10 | Anderson, *Colonial Pathologies*, 59.
11 | Anderson, *Colonial Pathologies*, 75.
12 | Packard, *White Plague, Black Labor*, 39.
13 | Packard, *White Plague, Black Labor*, 41.
14 | Packard, *White Plague, Black Labor*, 49.
15 | Packard, *White Plague, Black Labor*, 50.
16 | Fassin, *When Bodies Remember*.

17 | Swanson, "The Sanitation Syndrome," 382.
18 | Swanson, "The Sanitation Syndrome," 395.
19 | Packard, *White Plague, Black Labor*, 195–96.
20 | Packard, *White Plague, Black Labor*, 196.
21 | According to the French philosopher Michel Foucault, this mechanism is not unique to race demarcation. In *The Birth of Social Medicine*, Foucault suggests that the development of cities and the concurrent influx of large numbers of poor workers created a necessity for a type of medicine that he called "labor force medicine." As in South Africa or the Philippines, Foucault argues, it was the cholera epidemic of 1832 in France that crystalized a fear of the "proletarian or plebian population": Foucault, *The Birth of Social Medicine*, 152. This, he argues, was the driving force between dividing the urban space into rich and poor areas. It also was also the driver, he argues, behind the creation of welfare laws that, in providing health care to the poor, protected the wealthy.
22 | Mazower, *No Enchanted Palace*, 5.
23 | Mazower, *No Enchanted Palace*, 7.
24 | Mazower, *No Enchanted Palace*, 21.
25 | Mazower, *No Enchanted Palace*, 47.
26 | Mazower, *No Enchanted Palace*, 48.
27 | Mazower, *No Enchanted Palace*, 51.
28 | Dubow, "Smuts, the United Nations and the Rhetoric of Race and Rights," 62.
29 | Normand and Zaidi, *Human Rights at the UN*.
30 | Mazower, *No Enchanted Palace*, 56.
31 | Dubow, "Smuts, the United Nations and the Rhetoric of Race and Rights," 62.
32 | Normand and Zaidi, *Human Rights at the UN*, 111.
33 | Normand and Zaidi, *Human Rights at the UN*, 115.
34 | Getachew, *Worldmaking after Empire*, 72.
35 | Mazower, *No Enchanted Palace*.
36 | While the end of World War II and the coming of the UN system did lead to some changes—in fact, in subsequent years the General Assembly, led by India, would call into question South Africa's policies and take a stand on the country's apartheid policies—the organization, focused as it was on nation-states and Great Power politics, did not take any significant stands for the independence of colonies or for the rights of the colonized.
37 | Siddiqi, *World Health and World Politics*, 15.
38 | Siddiqi, *World Health and World Politics*.
39 | Farley, *Brock Chisholm, the World Health Organization, and the Cold War*.
40 | Cueto, *Cold War, Deadly Fevers*, 22.
41 | Keshavjee, *Blind Spot*.
42 | Keshavjee, *Blind Spot*.
43 | Comroe, "Pay Dirt."

44 | British Medical Research Council, "Streptomycin Treatment of Pulmonary Tuberculosis."

45 | Crofton and Mitchison, "Streptomycin Resistance in Pulmonary Tuberculosis."

46 | Dubos, "Microbiology."

47 | Fox et al., "Studies on the Treatment of Tuberculosis Undertaken by the British Medical Research Council Tuberculosis Units."

48 | Fox and Sutherland, "A Five-Year Assessment of Patients in a Controlled Trial of Streptomycin, Para-Aminosalicylic Acid, and Streptomycin plus Para-Aminosalicylic Acid, in Pulmonary Tuberculosis"; British Medical Research Council, "Treatment of Pulmonary Tuberculosis."

49 | Selikoff et al., "Treatment of Pulmonary Tuberculosis with Hydrazide Derivatives of Isonicotinic Acid."

50 | World Health Organization, *WHO/IUATLD Global Project on Antituberculosis-Drug Resistance Surveillance.*

51 | Cegielski, "Extensively Drug-Resistant Tuberculosis"; Manten and Wijngaarden, "Development of Drug-Resistance to Rifampicin."

52 | British Medical Research Council, "Emergence of Bacterial Resistance in Pulmonary Tuberculosis under Treatment with Isoniazid, Streptomycin plus PAS, and Streptomycin plus Isoniazid"; British Medical Research Council, "Treatment of Pulmonary Tuberculosis with Isoniazid"; Fox, "The Medical Research Council Trials of Isoniazid"; Mount and Ferebee, "United States Public Health Service Cooperative Investigation of Antimicrobial Therapy of Tuberculosis."

53 | Andrews et al., "Influence of Segregation to Tuberculous Patients for One Year on the Attack Rate of Tuberculosis in a Two-Year Period in Close Family Contacts in South India"; Andrews et al., "Prevalence of Tuberculosis among Close Family Contacts of Tuberculous Patients in South India, and Influence of Segregation of the Patient on Early Attack Rate"; Dawson et al., "A Five-Year Study of Patients with Pulmonary Tuberculosis in a Concurrent Comparison of Home and Sanatorium Treatment for One Year with Isoniazid plus PAS"; Fox, "The Problem of Self-Administration of Drugs"; Kamat et al., "A Controlled Study of the Influence of Segregation of Tuberculous Patients for One Year on the Attack Rate of Tuberculosis in a Five-Year Period in Close Family Contacts in South India"; Tuberculosis Chemotherapy Center, "A Concurrent Comparison."

54 | Fox, "Whither Short-Course Chemotherapy?"; Fox et al., "Studies on the Treatment of Tuberculosis Undertaken by the British Medical Research Council Tuberculosis Units"; Cegielski, "Extensively Drug-Resistant Tuberculosis."

55 | McMillen, *Discovering Tuberculosis.*

56 | Fox et al., "Studies on the Treatment of Tuberculosis Undertaken by the British Medical Research Council Tuberculosis Units," S231–79.

57 | On the claim about "attenuated strains" among guinea pigs, see Mitchison et al., "A Case of Pulmonary Tuberculosis due to Isoniazid-Resistant, Guinea-

Pig Attenuated, Mycobacterium Tuberculosis." On unfavorable treatment outcomes and higher rates of isoniazid resistance, see Andrews et al., "Influence of Segregation to Tuberculous Patients for One Year on the Attack Rate of Tuberculosis in a Two-Year Period in Close Family Contacts in South India"; Cegielski, "Extensively Drug-Resistant Tuberculosis"; Gangadharam et al., "Rate of Inactivation of Isoniazid in South Indian Patients with Pulmonary Tuberculosis"; Selkon et al., "Rate of Inactivation of Isoniazid in South Indian Patients with Pulmonary Tuberculosis"; Tuberculosis Chemotherapy Center, "A Concurrent Comparison."

58 | McMillen, *Discovering Tuberculosis*.

59 | Fox, "Realistic Chemotherapeutic Policies for Tuberculosis in the Developing Countries," 137.

60 | Kaplan et al., "Tuberculosis in Alaska, 1970."

61 | McMillen, *Discovering Tuberculosis*, 195.

62 | McMillen, *Discovering Tuberculosis*.

63 | World Health Organization and United Nations Children's Fund, *Primary Health Care*, 71, emphasis added.

64 | Cueto, "The Origins of Primary Health Care and Selective Primary Health Care"; Litsios, "The Christian Medical Commission and the Development of the World Health Organization's Primary Health Care Approach."

65 | Berman, "Selective Primary Health Care"; Gish, "Selective Primary Health Care"; Unger and Killingsworth, "Selective Primary Health Care"; Walsh and Warren, "Selective Primary Health Care."

66 | Unger and Killingsworth, "Selective Primary Health Care"; World Bank, *Health Sector Policy Paper*.

67 | Banerji, *Can There Be a Selective Health Care?*; Berman, "Selective Primary Health Care"; Gish, "Selective Primary Health Care."

68 | Walsh and Warren, "Selective Primary Health Care."

69 | Murray, "Quantifying the Burden of Disease."

70 | World Bank, *Investing in Health*.

71 | Kochi, "Tuberculosis Control."

72 | World Health Organization, *Treatment of Tuberculosis*.

73 | Coninx et al., "Drug Resistant Tuberculosis in Prisons in Azerbaijan"; Farmer and Kim, "Resurgent TB in Russia"; Farmer et al., "Recrudescent Tuberculosis in the Russian Federation"; Good, *American Medicine*; Kimerling, "The Russian Equation"; Kimerling et al., "Inadequacy of the Current WHO Re-treatment Regimen in a Central Siberian Prison"; US Centers for Disease Control and Prevention, "Primary Multidrug-Resistant Tuberculosis."

74 | Cegielski, "Extensively Drug-Resistant Tuberculosis."

75 | Wilkinson and Kleinman, *A Passion for Society*.

76 | Farmer, *Pathologies of Power*, 176–77.

The Moral Economies of Heart Disease and Cardiac Care in India

ON FEBRUARY 17, 1968, BOMBAY SURGEON P. K. SEN transplanted the heart of a twenty-year-old woman into a twenty-seven-year old shepherd bedridden with a progressive cardiomyopathy. As one participant told the *Times of India*, "The operation was technically a success. It was a perfect operation."[1] Sen received congratulatory telegrams from all over the world. He was the fourth surgeon in the world to attempt a heart transplant and the first in Asia. The editor of the *Journal of the Indian Medical Association* described Sen's feat as "a record for which the whole of India is proud."[2] Sen performed a second heart transplant in September.[3]

This story surprises many readers. It defies their expectations of health and health care in India. They imagine India in 1968 as a land of plague, smallpox, cholera, and leprosy. They assume that its doctors struggled to provide basic health care. They do not imagine a country afflicted by heart disease where surgeons competed on an international stage to perform the first heart transplant. Such assumptions have been widespread. In 1976, Halfdan Mahler, director-general of the World Health Organization (WHO), warned emerging economies against the temptation to invest in expensive medical technology. He argued that it was inhumane "to look after the privileged few, with all manner of expensive placebos, and leave the vast majority of the world's population without even essential care."[4] The World Bank reiterated this critique in 1993: "Many health services have such low cost-effectiveness that governments will need to consider excluding them from the essential clinical package. In low-income countries these might include heart surgery."[5]

The surprise about Sen's transplants and the rhetoric of appropriate technology reflect both Western beliefs about the conditions of life and the possibilities for health care in places such as India. These beliefs disregard the lived reality of patients, physicians, and policy makers. Why did Sen and his colleagues pursue heart transplants? Why did many in India, the United States, and the Soviet Union encourage and support their efforts? Arthur Kleinman's medical anthropology, in this case refracted through the history of medicine, demands that we take seriously the local worlds of patients and their caregivers.[6] His student, Paul Farmer, called on us to work in solidarity with the world's poor so that they could access health care.[7] Kleinman and Farmer provide perspectives that allow us to begin to understand the values and priorities that guided the pursuit of cardiac surgery in India.

Heart disease in India provides a valuable case study. In India, as in nearly every other country, heart disease has emerged as the leading cause of death. In India, as elsewhere, physicians and policy makers struggle to respond. A comprehensive response to heart disease required interventions at many levels. Prevention always made the most sense, especially as it became clear in the 1950s and 1960s that both coronary artery disease (CAD) and rheumatic heart disease (RHD) could be wholly prevented with appropriate—if difficult—reforms (whether smoking cessation, optimized diet and physical activity, or antibiotic management of streptococcal infections). For patients who did develop coronary disease, pharmacological management improved with each passing decade, enabling better management of blood pressure, cholesterol, and inflammation. Nonetheless, some patients reached such advanced stages of CAD or RHD that surgery offered the best prospects. But even if surgery was relevant only for a subset of patients, it attained the highest prestige. First in the United States, and then elsewhere in the world, cardiac surgeons represented the epitome of modern, technology-intensive health care. Their exploits received frequent media attention, leaving easy tracks for historians to follow. As the costs of cardiac surgery became an increasing concern, patients, physicians, hospitals, and ministries of health had to make difficult decisions about resource investment and allocation. Much was at stake. Should countries provide a basic standard of medical care for everyone or instead prioritize making the full range of care available to anyone who could figure out a means to access it? This question, contested early in the history of cardiac surgery, has become a recurring debate in global health.

Even as Sen worked to make transplants possible in India in the 1960s, surgeons throughout Asia, Africa, and Latin America worked to bring open heart surgery and the other dazzling technologies of late twentieth-century medical technoscience to their countries. Their efforts reflected both the globalization of heart disease and the allure of new medical technology. It was once easy to invoke the language of appropriate technology and condemn such efforts: the rhetoric justified withholding HIV therapy from the world's poor. Activists, anthropologists, and physicians challenged this consensus and redefined what was possible in global AIDS care. This reimagining of global health must continue, both because progress against AIDS remains incomplete and because serious effort has barely begun against heart disease, cancer, mental illness, and other constituents of the global burden of disease. Because of the work of Farmer and others, it has become unacceptable to invoke scarcity to deny AIDS care to populations worldwide. Advocates have seized on this precedent and now argue that it is equally unacceptable to deny mental health care, cancer treatment, or surgery. This promise, however, has not yet been fulfilled.

An exploration of the history of heart disease in India, with an eye on its future, serves this mission of reimagining well. Just as heart disease was the great epidemic of Europe and North America in the twentieth century, it will be the great epidemic of Asia and the rest of the world in the twenty-first. It offers valuable opportunities for historians and anthropologists who want to understand the social determinants of the shifting burden of disease, to explore the implications of these epidemiological transitions for caregiving, and to engage seriously with fundamental moral questions about practices, presumptions, and the possibilities of life. This work is also fundamental to the mission of social medicine. Kleinman and Farmer demonstrated the power of biopsychosocial analyses to diagnose disease not just in individuals, but also in societies.[8] They warned about the risk of "category fallacy" that occurs when Western researchers read other societies in Western terms and fail to recognize how local meanings influence everything from the manifestations of disease to health-care priorities. For instance, Western physicians, preoccupied by their assumptions about smallpox, plague, or cholera in India, failed to appreciate the growing significance—epidemiologically and culturally—of heart disease in India. When they deemed cardiac care an inappropriate technology, they denied the local reality for Indian physicians and patients. This motivated both of those groups to act on their own behalf to establish cardiac care in India.

Kleinman also rejected the narrow reductionism of biomedical science and called out the moral crises of structural violence. He scrutinized medical practice at many scales, from the human encounters of caregiving to the political economy of health care. Kleinman's social medicine is not merely an analytic perspective. He and Farmer argued that scholars must develop deliberate strategies to intervene in the worlds of disease and healing, attending to the economic, political, and moral stakes of every action. Such perspectives transform not just how we understand what Sen attempted to do, but also what we assume to be possible in the struggle against the epidemic of heart disease.

Narratives of Disease and Responsibility

Is there an epidemic of heart disease? Even that simple claim is fraught. *Epidemic* once had a clear meaning: an outbreak of an acute, contagious disease, classically smallpox or plague.[9] An epidemic was abrupt and disruptive, a crisis that demanded containment and response. However, as the burden of disease shifted toward chronic disease, whether tuberculosis, cardiovascular disease, cancer, or mental illness, usage of the term *epidemic* has shifted as well. The definition and usage of the category of epidemic has become fraught. The US Centers for Disease Control and Prevention allows *epidemic* to refer to an unexpected occurrence of any disease. Common usage has followed suit. A quick perusal of newspapers or magazines reveals an epidemic of epidemics: of suicide, sexual assault, gun violence, and even immunization refusal. Critics, however, worry that overuse of the term simply desensitized audiences to its impact. Every invocation of *epidemic* is deliberate. A declaration of an epidemic is a call for help, a demand that action be taken. Determination of what counts as an epidemic is as much a political act as a scientific one.

Just as the declaration of an epidemic is a call for aid, it is also an invitation for analysis. It is valuable to take an epidemic at face value and work to understand its causes. This leads to an analysis of social determinants and structural violence.[10] Social scientists also set their sights on discourse analysis and explore the meanings and functions of any claim of "epidemic," as well as the explanations and responses that follow.

Even though coronary atherosclerosis has been identified in ancient mummies, and even though British physicians had characterized the clinical syndrome of angina pectoris in the late eighteenth century, CAD first rose to prominence in Europe and North America in the twentieth century. It became the archetypal "disease of civilization."[11] An epidemic in slow motion, heart disease triggered a crisis in the United States in the mid-twentieth century. Physicians and journalists wrote with alarm about its increasing incidence. The federal government established the National Heart Institute in 1948 and dramatically increased funding for cardiac research and disease control programs. When President Dwight Eisenhower suffered a heart attack in September 1955, the nation was shocked and frightened; the stock market suffered its biggest drop since 1929. Yet even as concern continued to mount, the epidemic reached an inflection point and began to decline. Mortality from heart disease fell steadily from the 1960s into the 2010s. While this is one of the great public health triumphs of the twentieth century, it is too soon to declare victory. Epidemiologists have recognized concerning signs of an impending resurgence of heart disease. This enables competing narratives. Should they celebrate the triumph or warn of future catastrophes? Each position can be defended.[12]

Heart disease followed a distinct trajectory in India. Even as infectious diseases declined in Europe and North America, they persisted in India. India became a crucial battleground in the aborted effort to eradicate tuberculosis in the 1950s.[13] It was the test case for smallpox eradication in the 1960s.[14] It struggles with outbreaks of plague, with alarmist media coverage causing as much trouble as plague itself.[15] While the final toll of COVID remains contested, it is likely that India suffered more deaths than any other country.[16] Public health experts fear that India has become a breeding ground for antibiotic-resistant superbugs.[17] Amid such drama, it was easy for observers to overlook heart disease. Part of the problem is that heart disease is a hybrid category with many distinct pathological processes, each with its own epidemiologic profile. Some forms, such as syphilitic heart disease and RHD, are infectious. Others are inflammatory, degenerative, or congenital. Heart disease obscures the boundaries between communicable and noncommunicable disease.

Rheumatic heart disease was the first form to cause concern in India, albeit grudgingly. Experts in tropical medicine had considered RHD a creature of the temperate north. Only in the 1930s did they convince themselves that RHD actually did exist in India and other tropics.[18] This new consensus emerged as physicians recognized the links among streptococcal infection, rheumatic fever, and RHD. This new concept of infectiousness may have facilitated physicians' changing expectations about its presence in India. Doctors soon recognized not just that RHD existed in India, but also that it was more virulent: mitral valve stenosis developed at a younger age in India than in Europe or North America.[19] India once again appeared to be particularly susceptible, not just to plague, leprosy, and tuberculosis, but to heart disease as well.

Coronary artery disease had been recognized early on. Allan Webb, a professor of anatomy at the Medical College of Bengal in the 1840s, described "an old Bengallee" whose "coronary arteries are quite ossified, like quills."[20] In 1891, Patrick Hehir, staff surgeon in H. H. Nizam's Troops, described a man who collapsed with severe chest pain, shortness of breath, a feeble pulse, and clammy skin. Autopsy revealed a fatty heart with narrowed coronary arteries and a scar in the left ventricle.[21] The disease only slowly came to public attention. The *Times of India* first reported an Indian dying of a heart attack in 1926, when a retired judge in Hyderabad collapsed while visiting the Imperial Post Office.[22] Surveys from the 1920s to the 1950s found the disease to be rare. As late as 1959, Delhi cardiologist Sivaramakrishnan Padmavati could study hospital statistics, population surveys, and insurance data and conclude "that India has the lowest incidence of coronary artery disease in the world."[23]

Other Indian cardiologists, however, recognized CAD as a "growing menace."[24] Coronary disease, like rheumatic disease, seemed to have a heightened virulence in India, with the peak incidence occurring in people a decade younger in India than in Europe and North America. When I visited the Christian Medical Center in Vellore in March 2013, the impact of the growing burden of coronary disease was obvious. The principal of the hospital, cardiologist Sunil Chandy, explained that he saw patients with heart attacks in their late twenties, something almost never seen in the United States.[25] The hospital had recently opened a new emergency unit dedicated to acute chest pain. Signs for this unit and for the hospital's coronary care unit were prominent at the hospital's front entrance.

As CAD rose to prominence in India, doctors had two specific concerns. First, they feared that the disease would have its greatest impact on social and economic elites. Rustom Jal Vakil wrote from Bombay in 1956, "Since cardiac invalids are often in the prime of life and high up on the social or intellectual ladder, their rehabilitation or return to 'the maximum physical, mental, emotional, social, vocational, and economic usefulness' becomes a matter of great importance and urgency."[26] Second, they assumed that the incidence would grow as India modernized. Boston cardiologist Paul Dudley

White warned his Delhi colleague Sujoy Roy in 1961 that "coronary heart disease will be on the increase as India gradually becomes more prosperous."[27] Indian physicians had to manage a disease not simply as it existed, but also as they feared it might become. White's fears were soon realized. In May 1964, India's Prime Minister Jawaharlal Nehru collapsed and died. Even though his doctors believed that he had suffered a ruptured aortic aneurysm, the press reported it as a heart attack.[28] In either case, cardiovascular disease had become a force that shaped India's history.

As Western and Indian epidemiologists paid increasing attention to coronary disease in India, it confounded them—another category fallacy. Based on what they had learned from the Framingham Heart Study, they predicted that CAD would be more prevalent in the north of India than in the south, where most adults were nonsmoking vegetarians. Much to their surprise, rates of CAD were actually seven times higher in the south than in the north.[29] Fifty years of research has now sought to understand what is

FIGURE 5.1 | View from the entrance of the hospital of the Christian Medical College in Vellore, India. Signs directing patients to the Coronary Care Unit and the dedicated Chest Pain Unit in the Emergency Department feature prominently, a reflection of the changed burden of disease in India. Photograph by David S. Jones.

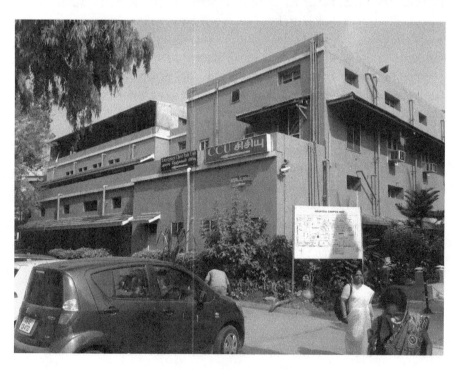

happening, yet key questions remain unresolved. The lingering confusion allows historians and medical anthropologists to explore not just the illness narratives told by the sick, but also the explanatory models offered by clinicians and researchers.[30]

Many studies in the 1960s and 1970s focused on Indian migrants and found high rates of CAD in Indians living outside India. Prior studies of Japanese migrants to Hawaii and California found that their CAD risk increased as they adopted American diets and lifestyles. In the Indian diaspora, however, elevated rates of CAD were seen regardless of whether the migrants maintained traditional practices or adopted new diets and tobacco use.[31] Researchers concluded that there must be some intrinsic factor to account for the high rates of CAD seen in South Asians worldwide. Some argued that the susceptibility arose from developmental factors, such as a mismatch between fetal and adult nutritional environments.[32] Others argued that Indians have small coronary arteries that leave them more susceptible to atherosclerotic coronary occlusions.[33] Researchers actively sought genetic explanations of Indian susceptibility, a pursuit that often glossed over the ethnic complexity of South Asian populations.[34]

Assertions of South Asian susceptibility to CAD now appear often in popular media.[35] Ambitious (or appropriately concerned?) physicians have carved out a new niche in a competitive medical marketplace: Stanford Health Care offers a specialty clinic for South Asians with heart disease.[36] According to its website, "South Asians (people from India, Pakistan, Bangladesh, Nepal, Bhutan, Maldives, and Sri Lanka) have a higher risk of heart and vascular disease than any other ethnic group. Our treatment and research center help South Asians better understand their risk factors and develops targeted treatment plans for each patient." The website's "Q&A," however, makes clear that the clinic's physicians worry about the same risk factors and employ the same treatments that are used with other coronary disease patients. This pattern of marketing race-based claims in the absence of robust evidence of significant racial differences in pathophysiology or treatment response is part of what Anne Pollock has identified as medicine's "durable preoccupation with difference."[37]

India now has the second highest number of heart attack deaths in the world, with roughly 1,519,000 each year.[38] India does not have the highest rate of coronary disease, but its rising rate (109.2 deaths per 100,000) now approaches the falling rate in the United States (170.0 deaths per 100,000), a testament to multiple epidemiological transitions. The rising burden of coronary disease in India—an epidemic by most meanings of the word—now fuels heated debates about responsibility and policy. K. Srinath Reddy, India's preeminent cardiologist, has advocated a stronger response by the national government. He blames the government's lack of response on the mistaken belief that cardiovascular disease (CVD)—a broader term for heart diseases that encompasses one of the most common, CAD—"is largely a problem of the urban rich." He warns that "the social gradient is now reversing, for many CVD risk factors and CVD related events, with the poor becoming the dominant victims as health transition advances the CVD epidemic."[39] The government must respond.

Epidemiology, however, is rarely clear-cut. A "comprehensive review" by researchers from India, England, and the United States found that the incidence of coronary disease was much higher among Indian elites than among the poor. The authors argued that the Indian government should continue to prioritize health problems that are "health concerns of the majority of the population" (e.g., infectious disease, maternal and child health) and that CAD was not one of them.[40] The unstated assumption is that the middle- and upper-class Indians who suffer from the disease can afford to engage private health-care services, allowing public hospitals to focus on the diseases of the poor. This is part of a broader critique of global health policy spearheaded by the cardiologist-anthropologist Gene Bukhman. He has argued that the WHO's focus on just four noncommunicable diseases (i.e., cardiovascular disease, diabetes, cancer, and chronic respiratory disease) and four risk factors (i.e., tobacco use, unhealthy diet, physical inactivity, harmful use of alcohol) prioritizes middle-income populations. He wants the WHO to focus instead on the noncommunicable diseases (NCDs) of the "bottom billion," which include RHD, cervical cancer, and chronic lung disease, but not CAD.[41]

Is heart disease an unmitigated crisis in India or something that will soon begin a dramatic decline, as happened in the West? Is it a disease of the elites, something that does not demand government intervention, or has it spread into all reaches of society? Is it the result of lifestyle "choices," such that individuals bear responsibility, or is it yet another mode of structural violence in which an unjust burden of social stress and air pollution focuses the global burden of CAD on the world's poor? Answers to these questions should be matters of fact that offer clear guidance for policy. Data, however, remain incomplete and ambiguous. This leaves researchers with discretion to craft competing narratives and policies.

The moral stakes are clear. Who or what is responsible for the disease? What obligations do patients, families, and societies have to provide care? If South Asians have an intrinsic susceptibility to CAD, one might conclude that they have a particular obligation to live fastidious lives. But if CAD is actually a product of structural violence—violence that preys on the poorest, most marginalized members of society—then responsibility might reside in governments to allocate resources to prevent and treat the burden of heart disease. It remains to be seen which narratives of CAD will dominate Indian discourse and what actions these narratives will motivate. Medical anthropologists can continue to work at the interface of disease and society to excavate the meanings, interests, and stakes of epidemics and to reveal their profound consequences for peoples' lives.

Narratives of Therapeutic Capability

As the first generation of Indian cardiologists worked to direct attention toward the looming problem of heart disease, they recognized competing priorities. R. P. Malhotra and N. S. Pathania acknowledged in their 1958 study of coronary disease that "we in India at present have to continue to think in terms of more important problems, such as those in infant mortality, infectious disease, nutritional disorders, overpopulation, and a host of other public health problems."[42] Attitudes began to shift in the 1960s. Paul Dudley White, a proponent for heart disease research and prevention worldwide, worked with colleagues in India to establish the All India Heart Foundation as a center for cardiac advocacy. He encouraged Indians to focus their attention on prevention: "When I see a patient fifty years old with angina pectoris or a heart attack coming much too young, I do not stop with him: I ask about his sons, too. What is their state of health? Are they putting on too much weight? Are they smoking? Have they settled down early in life to an existence of physical indolence?"[43] White sought simultaneously to treat the patient, the family, and even society.

Physicians in India, as elsewhere, were never satisfied with prevention. Medical services, especially new technoscientific dreams, held irresistible allure. The political and medical leaders of independent India pushed aggressively to develop medical expertise. If India was to be a modern nation, it had to be capable of all that modern nations could do. Amrit Kaur, White's friend and India's first minister of health, pushed for broad investments in medicine, including surgery: "Living as we are in a scientific and machine age there is no knowing what the surgeon of the future may be called upon to do." Surgery of the brain and "even the heart" was within reach.[44] To make the case for basic surgical services, Kaur argued that surgery could help alleviate important public-health problems, especially obstetric complications.

The case for cardiac surgery was more complex. It began with tuberculosis. The development of thoracic surgery in England and the United States in the 1940s allowed surgeons to offer partial relief to patients with severe tuberculosis by collapsing or removing the most infected portions of their lungs. Hospitals in India, where tuberculosis remained rampant, sought to provide this new surgical treatment. Reeve Betts, a Boston-trained thoracic surgeon who moved to India as a missionary surgeon in 1948, recognized the tension between the need to train general surgeons and the value of surgical specialists: "In India, up to the present time, the emphasis has been placed rightly on training doctors with a well-rounded general knowledge and experience. The time has arrived, however, when consideration should be given to training other doctors in special fields of endeavour."[45] When the Christian Medical College at Vellore formally established its Department of Thoracic Surgery in 1949, under Betts's leadership, the government of India designated it "the center for training for chest surgeons for all India."[46] Thoracic surgery spread quickly to Bombay, Calcutta, and a few other centers in India.

India's success with thoracic surgery put cardiac surgery within reach.[47] Many of the early cardiac procedures, such as ligation of a patent ductus arteriosus, could be done by any trained thoracic surgeon. Simple valve repairs required a bit more bravery, but no specialized training or devices. As the prevalence of RHD in India was recognized in the 1950s, surgeons had a growing justification for investments in cardiac surgery: they offered palliation to children and young women, "innocent victims" of rheumatic (and congenital) heart disease. Cardiothoracic surgery could join social medicine in its crusade against tuberculosis and RHD.

To bring cardiac surgery to India, surgeons navigated India's complex relationships with England, the United States, and the Soviet Union. They welcomed support from the Rockefeller Foundation, the US government, and others who sought to win India's allegiance. This created opportunities for aspiring Indian cardiac surgeons, such as P. K. Sen, to travel to Minneapolis, Houston, and Cleveland to learn new cardiac techniques.[48] India, however, resisted falling under the sway of the United States during the Cold War.[49] A. V. Baliga, one of Sen's senior surgical colleagues at King Edward Memorial (KEM) Hospital, led the Indo-Soviet Cultural Society and spearheaded outreach efforts to the Soviet Union.[50] Sen made trips to Moscow in 1962 and 1965 to learn techniques of experimental cardiac surgery from V. P. Demihkov, who had achieved notoriety for his innovative and macabre animal experiments, including heart transplants and operations that produced dogs with two heads.

Much of the early research in open heart surgery in India relied on heart-lung machines imported from England, Denmark, and the United States. However, some surgical teams worked assiduously to develop their own, indigenous devices. Kersi Dastur, a self-trained cardiac surgeon, worked at B. Y. L. Nair Hospital in Bombay. Unable to import a foreign-made machine, he studied American designs, recruited local engineers and machinists, and built his own device. When he completed an open-heart operation in February 1961, the first in India, the *Times of India* specified that he had used "the first Indian-made 'heart-lung machine.'"[51] These machines had politics.

The complex motivations for cardiac surgery can be seen in the commentary on Sen's heart transplants provided by the editor of the *Journal of the Indian Medical Association*:

> The question so commonly asked, whether India should also undertake these risky and expensive operations, needs only one answer—India must. If India has sought the atomic reactor, built huge industrial complexes of steel, communicated through Telstar, and has advanced jets for its defense, there must also be in the country a few top-class medical centers given the full freedom, finance and personnel where a quality of work equal to the best in the world can be carried out without interference. It is the only way to develop a consciousness for the high quality of work which is essential in this medical field today, or else the technological and scientific gap will be so large that it will never be bridged.[52]

It did not matter whether heart surgery was appropriate or not. India simply had to try.

Such investments left a complicated legacy. India remains a country with profound health-care inequities. Nearly fifty years after Sen's transplant, and despite the new promise of "Modicare," many in India lack access to basic health care. Meanwhile, extensive investment in the private sector has produced some of the world's very best cardiac care. Devi Shetty's Narayana Health hospital system has won accolades for providing state-of-the-art surgery at low prices.[53] Elite surgeons in Chennai, Bangalore, and Mumbai rival the experience of the best surgeons in Cleveland or Houston. As has happened with the reproduction clinics described by Marcia Inhorn in this volume, India has become a site of medical cosmopolitanism, with cardiac tourists coming from all over the world. In an aggressive inversion of colonial legacies, Shetty has even established a satellite hospital in the Cayman Islands to compete directly for patients from the United States. The idea that a patient from Michigan might choose to fly to the Caribbean to have bypass surgery performed by an Indian surgeon surprises many in the United States. Their surprise reflects a misunderstanding of how cardiac capability is distributed in the world today. As David Harvey and other geographers of postmodernity have shown, the contraction of space and time brought about by capitalist economies has collapsed distances between people and places.[54] But this has not eliminated profound inequalities; in many cases it has actually increased them.

Moral Economies of Care and Experiment

Sen's team completed its first heart transplant in the early hours of the morning on February 17. Initially everything looked fine: the transplanted heart beat in the recipient's chest. Success was fleeting. The heart beat just three hours, then failed. The patient died. Sen's team, however, proceeded to describe the operation as "technically a success."[55] To understand how a failed operation could be considered a success, it is necessary to follow Kleinman's advice and attend to the local stakes of the operation.[56] What was the moral world in which these surgeons worked and in which their patients lived, received transplants, and died? This is a core task of medical anthropology. Astute ethnographers can recognize latent structures and call out the forces that generate suffering and inequality. Historians, in contrast, have only partial access to the events that they study and can only speculate about their actors' motivations. The luxury of hindsight provides some compensation for this deficit and allows historians to offer perspectives that might not be evident in contemporary analyses. Sen's transplant demonstrates this well.

Cardiac surgeons were familiar with death. When John Gibbon made the first attempts to use a heart-lung machine, three of his four patients died; he did not try again. Kersi Dastur, the first surgeon to attempt open-heart surgery in India, lost six of his first ten patients. Sen's first open-heart patient also died, but his team saw a silver lining: "From this one single case we learnt much more than the hundreds of animal experiments that we had performed."[57] They revised their techniques, practiced more, and eventually succeeded. While the death of Sen's first transplant patient was surely a disappointment, it was not a surprise, and it would not have diminished his hopes for the procedure.

This reflects an attitude toward experimentality that has been pervasive in medicine.[58] Anthropologists and historians have shown that there are many ways to judge the efficacy of a therapeutic intervention.[59] Surgeons often have multiple goals for each operation. While they hope that the patient will benefit, they know that they can also improve their understanding of the body, refine their own skills, or gain more evidence about the merits of the surgical procedure. Surgeons have seen themselves as explorers, bolding going where no one had gone before.[60] They knew that they walked fine lines between experiment, innovation, and care. Sen had many critics who accused him of straying too far. As the pace of heart transplants increased in May 1968, often with disappointing results, a Bombay doctor advised surgeons to go back to the laboratory to perfect their techniques lest the public begin to fear that surgeons were conducting "experiments on human guinea pigs."[61] After Sen's second transplant failed after just fourteen hours, another critic argued that "it seems criminal to waste so much on operations that are almost predictable failures." India should wait: "It seems more practical to allow the better equipped and financed and more advanced Western centers to carry out these pioneering procedures, perfect the techniques involved and then, and then only, adopt them modifying them as necessary."[62] A third writer warned that Sen's rush to transplant, his "enthusiasm to put India on the cardiac map of the world," was "tantamount to playing with human lives."[63]

Some commentators did come to Sen's defense. One argued that it was better to try and fail than not to try: "We should appreciate the display of a pioneer spirit by anyone in this routine-minded country."[64] Sen celebrated his own willingness to take risks, noting that it was "this desire to break away from colorlessness into the ambit of the unknown which makes scientific buccaneers of us."[65] His confidence never flagged. After his second transplant patient died, he emphasized that his team was "getting nearer complete success. It is very encouraging."[66] Sen knew that innovation inevitably carried risk. He also realized that the transplant had meanings beyond the patient. His team had been working to develop open heart surgery and cardiac transplantation since 1954. The simple fact that they could perform a transplant in February 1968, just eleven weeks after Christiaan Barnard's first attempt, was a tremendous accomplishment. It demonstrated that his team had engaged with the state-of-the-art of cardiac surgery and adapted it to local circumstance.

It is also possible that no one actually expected the patient to survive. Sen's team knew who the ideal candidate would be: someone with incurable, incapacitating heart disease but "reasonably healthy pulmonary, renal, hepatic and central nervous system function."[67] Their twenty-seven-year old shepherd certainly had incurable, incapacitating cardiac disease. Despite five months of intensive medical care, he could walk only twenty meters before becoming short of breath. But he also suffered from kyphoscoliosis, restrictive lung disease, emphysema, and likely pulmonary hypertension. This set of comorbidities—in hindsight—made survival after a transplant nearly impossible. So why did Sen choose him? A cynic might argue that the shepherd's life had become so thoroughly compromised, both medically and socially, that he could be co-opted into a surgical demonstration project.

Sen's team exhibited a similarly stark attitude toward potential organ donors. Their first donor received little comment in the official case report: she was a twenty-year-old woman admitted to KEM Hospital on a Friday afternoon with "a severe head injury following a railway accident."[68] She was reduced to an anonymous member of a class of valuable medical resources: otherwise healthy young humans who had suffered irreparable brain injuries. As Sen's colleagues explained, the ideal donor had to be "reasonably healthy prior to death." As a result, "Young people dying from sudden trauma are therefore the best donors." Such people were readily available in Bombay: "In an urban community, accidents like train accidents often cause fatal . . . injuries providing the donor-organ material."[69] The problem, in Sen's view, was that these potential donors were not available for use by would-be transplant surgeons. Societal discomfort with the idea of brain death slowed the development of transplant surgery in India and elsewhere. In November 1968, two months after his second transplant, Sen decried the "'world-wide neurosis'" that had arisen about heart transplants. He thought that overblown concerns prevented more transplants from being done. He saw this as a missed opportunity, especially given India's seemingly abundant supply of donors.[70] This frustrated him immensely.[71] India did not enact the brain death policies that heart transplantation required until 1994.

Such considerations support a cynical interpretation that resonates with Giorgio Agamben's analysis in *Homo Sacer*.[72] The rural and urban poor in India lacked the basic civic rights of ordinary people. They had become "bare life," vulnerable to violation and exploitation as would-be Indian cardiac transplant surgeons pursued cardiovascular modernity.

But we must judge with care. Other readings of this episode offer more sympathy to the doctors. In June 2016 I traveled to Mumbai and interviewed A. P. Chaukar.[73] In 1968 he was the surgical registrar who assisted Sen with his first heart transplant. When I asked Chaukar about the first patient's co-morbidities, he agreed that, in retrospect, the fatal outcome was a foregone conclusion. He insisted, however, that the consequences of comorbid disease were not appreciated at the time. No physicians, in India or anyplace else, had experience with heart transplantation in sick adults; all of their prior experimental work had used healthy dogs. They did not know the extent to which pulmonary disease undermined prospects for post-transplant survival. They did not know the extent to which the donor heart weakened as it underwent the natural dying process required then by Indian law. When the compromised heart was transplanted into the compromised recipient, it could not sustain the extra work required by the recipient's pulmonary disease. While the likelihood—even the inevitability—of failure in this case is explicable after the fact, Chaukar explained that it had not been anticipated at the time. What tilted their imaginations toward optimism or pessimism? S. V. Joglekar, dean of Sen's medical school and a longtime supporter of his efforts to develop cardiac surgery, attributed Sen's optimism to the drama of Barnard's accomplishment. Whatever pessimism had existed before the first transplant dissipated in December 1967: "It can now be said with emphasis that there is every possibility of success."[74] Surgeons had high hopes about what might be possible.

Should Sen and Chaukar have realized that their patient's prognosis was poor? Surgeons who imagined that a transplant was possible could also have imagined what might go wrong. I have often been tempted to judge such motives and actions, but Kleinman has warned me about the elusiveness of such judgments. Psychiatrists struggle to understand patients whom they have seen weekly over many years. How can historians understand their informants from incomplete archives? Is it possible to know what was in the mind (and heart) of these surgeons, to understand what really mattered to them (or their patients)? Sen led the surgery service of a large urban hospital in Bombay in the 1950s. He knew well the challenge of stretching scarce health-care resources to respond to the massive needs of Bombay's growing population. He had recognized the growing burden of heart disease. He had witnessed the deaths of countless patients, people who could have been saved had his hospital had the full capabilities of a medical center in Europe or the United States. I do not know whether Sen actually decried the geographic inequities that condemned his patients to death, but such thinking motivated patients and their physicians in the 1990s to fight against geographic barriers to AIDS care.

Seen in this light, Sen might have felt an obligation to future patients to do what he could to make new kinds of surgery possible in Bombay, even if that involved experimental surgery on current patients. He may have been making sincere if unrealistic efforts to provide health care amid scarcity. Does this justify the risks he took? Paul Farmer has described how physicians face a choice between accepting the profound inequalities that exist or doing something about them despite seemingly impossible odds.[75] Sometimes this requires compromise and improvisation.[76] Only by attempting what is deemed unwise, or even impossible, is it possible to redefine what is possible.

Conflicts between idealism and pragmatism are inevitable. In 2007, I proposed a thought experiment to my colleagues in the Department of Social Medicine at Harvard Medical School, many of whom—especially Farmer—had worked to change what was possible in global AIDS policy. That year more than one million people in India had died from heart attacks. In the United States, physicians can reduce mortality from heart attacks by reopening obstructed coronary arteries with angioplasty within an hour of onset of symptoms. I asked whether our commitment to global health equity obligated us to work to make angioplasty available to the people of India. Farmer and our other colleagues scoffed, despite their deep commitment to global health equity for HIV and tuberculosis. They questioned the value of coronary angioplasty (despite a very strong evidence base), the feasibility of implementation in India (e.g., urban traffic gridlock makes it difficult to transport patients quickly to hospitals), and the enormous costs—and opportunity costs—that an investment in interventional cardiology would require. Such resistance had once blocked global access to antiretroviral therapy. Farmer and the others recognized the irony of their resistance to global access to interventional cardiology, but they did not back down. Should we accept the obstacles as inevitable, or should we challenge them as socially constructed presumptions? Should we accept pragmatic realities or advocate to change what is possible?

Fifty years after Sen's first transplant, his students and their students have achieved outstanding outcomes with cardiac surgery in India. They have also made much progress controlling costs: cardiac surgery can be had at a fraction of US prices.[77] Despite this success, cardiac care remains out of reach for many in India. Heart transplants have faced additional obstacles. Only in 1994 did India's Parliament sanction the concept of brain death. Surgeons at the All-India Institute of Medical Sciences performed India's first successful heart transplant that year. Surgeons in Mumbai, however, were slow to follow. The first successful heart transplant there did not take place until August 2015, and this required elaborate arrangements. The donor died in Pune, normally a four-hour drive from Mumbai. To transport the heart quickly, authorities cleared traffic off a route from the hospital to the Pune airport. A Navy plane flew the heart to Mumbai, where traffic officials again cleared the roads to Fortis Hospital. This "well-orchestrated symphony between the two cities and its local administrations" allowed the heart to arrive after only an hour. The joint commissioner of police for traffic thought that such effort was justified: "Saving a valuable life made it well worth the effort and we are grateful that the citizens of Mumbai co-operated willingly in this humane endeavour."[78] Fortis Hospital quickly scaled up its program and by summer 2016 had completed twenty more heart transplants, again with help from police and city officials to clear traffic off Mumbai's congested streets.[79] Is this investment in resources appropriate? This is a question that must be answered not just by physicians and public officials in Mumbai, but in every place that seeks to deploy resource-intensive medical technologies.

Physicians in India face a transformed global burden of disease. Old epidemics persist as new ones emerge, and the meanings of the term *epidemic* itself remain constantly in flux. Would-be caregivers grapple with fundamental challenges. How can they provide better care for the persistent infections (e.g., malaria, tuberculosis, HIV), while providing care for the emerging chronic conditions (e.g., heart disease, diabetes, mental illness)? How can they invest in medical care without losing sight of the enormous benefit promised by investments in prevention? How can they invest in medicine and prevention without losing sight of the need to critique and transform the structural violence that produces the burden of disease? Many people say that this is impossible and that the needed resources simply do not exist. Kleinman and Farmer inspired many of us to try. Perhaps that is what Sen did: attempt a transplant to demonstrate what was possible without concern for what was appropriate or sustainable. Figuring out how (and where and when) to make the possible a reality to combat the epidemics of the twenty-first century will be one of the great challenges of our time.

Notes

1 | "First-Ever Heart Transplant in India," 1.
2 | Banerjee, "Cardiac Transplantation," 539.
3 | Jones and Sivaramakrishnan, "Transplant Buccaneers."
4 | Mahler, "Report of the Director-General," in Cooper, *Report of the United States Delegation to the World Health Assembly*, 63.
5 | World Bank, *Investing in Health*, 10.
6 | Kleinman, *Patients and Healers*; Kleinman, *The Soul of Care*; Kleinman, *What Really Matters*.
7 | Farmer, *Partner to the Poor*.
8 | Kleinman, *The Illness Narratives*; Kleinman, *Social Origins of Distress and Disease*; Farmer, *Partner to the Poor*.
9 | Rosenberg, "What Is an Epidemic."
10 | Farmer, *AIDS and Accusation*.
11 | Rosenberg, "Pathologies of Progress."

12 | Jones and Greene, "The Decline and Rise of Coronary Heart Disease."

13 | McMillen, *Discovering Tuberculosis.*

14 | Bhattacharya, *Expunging Variola.*

15 | Sivaramakrishnan, "The Return of Epidemics and the Politics of Global-Local Health."

16 | Biswas, "Why India's Real COVID Toll May Never Be Known."

17 | Harris, "'Superbugs' Kill India's Babies and Pose an Overseas Threat."

18 | Kutumbiah, "A Study of the Lesions in Rheumatic Heart Disease in South India."

19 | Roy et al., "Juvenile Mitral Stenosis in India."

20 | Webb, *Pathologia India*, liv.

21 | Hehir, "Angina Pectoris with Post-mortem Examination," 268.

22 | "Obituary."

23 | Padmavati, "The Cardiac Patient in Underdeveloped Countries," 423.

24 | Vakil, "Modern Approach to Cardiovascular Problems," 521.

25 | Sunil Chandy, interview by the author, Vellore, March 2013.

26 | Vakil, "Cardiology—Past and Present," 10.

27 | Paul Dudley White to Sujoy B. Roy, letter, April 7, 1961, Paul Dudley White Papers, H MS C36, Francis A. Countway Library of Medicine, Harvard Medical School, Boston.

28 | "Jawaharlal Nehru Is Dead"; Sharma, "Panditiji Bled to Death in a Medical Mess."

29 | Malhotra, "Geographical Aspects of Acute Myocardial Infarction in India with Special Reference to Patterns of Diet and Eating."

30 | Kleinman et al., "Culture, Illness and Care."

31 | McKeigue and Marmot, "Mortality from Coronary Heart Disease in Asian Communities in London."

32 | Stein et al., "Fetal Growth and Coronary Heart Disease in South India."

33 | Dhawan and Bray, "Are Asian Coronary Arteries Smaller than Caucasian?"

34 | Mastana, "Unity in Diversity."

35 | Vara, "Heart Disease Snares South Asians."

36 | See Stanford Health Care's Stanford South Asian Translational Heart Initiative website, https://stanfordhealthcare.org/medical-clinics/stanford-south-asian-translational-heart-initiative.html.

37 | Pollock, *Medicating Race.*

38 | See the Institute for Health Metrics and Evaluation's GBD Compare data-visualization tool, at https://vizhub.healthdata.org/gbd-compare/.

39 | Reddy, "India Wakes Up to the Threat of Cardiovascular Diseases," 1370.

40 | Subramanian et al., "Jumping the Gun," 1410.

41 | Bukhman et al., "Reframing NCDs and Injuries for the Poorest Billion"; Schwartz et al., "The Origins of the 4 × 4 Framework for Noncommunicable Disease at the World Health Organization."

42 | Malhotra and Pathania, "Some Aetiological Aspects of Coronary Heart Disease," 531.

43 | White, *Coronary Heart Disease*, 14.

44 | Kaur, quoted in "Proceedings of the XII Annual Conference of the Association of Surgeons in India," iii.

45 | Betts, "Thoracic Surgery," 168.

46 | Christian Medical College and Hospital, "Vellore's Surgeons Trained in North America Add Two Specialties Needed in India," 1948, Andover-Harvard Theological Library, Harvard University, Cambridge, MA, "Christian Medical College and Hospital, Vellore," folder. See also Basu, "Origin and Development of the Association of Thoracic and Cardiovascular Surgeons of India."

47 | Sen, "The Present Status of Surgery of the Heart."

48 | Jones and Sivaramakrishnan, "Making Heart-Lung Machines Work in India."

49 | Engerman, *The Price of Aid*.

50 | Bakaya, *A.V. Baliga*.

51 | "Heart Operation in Bombay"; Jones and Sivaramakrishnan, "Making Heart-Lung Machines Work in India."

52 | Banerjee, "Cardiac Transplantation," 541.

53 | Altstedter, "The World's Cheapest Hospital Has to Get Even Cheaper"; McCarthy, "India's Philanthropist-Surgeon Delivers Cardiac Care Henry Ford Style."

54 | Harvey, *The Condition of Postmodernity*.

55 | "First-Ever Heart Transplant in India."

56 | Kleinman, *What Really Matters*.

57 | Parulkar, "Developments in Cardiovascular Surgery in India during Last Five Decades," S24.

58 | Fox and Swazey, *The Courage to Fail*; Petryna, "Experimentality."

59 | Jones, *Broken Hearts*; Kleinman, *Patients and Healers in the Context of Culture*; Rosenberg, "The Therapeutic Revolution."

60 | Lawrence and Brown, "Quintessentially Modern Heroes."

61 | Mani, "Letter to the Editor," 5.

62 | Morehead, "Transplants in India," 8.

63 | Pant, "Heart Transplants," 8.

64 | Nadkarni, "Transplants in India," 10.

65 | Sen, "Heart Transplantation—The Triumph and the Muddle," 71.

66 | "Dr. Sen Does His Second Heart Graft."

67 | Datey et al., "Cardiac Assessment and Selection," 547. See also Kinare, "Autopsy," 558.

68 | Sen et al., "The Operation," 549. See also Joglekar, "Heart Transplant—Ethical and Legal Aspects," 558.

69 | Bhalerao and Patil, "Donor Selection and Management," 556.

70 | "More Donors than Recipients for Heart Transplants," 11.

71 | Sen, "Heart Transplantation—The Triumph and the Muddle," 71.

72 | Agamben, *Homo Sacer*.

73 | A. P. Chaukar, interview by the author, Mumbai, June 2016.

74 | Joglekar, "Heart Transplant—Ethical and Legal Aspects," 557.

75 | Farmer, *Infections and Inequalities*.

76 | Livingston, *Improvising Medicine*.

77 | Altstedter, "The World's Cheapest Hospital Has to Get Even Cheaper."

78 | "First Ever Successful Heart Transplant Conducted in Mumbai Thanks to Efforts of Police."

79 | "Aurangabad Engineer's Heart Give Thane Resident New Life."

Intimate and Social
Spheres of Mental Illness

ENTERING THE RECEPTION AREA, I moved quickly to shake off the sub-freezing wind chill of late winter. The glint of New Mexican sunlight shone through the windows of the pueblo-style residential treatment cottage where I met Taciana. This was her first psychiatric hospitalization, and she had arrived the previous week. Petite and soft-spoken, she seemed younger than her fourteen years of age. She had agreed to meet with me, and I began by letting her know that I was not part of the treatment team but part of a research team trying to learn how young people come to the hospital. After giving her consent to participate in the study, she launched immediately into a forceful narrative: "I am Zuni. . . . I came here because bad things happened to me and some people told me I could come here to rest. People could take care of me. This is my first time coming here, or in trying to commit suicide. I hate myself. Because I hear voices, like voices telling me what to do, or 'hang yourself, do it, become like one of us.'"

She explained that hanging herself seemed like it was "worth it" and that she had no idea how long she'd been hanging before her father found her. He told her that she needed help. She agreed and subsequently told her school counselor that she wanted help because she was "having trouble dealing with anger." The counselor responded by saying that "there were some real nice people at a hospital who can help." She underscored that she had "volunteered" to come to the hospital "for depression" and because "I was dealing with a lot of things." This included the recent death of her grandfather. There seemed no point in going to school any longer. She smoked marijuana, drank alcohol, and used other drugs with greater frequency. She sought out her oldest brother. He told her that she had been "hanging around the wrong people," "getting angry," and needed to follow the light "to get out of your trouble." Looking down at the floor, she continued with how, at an early age, social workers had removed her from her home because, while there was always plenty of alcohol, drugs, and fighting, there was little food or care. Looking up, she said that coming to the hospital had really helped her and that she was glad she came. Without interview questions or prompting, she continued her story of a young life ravaged by assaults on her bodily and psychic integrity.[1]

The circumstances of Taciana's life and suicide attempt were not uncommon as precipitating events of admission to the hospital among participants in an ethnographic study of children living on the edge of experience under conditions of structural violence. This particular study, as with several I have conducted as a medical anthropologist, was an endeavor that brought together a research team of medical anthropologists, psychiatrists, and psychologists working collaboratively with a clinical team of providers in a children's psychiatric hospital in New Mexico. The state ranks extremely high in child poverty as well as in ethnic diversity (48.5 percent Hispanic/ Latinx and 10.5 percent Native American/First Nation peoples).[2] Poverty and fragmentation of kin networks mark the lived experience of many youth living under conditions such as Taciana's.

In this chapter, I reflect on the needs, capacities, and conditions surrounding mental illness. As Taciana's narrative makes clear, this endeavor requires attention to intersecting spheres. First is the primacy and immediacy of experience as the starting point for moral modes of inquiry.[3] For Taciana, this begins with her Zuni identity, self-hate, bereavement, anger, and drug use. Second is attention to cultural meaning and expression. These are essential to avoiding the epistemological error of "category fallacy," wherein psychiatric diagnostic categories can be applied in the absence of cultural validity.[4] While Taciana reported that she came to the hospital "for depression," she makes clear that far more is going on in her social world in relation to danger and uncertainty and her experience of what really matters.[5] Third is the palpable centrality of suffering in human lives that can conduce to conditions of mental illness. Taciana felt lost and in anguish, struggling to figure out how to be, or not be, in this world. Across these spheres of experience, meaning, and suffering, I have identified struggle as a central process of mental health and illness. This point is vital since many approaches in cultural anthropology, and medical anthropology, can appear to be tone-deaf to the considerable agency and effort of people with whom they work and about whom they write. Attention to struggle across these spheres can also emphasize the high human stakes involved in their intersection, as well as their relevance for the movement to scale up global mental health care. Accordingly, I conclude this essay with a reflection on the importance of ethnographic approaches as foundational for this emerging field.

Ethnographic Foundations and Extraordinary Conditions

Thinking about intimate and social spheres of mental illness ideally entails multiple vantage points from health sciences and social sciences to bring together what I think of as sets of "extraordinary conditions."[6] Common use of the term *extraordinary* implies circumstances or capabilities that are exceptional or unusual. This makes sense in certain contexts, of course, but is not my concern. Condensed into my use of this phrase is a double meaning referring to (1) personal experiences of bodily and psychic alteration that are culturally diagnosed as various forms of serious mental illness; and (2) social conditions of precarity as recurring or sustained forces of violence, poverty, misogyny, racism, abuse, or neglect.[7] These dual sets of extraordinary conditions are reciprocally produced. They might come to feel "ordinary" in the sense of becoming routinized, recurrent, or expectable. However, as experiential modes of suffering and conditions of social pathology, they are not in this formulation properly regarded as either unusual or normative but instead as sites for engaged listening, care, and social change.[8]

To illustrate such extraordinary conditions, I draw on my collaborative research on culture and mental health. The studies have focused on key issues in the field, including the course and outcome of schizophrenia in kin-based households; psychic trauma and depression among immigrants, migrants, and refugees fleeing political violence; clinical ethnographies of inpatient and outpatient settings; the mental health of children and families marked by neighborhood and drug-related violence; and carceral immigration policies as a sociopolitical determinant of mental health. These studies are situated within the now substantial body of work by medical anthropologists investigating multiple forms of affliction such as depression, schizophrenia, bipolar, anxiety, neurodegenerative, substance misuse, and eating disorders, yielding fine-grained ethnographic views of psychopharmacology, biomedical technologies, (un)natural disasters, institutions and incarceration, and transnational forces.[9]

The background for the ethnographic study of mental illness concerns an enduring problem within anthropology, psychiatry, and the philosophy of science: how to conceptualize the normal and abnormal, the healthy and the pathological. Early twentieth-century challenges by anthropologists and psychiatrists who were ethnographically and psychologically minded went against the grain of conventional thinking about mental illness. The substantial diversity of cultural and psychological experience was identified through comparative method, as deployed in Ruth Benedict's analysis of the unstable boundary between the normal and the abnormal.[10] Writing against racialized and sexist thinking that has institutionalized inequality, her attention was trained on the multiplicities of experience and identity not as aberrant deviations but as existing across a cultural range of gendered and sexual being. The psychiatrist Harry Stack Sullivan insisted on the "normality" of schizophrenia. Arguing from a continuous model for conceptualization, Sullivan maintained there was little difference between the slip of the tongue or inability to recall the name of a close colleague and the fixed delusion that one was Napoleon III. The anthropological linguist and psychological anthropologist Edward Sapir was resolute that "cultural anthropology, properly understood, has the healthiest of all scepticisms about the validity of the concept of 'normal behavior'" and is "valuable because it is constantly rediscovering the normal."[11] A series of ethnographic-psychiatric projects directed toward dismantling dire limitations of European thinking about mental illness ensued, including works by Gregory Bateson, Cora Du Bois, George Devereux; A. Irving Hallowell, and Abram Kardiner.[12] This body of work paralleled formulations of philosophers of science who argued for separation of the "abnormal" and the "normal" as untenable.[13] Beginning at the end of the 1970s, a series of publications by Arthur Kleinman both consolidated these advances and launched a paradigm shift, renovating the field of transcultural psychiatry and energizing a new generation of medical anthropologists.[14] This transformation endures as straightforward and incisive and undergirds which questions are asked and which are overlooked in anthropology.

The Primacy of Experience

The theoretical move to foreground experience *qua* experience is vital within anthropology, since the very notion has generally been missed or ruled as outside the parameters of the field.[15] In the 1980s, explicit anthropological foray into the question of experience was framed as likely peculiar to modernity and of limited application. Further, experience was defined incongruously as "cultural performance and display."[16] Thus, this curdled into pretty much the same old thing: experience is a suspect notion.

Kleinman's case for the primacy of experience as the *starting point* of anthropological investigation remains innovative since attention within medical anthropology has largely been trained on critiques of biomedical reductionism.[17] This merely supplants biomedical reductionism with cultural reductionism:

> The [anthropologists'] interpretation of some person's or group's suffering as the reproduction of oppressive relationships of production, or the symbolization of dynamic conflicts in the interior of the self, or as resistance to authority, is a transformation of everyday experience of the same order as those pathologizing reconstructions within biomedicine. Nor is it morally superior to anthropologize distress, rather than to medicalize it. What is lost in biomedical renditions—the complexity, uncertainty and ordinariness of some man or woman's unified world of experience—is also missing when illness is reinterpreted as social role, social strategy, or social symbol . . . anything *but* human experience.[18]

Arthur Kleinman and Joan Kleinman hastened to point out that human experience can never be acultural, ahistorical, or understood apart from social power. The principal problem of experience-distant anthropological interpretation is the risk of "delegitimating their subject matter's human conditions. The anthropologist thereby constitutes a false subject; she can engage in a professional discourse every bit as dehumanizing as that of colleagues who unreflectively draw upon the tropes of biomedicine or behaviorism to create their subject matter. Ethnography does participate in this professional transformation of an experience-rich and near human subject into a dehumanized object, a caricature of experience."[19]

The value of an epistemological weighting of experience for ethnographic study of mental illness can be demonstrated by pointing to key issues concerning psychosis. First is how a concentration on experience sheds light on models of the normal and the pathological as continuous phenomena.[20] This has been demonstrated for an understanding of schizophrenia in an interdisciplinary volume edited by me and the late psychiatrist-anthropologist Robert Barrett.[21] In that book, contributors bid adieu to approaches derived solely from descriptive psychopathology and classificatory psychiatry in favor of interrogating the nexus of subjectivity, culture, and psychosis through multiple ethnographic filters. Second, the subjective experiences of people diagnosed with schizophrenia appear as matters of bodily alteration and social disruption.[22] These include alterations in—but not the negation of—embodied selves, emotional experience, sexual desire and identity, cultural interpretation, and social relations as fundamental human processes.[23]

In these two respects, using an experience-near ethnographic approach with people and kin who actually live with conditions of mental illness in "real world," everyday environments brings into view what I have argued is the sine qua non of an anthropological understanding of mental illness: people living "with" conditions of serious mental illness differ little in fundamental human capacities from those "without" mental illness.[24] Yet people with mental illness have curiously been regarded as somehow lacking culture and lacking in emotion or social attachments and, at best, are treated as footnotes for anthropological theorizing.[25] Such sequestration not only "does damage to the integrity of non-ordinary subjects but also leads to intellectual peril for scholarly of fields that indulge in it."[26]

When we compare different kinds of disorders—say, depression and schizophrenia in my studies—an ethnographic surprise emerges in relation to the interpretation of lived experience. What appears ineffable, yet subjectively perceptible, is an alteration of what can be termed the *rhythm of life*. Often there appeared to be a moral struggle either to maintain or find anew one's sense of rhythm or involvement in the flow of everyday activities. Patients articulated their suffering over having lost or been thwarted from ever finding a sense of rhythm, given the persistent or recurring context of major mental disorder.[27]

Without devaluing the utility of identifying symptoms and making psychiatric diagnoses, my ethnographic studies of the experience of and response to mental illness reveal not the centrality of symptoms but, instead the centrality of processes of *struggle* against this disruption of rhythm. Struggle is intrinsic and is seldom eclipsed in the often weighty and intrepid social engagement with living, working, and caring for others despite an onslaught of debilitating and frightening experiences of mental affliction. In this respect, my research suggests that the lived experience of mental illness is described more precisely not by the conceptual pairing of vulnerability and resilience but, rather, by replacing that pairing with the more active processes of precarity and struggle.

The ethnographic value of studying experience looms large also for the intersubjective specification of alterity, the cultural delineation of those with and without mental illness as "us" and "them." As cultural and political processes, otherizing often renders subjects not fully human. The construction can be observed in the difference between experience-distant and first-person accounts of mental illness, as well as everyday discourse on perceived kinds of people and nonpeople. This occurs across nearly all social sectors, including academic professions such as anthropology and psychiatry.

I vividly recall speaking with an eminent psychiatrist who specializes in schizophrenia one Sunday morning after brunch in New York City. The psychiatrist was a consultant on one of my studies funded by the National Institute of Mental Health, and we had spent two hours going over the study design and procedures. In a relaxed moment while saying goodbye on the street as I caught a cab, he confided, "Really, Jan, I'll be very surprised if you find anything like you seem to be looking for in those people, certainly nothing of a real psychological life. I've never seen it." I was shocked: how could someone who worked so closely with people not know more about experiential realities? Two decades since, having heard the same refrain in different ways across many quarters, professional and nonprofessional alike, the surprise has long since worn off. The shock, however, has not.

On the basis of decades of ethnographic and longitudinal studies that I have collaboratively undertaken, there is no empirical or ethical basis for the otherizing of people living with conditions of mental illness. Such otherizing takes place because mental illness concerns fundamental human processes that are ignored, denied, or downgraded by people who imagine themselves as different from, and morally superior to, their objects of derision. Modulations in the rhythm of life and engagement in struggle are experienced by both the afflicted and unafflicted. Thus, distinctions—explicit and implicit—between "us" and "them" are untenable.[28] Moving away from pathologizing categories of incapacity and inferiority and toward capacity and similarity is important. Sebastián, one of the many hundreds of persons with whom I have worked, put it well when he told me, "I'm just like everyone else, except I hear voices."[29]

Cultural Validity: Traversing the Category Fallacy

Working to develop an alternative to decades of universalist assumptions in psychiatry, Kleinman identified the practice of making clinical diagnoses in the absence of cultural validity as predicated on a "category fallacy."[30] The observation and interpretation of the behavior and expression of symptoms is problematic in the absence of considering culturally communicative meanings. The risk is that reliance on standardized diagnostic criteria can fail to recognize substantial cultural variation in the expression of symptoms in relation to gender, social class, ethnic identification, linguistic and paralinguistic expression, and somatic modes of attention. The notion of "somatic modes of attention," formulated by Thomas Csordas, draws attention to the "culturally elaborated ways of attending to and with one's body in surroundings that include the embodied presence of others."[31] Ethnographic examples include somatization among Chinese patients, Fijian bodily experience not in relation to the individual self but more as matters of community practice, and Salvadoran embodiment of fear and anxiety experienced as intense heat (*calor*) that pervades the body.[32] Neglecting such culturally constituted phenomena can lead to misdiagnoses or improper treatment. For instance, in the Salvadoran case, *calor* has been diagnosed in emergency room settings as acute psychosis or panic attacks for which psychiatric hospitalization is required. A core problem remains one of ethnocentrism built into diagnostic categories developed for European or Euro-American populations and not infrequently skewed toward men of middle-class backgrounds. Thus, the problem concerns the question of what can validly constitute the "normative baseline" and how, when misapplied, the description and classification of categories of disorder (psychotic, mood, anxiety, etc.) can be misleading or useless.

While for research purposes reliable psychiatric diagnostic categories can be useful as starting point for identifying and sorting kinds of illness, in ethnographic work they can never be an end point of inquiry.[33] To return to the case vignette of Taciana, there appears to be clinical utility for the diagnostic category of depression that she herself endorsed. But as we saw from her perspective, far more was going on in relation to "bad things" happening to her. In the New Mexican study, we used the child version of the Structured Clinical Interview for the *Diagnostic and Statistical Manual of Mental Disorders*, Fourth Edition (*DSM*-IV), or the KID-SCID, administered by a clinical research team member, to ascertain research diagnostic criteria (versus clinically deployed diagnoses).[34] The child psychiatrist working with our team is highly experienced and has worked with Native Americans for decades. Thus, he is highly attuned to culturally and ecologically specific conditions of life in the region. Results show that Taciana met research diagnostic criteria for several diagnoses: attention-deficit/hyperactivity disorder (ADHD), with culturally specific qualifications and equivocations; major depressive disorder (with mood concurrent psychotic features); separation anxiety disorder; posttraumatic stress disorder; alcohol dependence; drug dependence (several, including cannabis, cocaine, inhalants); and subthreshold bulimia nervosa. This is a dizzying array of diagnoses that are unstable not only as clinical categories but also as a function of age. Clinicians generally agree that it is difficult to diagnose children and young adolescents in light of developmental processes of change. Yet according to SCID research diagnostic criteria, which entail high levels of symptom severity, nearly all in the study met criteria for two to three psychiatric diagnoses. This particular research project has led me to look askance at psychiatric diagnoses in the case of children living under conditions of structural violence. However, from Taciana's perspective it seemed that she herself considered depression, trauma, drugs, and parental abandonment as highly relevant to her situation.

As she insisted, however, this was not the whole story. She simultaneously considered that she needed protection from the "bad things" that had happened to her. The matter also entails the question of temporal validity insofar as this was her interpretation at the outset of her first psychiatric hospitalization. Two months after being discharged from what our research team and the research participants regard as a relatively high-quality care facility, the situation had become even more complex and layered. Taciana's narrative departed sharply from that introduced above ("I am Zuni.... I came here because bad things happened to me") to a neoliberal rhetoric of the for-profit behavioral-health residential facility to which she was transferred: "I'm here because I fucked up my life. I did it to myself. I can't really do anything right. I need to use my coping skills." Yet Taciana combined this institutional concentration on her wrongdoing with a sustained conviction that Zuni ritual healing (dancers) and religious power (corn pollen) were effective in "sucking these little bad things outta you" and "taking the stress, anger, and depression out of one's system." She clung to her corn, which she felt had protected her since she was a baby. Yet in the pauses and silences in the telling of that narrative, there was a palpable intersubjective sense of confusion of the unsaid: if the corn was protective, if the gods were powerful, how could she feel so terribly lost and abandoned in such an awful place with so little care?

Thus, cultural definitions of and explanations for mental illness can shape experience as matters of internalization, acceptance, or rejection, varying over time and across settings. While the change in Taciana's narrative from one based on cultural identity and harm by others to self-accusation and individualized responsibility is disturbing, caution should be exercised by researchers and clinicians alike before discarding *psychiatric diagnoses* as irrelevant or harmful. Important to note in this instance is that the changed narrative is focused not on a cultural diagnostic category (e.g., depression) but, instead, on ethnopsychologically imagined individual flaws deployed by low-paid staff with little professional training who work in residential facilities largely in a carceral capacity. The attribution of individual moral blame would be staunchly denied by professional psychiatrists or clinical psychologists, who instead endorse a disease model. For them, the question of individual characteristics and responsibility is present, albeit in subtler and more deeply seated forms.[35]

Historically, there is ample evidence of the harm that can come from thinking psychiatric diagnoses apply to some people and not others. This is the case in racialized accounts of mental illness crafted through colonial psychiatry. Working for the British government in Kenya, for example, the physician J. C. Carothers made sweeping claims that "African" peoples were innately lacking in moral sensibilities of guilt, shame, and responsibility. This claim was used to promote the a priori presumption that "Africans" could not, and therefore did not, suffer from depression.[36] Working ethnographically during that same period, the anthropologist-psychiatrist M. J. Field drew an entirely different conclusion based on detailed ethnographic and clinical materials. Field reported major depression to be common in rural Ghana, with symptoms remarkably similar to those she had observed clinically in London. Through meticulous case studies documenting sentiments of guilt and clinical syndromes of depression, Field established not only that depression was common in rural Ghana, but also that it was particularly notable among women of seniority who had lost social power in the context of patriarchal privilege.[37]

It is difficult to imagine how flawed thinking about depression would ever have been significantly challenged in the absence of ethnographic studies. While there is a growing recognition of somatic complaints as possibly indicative of depression in some primary care settings, everyday clinical discourse on types of depression as "sophisticated" (psychological and verbal emotional presentations) or "unsophisticated" (somatic and bodily presentations) has hardly disappeared.[38] Kleinman's works from Taiwan and China demonstrated that depression is experienced and expressed primarily not as dysphoric affect but, rather, in somatic terms that is not reducible to differences in formal education or economic status.[39] Yet somatic experience and expression of depression are in varying degrees prevalent worldwide, including in much of the United States.

Centrality of Suffering as Existential and Social Experience

Within medical anthropology, a research focus on suffering mirrors the human condition broadly and specifically under duress. The identification of social and personal suffering in Kleinman's formulation entails the recognition of "suffering [as] one of the existential grounds of human experience; it is a defining quality, a limiting experience in human conditions." This identification is simultaneously qualified with a caution against "essentializing, naturalizing, or sentimentalizing suffering in its many forms, both extreme and ordinary."[40] Moreover, the invocation of "suffering" can be misdirected through popular appropriations or as an objectification of people.

Perhaps unsurprisingly, given the prominence of scholarship in medical anthropology concerned with pain, suffering, and affliction as critical domains of anthropological analysis, this area has been critiqued in some quarters as a delimited pursuit.[41] Such is the case with Joel Robbins's infelicitous characterization of anthropological studies that address suffering as the discursive replacement of the historically fraught "savage slot" with that of the "suffering slot."[42] This rendering of medical anthropological scholarship is destitute by virtue of imprecision and conflation, as "a problematic instance of equating an anthropological focus on the various forms of human suffering with the erstwhile anthropological interest in conceptions of the savage. Such a caricature erroneously compares a mode of experience (suffering) with a category of being (savagery) and confuses description (of savagery) with critique (of suffering)."[43]

Robbins, arguing that medical anthropology is dominated by a concentration on affliction and suffering, provides a wholesale characterization of the field as a largely sentimental pursuit, leading us astray from the rightful direction for anthropology. Without irony, there is a call for a "return" to moral theory and philosophy in pursuit of an "anthropology of the good."[44]

Given the legacy of inattention to mental illness that has now been supplanted by a considerable body of work by medical anthropologists, a call for such a "return" appears to be a move to delegitimize people who live with such conditions and render them peripheral to the cultural theorizing of society, institutions, and human value. Quite the opposite has been true for seminal thinkers in the history of medicine who have examined the broader relevance of mental illness.[45] The intersection of society, institutions, and madness is well known in the work of Michel Foucault, and it is particularly compelling in his essay on the interconnections of passion, delirium, and madness.[46] Within medical anthropology, this brings to mind the now classic volume on depression as emotion and disorder edited by Kleinman and Byron Good that collected ethnographic and clinical studies bridging the fields of ethnopsychology and cross-cultural psychiatry.[47] Studies of psychological trauma have also drawn on historical and cultural treatments of emotion and illness, such as the publication of "Psychological Automatism" in 1889 in which Pierre Janet formulated trauma in the wake of an event experienced as "vehement emotion" followed by dissociation or attachment to the trauma such that people cannot easily go on with their lives.[48] Treatments for trauma in specific contexts of political violence and warfare have also concerned the interface of or continuum between psychic disease processes and dysphoric affects.[49]

Thus, however a political academic move to downgrade the anthropological study of suffering is intended, it is offensive by distorting not only the lives of many worldwide but also the wealth of ethnographic works that critically examine the lifeworlds of people, communities, and institutions under geopolitical forces of repression. A commentary by Seth Holmes on this most recent iteration of cultural reductionism identifies it as an "ethnographic refusal in which anthropology students are counseled or ridiculed away from theorizing and representing realities their research participants may experience and narrate as suffering and violence."[50] In Holmes's ethnographic case, as well as in many of my studies, writing and speaking about suffering is not the idiom of the anthropologist but precisely the language of the people with whom we live and work. The denial of suffering is just that: denial. And, perhaps, as Holmes suggests, ethnographic refusal. Anything *other than* experience.

Global Mental Health and Medical Anthropology:
Possibilities and Impediments

The field of Global Mental Health (GMH) emerged with the battle cry, "No health without mental health."[51] The move to prioritize mental health seeks to balance the great disparity of attention and funding for infectious and other diseases at the expense of what are classified as "noncommunicable" diseases.[52] Typically, the disproportionate emphasis on infectious disease is presumed to be justified in terms of grave risk to mortality and biosecurity. This is problematic, however, in light of the high proportion of populations living with disabilities associated with mental disorders. Further, when comparing the general population and those with mental disorders through meta-analysis models, the risk of mortality is significantly higher among people with mental disorder. The median number of years of life lost is estimated at ten years worldwide, with eight million (14.3 percent) deaths attributable to mental disorders annually.[53]

For the development of a theoretical and methodological foundation for the field of GMH, there is a prodigious body of interdisciplinary work produced by cultural psychiatrists, by medical anthropologists, and in allied fields. However, this would hardly be observable from review of GMH publications of the past two decades. Currently, there appears to be a lack of either familiarity with or serious interest in integration of anthropologically infused thinking within the GMH enterprise. This circumstance evokes a distinct sense of déjà vu with respect to what transpired in the wake of the International Pilot Studies of Schizophrenia (IPSS) conducted by the World Health Organization (WHO) in the 1970s.[54] An ambitious study across five continents complemented by additional longitudinal follow-up studies, the IPSS released initial findings for transnational differences in course and outcome that remain robust.[55] The IPSS design was conceived and carried out in the absence of collaboration with anthropologists. This oversight had substantial consequences, since the studies' findings were both unexpected and significant. Poorer therapeutic outcomes were observed in European and North American countries than in nations of the Global South.[56] The transnational studies also revealed unexpected variation in what had been considered pathognomonic or "signature" symptoms across sites. However, in the absence of ethnographic materials collected in tandem with clinical assessments, there was no empirical route to investigate the meaning of such results.

It was left to subsequent research to develop hypotheses and investigate possible sources of variation to account for the observed differences in the course and outcome. Among the most significant of these sources has been familial response or "expressed emotion"—emotions, attitudes, and behavior of kin toward ill relatives. Levels of expressed emotion likely account for some of the variation in who improves and who does not over time, and variation in levels of expressed emotion, in turn, can be accounted for partly by *conceptualizations* of mental illness—for example, personality defect, moral transgression, witchcraft, or cultural chemistry.[57] Another source of variation in course and outcome is the role of psychopharmacology, often the primary or only treatment available in some global settings, while other settings lack availability entirely. People who take psychotropic medications (and their kin) may seek medications for therapeutic benefits while at the same time grapple with paradoxes of the lived experiences of taking them.[58] Psychopharmacological practices blur the "conjunction of magic, science, and religion with respect to pharmaceutical markets and global capitalism, on the one hand, and culture and lived experience of pharmacological agents, on the other."[59]

Many of the controversies surrounding the production, marketing, use, and misuse of psychopharmaceuticals are well rehearsed within medical anthropology. In the absence of working with people who actually live with mental illness and take medications to alleviate their condition, many critiques that target psychiatric biomedicine are remarkably distal or uninformed when applied to people who are afflicted.[60] While the argument in medical anthropology leans generally against psychopharmacology, the presumption in biological psychiatry often leans uncritically in favor. Both of these generalized stances are unproductive. The neglect of attention to culture and experience is particularly acute for practices of dispensing and taking psychotropic medications. Application of the concepts of experience and cultural validity in the realm of psychopharmacology has largely been precluded by the presumption that, as bioactive compounds, psychotropic drugs are "culture-free" and thus require little cultural and social attention. Recent ethnography shows that this is plainly wrongheaded. Our research makes clear that, while patients and kin value them for specific purposes, the meanings and practices surrounding these drugs produce what I have called medication-related paradoxes of lived experience. These conundrums can entail the valuation of improvement or symptom control while at the same time ambivalence about taking the medication.

While there is no shortage of controversy, or dilemmas, surrounding treatment with medications, it is clear that the drugs are actively sought worldwide by kin and those afflicted. Across low-, middle-, and high-income countries, people are generally aware of these drugs. For example, as Ursula Read has documented in Ghana, people not only actively seek out "hospital medicine" for mental illness but also sometimes use it in preparation for consultation with a religious healer.[61] At the same time, there is a deep longing for cure and dissatisfaction with side effects that may not help with work or social functioning.[62] The limitations surrounding psychopharmaceuticals affect people and their kin in ways that are remarkably similar and distinctive worldwide, as is detailed ethnographically in case studies from Ghana, India, Indonesia, Mexico, Tanzania, and the United States.[63]

There are opportunities to advance GMH in a way that takes seriously "No health without mental health," but this would require serious anthropological involvement at a collaborative design table. Within medical anthropology, there is debate and critique regarding the GMH endeavor, and it remains to be seen how this actually will be taken up.[64] The work of medical anthropologists is not delimited to providing "vignettes" from, or clean-up of, jobs gone awry. As I have stressed in conferences with GMH leaders, the work of medical anthropology must be foundational to the entire enterprise. Failure to make it so will result in less than efficacious or sustainable partnerships in the service of improved mental health for all. Ethnographically and experientially attuned approaches to GMH can provide empirical grounding for doing away with the long-standing dichotomous mind-body separation and truncated attention to mental health merely as an "add-on" for infectious diseases (such as HIV/AIDS and tuberculosis).

Accomplishing this necessitates real collaboration, but it hardly requires going back to the drawing board, given the rich legacy of anthropological scholarship at the interface of anthropology and psychiatry that I referenced at the beginning of this chapter. But the legacy of social hierarchy within academic disciplines remains an obstacle to creating sustainable partnerships among primary stakeholders (patients, kin, providers) in local communities and among health policy officials. Without doubt, the core issues of sustainability and efficacy of partnerships and therapeutic care must be grounded in ethnographic knowledge and practice.[65]

A breakthrough to foster such an effort came in the spring of 2016 at a series of meetings in Washington, DC, cosponsored by the World Bank Group, the WHO, the National Institutes of Health, and Georgetown University. Entitled "Out of the Shadows: Making Mental Health a Global Priority," the meetings were an auspicious raising of political and social consciousness for mental health in its own right as a matter of human need and social justice. In an opening plenary address at the World Bank Group, Kleinman challenged three pervasive "myths": that mental illness is untreatable; that it is unimportant; and that caring for it is not cost-effective. Speaking from the nexus of psychiatry and anthropology, he asserted that "behind every data point there is real suffering."[66] At the end of the week, at a closing symposium, the powerful overall message was that we will get nowhere in the absence of generative theoretical models to guide our efforts. I have argued that any theoretically informed approach to GMH must take into consideration the decades of research in medical/psychiatric anthropology. Anthropological theory is critical to strengthen the intellectual and political platform from which to bridge the therapeutic concerns of GMH and the interpretive concerns of medical anthropology.[67] Constructing this bridge will require less formulaic and more nuanced anthropological analyses of the complex and paradoxical features of health care, considering experiential modes of suffering and institutional processes for the provision of health care in a globalizing world. As Vikram Patel remarked in the above noted 2016 symposium's closing session, "When it comes to mental health, we are *all* developing countries."

As I have argued, efforts targeted at the "scaling up" of mental health care must be focused, effective, and sustainable. While economic and political constraints constitute the first obstacle to obtaining care, other obstacles are embedded in mental health policy worldwide that lacks sufficient political will for transformation. What is needed are tailored approaches to incorporate the social, cultural, and psychological contexts of mental illness and its treatment, on the one hand, and the socioecological context of environments in relation to socioeconomic and political conditions that can produce and exacerbate mental illness, on the other.[68] In the absence of in-depth and extended anthropological engagement, the GMH field could easily reproduce earlier follies within contemporary implementation and intervention sciences. "Culture lite" (as an example, through simplified or formulaic reference to idioms of distress) will not suffice for tackling core issues of cultural validity and therapeutic efficacy. Neither will indiscriminate discarding of psychiatric knowledge by some psychiatrists who, ironically, take cultural relativism further than most contemporary psychiatric anthropologists.[69]

Against the background of concern for what I have outlined as extraordinary conditions, we now have several decades of studies to demonstrate the breadth and depth of cultural and social processes as fundamental to the shaping of nearly every aspect of mental illness:[70]

- Risk/vulnerability factors (precarity)
- Type of onset (sudden or gradual)
- Symptom content, form, constellation
- Clinical diagnostic process
- Subjective experience and meaning of problem/illness
- Kin identification and conception of and social-emotional response to illness
- Community social response (support, stigma)
- Healing modalities and health-care utilization
- Experience, meaning, and utilization of health care/healing modalities (including psychotropic drugs)
- Resources for resilience and recovery
- Course and outcome

In practice, these factors, of course, are not only culturally shaped but form a matrix in which each factor can be inflected by the others. Severity of symptoms is inflected by cultural perception and attention to the symptoms; degree of disability/impairment is inflected by severity; and so forth. Behind all of this is the cultural definition of what counts as a problem in the first place.

In sum, just as there can be "no health without mental health," there can be "*no understanding of mental health without culture.*" The concept of culture, largely out of fashion in cultural anthropology, as well as to medical anthropology, cannot be a casualty of translation or vogue. Cultural orientations and processes are more at issue than places or peoples, "beliefs" or behavior.[71] As Sapir set forth nearly a century ago, the locus of culture is dynamically created and re-created in the process of social interaction.[72] Cultural orientations are also critical for subjectivity and processes of attention, perception, and meaning that shape personal and public spheres. Such orientations are embedded generally in what Bateson called a community's ethos and what I more specifically have called a political ethos.[73] Through my studies I have found that a sustained ethnographic approach to the experience of mental illness should productively focus on engaged processes of struggle rather than symptoms. Struggle is intrinsic experiences of mental and neurological affliction, including the pernicious problem of discrimination (often referred to as social stigma).[74] Given this situation, it is necessary to advocate for continued research at the juncture of anthropology and psychiatry.

Notes

I appreciate the research collaboration extended by the medical director and clinical staff of the hospital. I stand in admiration of the dedication of providers in the face of limitations by state and nationwide behavioral health corporations that restrict therapeutic practice. An earlier version of this chapter was presented at the conference A Special View of Asia and the World, Asia Center, Harvard University, Cambridge, Mass.

1 | Case study excerpted from Jenkins and Csordas, *Troubled in the Land of Enchantment.*

2 | US Census Bureau, 2017, https://talkpoverty.org/state-year-report/new-mexico-2017-report/.

3 | Kleinman, *Experience and Its Moral Modes.*

4 | Kleinman, *Rethinking Psychiatry.*

5 | Kleinman, *What Really Matters.*

6 | Jenkins, *Extraordinary Conditions.*

7 | Jenkins, *Extraordinary Conditions*.

8 | Neely Myers and Kristin Yarris have recently drawn together a collection of ethnographic works on the intersection of extraordinary conditions, psychiatric care, and moral experience: see Myers and Yarris, "Extraordinary Conditions."

9 | Jenkins and Barrett, *Schizophrenia, Culture, and Subjectivity*; Basu, "Listening to Disembodied Voices"; Becker, *Body, Self, and Society*; Biehl, *Vita*; Biehl et al., *Subjectivity*; Brodwin, *Everyday Ethics*; Carpenter-Song, "Children's Sense of Self in Relation to Clinical Processes"; Carpenter-Song, "The Kids Were My Drive"; Chen, *Breathing Spaces*; Csordas, "The Navajo Healing Project"; Csordas and Jenkins, "Land of a Thousand Cuts"; Das, *Life and Worlds*; Desjarlais, *Shelter Blues*; Dumit, *Drugs for Life*; Duncan, *Transforming Therapy*; Ecks, *Eating Drugs*; Farmer, "An Anthropology of Structural Violence"; Farmer, *Pathologies of Power*; Good, *Medicine, Rationality, and Experience*; Good et al., *Shattering Culture*; Hinton and Good, *Culture and Panic Disorder*; Hinton et al., "PTSD and Key Somatic Complaints and Cultural Syndromes among Rural Cambodians"; Holmes, *Fresh Fruit, Broken Bodies*; Jenkins, *Pharmaceutical Self*; Jenkins and Carpenter-Song, "The New Paradigm of Recovery from Schizophrenia"; Jenkins and Carpenter-Song, "Stigma despite Recovery"; Kleinman and Good, *Culture and Depression*; Kleinman, *Social Origins of Distress and Disease*; Lovell, "The City Is My Mother"; Lovell, "Tending to the Unseen in Extraordinary Circumstances"; Martin, *Bipolar Expeditions*; Martin, "Sleepless in America"; Myers and Yarris, "Extraordinary Conditions"; Read, "I Want the One That Will Heal Me Completely so It Won't Come Back Again"; Read et al., "Local Suffering and the Global Discourse of Mental Health and Human Rights"; Reyes-Foster, *Psychiatric Encounters*; Rhodes, *Emptying Beds*; Rhodes, *Total Confinement*; Whyte, "Health Identities and Subjectivities"; Whyte et al., *Social Lives of Medicines*; Yahalom, *Caring for the People of the Clouds*; Yarris, "The Pain of 'Thinking Too Much.'"

10 | Benedict, "Anthropology and the Abnormal."

11 | Sapir, "Culture, Genuine and Spurious," 235.

12 | Bateson, "Minimal Requirements for a Theory of Schizophrenia"; Devereux, "Normal and Abnormal"; Du Bois, *The People of Alor*; Hallowell, *Culture and Experience*; Sapir, *Culture, Language and Personality*; Kardiner, *The Traumatic Neuroses of War*.

13 | Canguilhem, *On the Normal and the Pathological*; Foucault, *Madness and Civilization*.

14 | Kleinman, "Depression, Somatization and the 'New Cross-Cultural Psychiatry'"; Kleinman, *The Illness Narratives*; Kleinman, *Patients and Healers in the Context of Culture*; Kleinman, *Rethinking Psychiatry*; Kleinman, *Social Origins of Distress and Disease*.

15 | White, "Culturological versus Psychological Interpretations of Human Behavior," 686–87. Whether reading the tables of contents within books or

full ethnographies published prior to the 1970s, one is hard pressed to find accounts of, or even footnotes about, people with mental illness. As cultural actors, they scarcely make an appearance.

16 | See, e.g., Abrahams, "Ordinary and Extraordinary Experience," 45–48; Turner and Bruner, *The Anthropology of Experience*.

17 | Kleinman, *Experience and Its Moral Modes*; Kleinman, *What Really Matters*.

18 | Kleinman and Kleinman, "Suffering and Its Professional Transformation," 276, emphasis added.

19 | Kleinman and Kleinman, "Suffering and Its Professional Transformation," 276.

20 | This approach represents an intellectual departure from conventional approaches to psychosis, as represented in Aulagnier, *The Violence of Interpretation*; Kring and Johnson, *Abnormal Psychology*.

21 | Jenkins and Barrett, *Schizophrenia, Culture, and Subjectivity*, 7.

22 | Jenkins and Barrett, *Schizophrenia, Culture, and Subjectivity*, 7.

23 | Jenkins, "Schizophrenia as a Fundamental Human Process."

24 | Jenkins and Barrett, "Introduction."

25 | Jenkins, *Extraordinary Conditions*, 3.

26 | Jenkins, *Extraordinary Conditions*, 3.

27 | Jenkins, "Subjective Experience of Persistent Schizophrenia and Depression among Latinos and Euro-Americans," 23.

28 | Jenkins, *Extraordinary Conditions*.

29 | Jenkins, *Extraordinary Conditions*, 80.

30 | Kleinman, *Rethinking Psychiatry*, 15.

31 | Csordas, *Embodiment and Experience*, 38.

32 | Kleinman, *Social Origins of Distress and Disease*; Becker, *Body, Self, and Society*; Jenkins and Valiente, "Bodily Transactions of the Passions."

33 | Byron Good makes this argument in "Culture and Psychopathology."

34 | The project psychiatrist and the clinical psychologist on the research team were trained in administration and research reliability for this procedure in Jenkins and Csordas, *Troubled in the Land of Enchantment*.

35 | Jenkins and Kozelka, "Global Mental Health and Psychopharmacology in Precarious Ecologies."

36 | Carothers, "Frontal Lobe Function and the African."

37 | Field, *Search for Security*.

38 | Kirmayer and Robbins, "Three Forms of Somatization in Primary Care"; Tylee and Gandhi, "The Importance of Somatic Symptoms in Depression in Primary Care."

39 | Kleinman, "Depression, Somatization and the 'New Cross-Cultural Psychiatry'"; Kleinman, *Patients and Healers in the Context of Culture*; Kleinman, *Social Origins of Distress and Disease*.

40 | Kleinman and Kleinman, "The Appeal of Experience," 2.

41 | Kleinman, *The Illness Narratives*; Kleinman, *Social Origins of Distress and Disease*; Kleinman et al., *Social Suffering*.

42 | Robbins, "Beyond the Suffering Subject."

43 | Jenkins, *Extraordinary Conditions*, 266.

44 | Robbins, "Beyond the Suffering Subject."

45 | Canguilhem, *On the Normal and the Pathological*; Foucault, *Madness and Civilization*.

46 | Foucault, *Madness and Civilization*, 85.

47 | Kleinman and Good, *Culture and Depression*.

48 | Kolk and Hart, "Pierre Janet and the Breakdown of Adaptation in Psychological Trauma."

49 | Kardiner, *The Traumatic Neuroses of War*; Rivers, "The Repression of War Experience."

50 | Holmes, "Discussing 'Suffering Slot Anthropology' with Migrant Farm Workers."

51 | Prince et al., "No Health without Mental Health."

52 | Kozelka and Jenkins, "Renaming Non-communicable Diseases," e655.

53 | Walker et al., "Mortality in Mental Disorders and Global Disease Burden Implications," 334.

54 | World Health Organization, 1973, 1979.

55 | Sartorius et al., "Long-term Follow-up of Schizophrenia in Sixteen Countries"; Hopper, "Interrogating the Meaning of 'Culture' in the WHO International Studies of Schizophrenia."

56 | World Health Organization, *Schizophrenia*.

57 | Jenkins, *Extraordinary Conditions*; Jenkins and Karno, "The Meaning of Expressed Emotion."

58 | Jenkins and Carpenter-Song, "The New Paradigm of Recovery from Schizophrenia."

59 | Jenkins, *Pharmaceutical Self*, 3.

60 | Summerfield, "Afterword."

61 | Read, "I Want the One That Will Heal Me Completely so It Won't Come Back Again," 441.

62 | Jenkins and Carpenter-Song, "The New Paradigm of Recovery from Schizophrenia."

63 | Read, "I Want the One That Will Heal Me Completely so It Won't Come Back Again"; Ecks, *Eating Drugs*; Basu, "Listening to Disembodied Voices"; Duncan, *Transforming Therapy*; Good, "The Complexities of Psychopharmaceutical Hegemonies in Indonesia"; Whyte, "Family Experiences with Mental Health Problems in Tanzania"; Jenkins, *Extraordinary Conditions*.

64 | A recent summary of key issues and critiques is in White et al., *The Palgrave Handbook of Sociocultural Perspectives on Global Mental Health*.

65 | Kim et al., "Scaling Up Effective Delivery Models Worldwide."

66 | Arthur Kleinman, summarized in Mendenhall, "The Georgetown Symposium on Global Mental Health."

67 | Good, *Medicine, Rationality, and Experience*.

68 | Jenkins and Kozelka, "Global Mental Health and Psychopharmacology in Precarious Ecologies."

69 | Summerfield, "Afterword."
70 | The list is reproduced from Jenkins, *Extraordinary Conditions*.
71 | The concept of belief in medical anthropology imploded more than twenty-five years ago the wake of meticulous critique in Good, *Medicine, Rationality, and Experience*.
72 | Sapir, "Cultural Anthropology and Psychiatry," 236.
73 | Bateson, *Naven*; Jenkins, "The State Construction of Affect."
74 | Jenkins and Carpenter-Song, "Stigma despite Recovery."

PART III

Worlds *of* Biotechnological Promise *and* the Plasticity *of* Self *and* Power

AS TECHNOLOGICAL ADVANCES IN CLINICAL MEDICINE, genomics, and "smart" technology increasingly complicate and blur definitions of the self, the social, and the multiplicity of the biological, what are the possibilities for rethinking both human conditions and the arts of care?

In his work as a social scientist and as a psychiatrist and caregiver, Arthur Kleinman has consistently brought into view the relationship among medical technologies, diagnostic categories, and the experience of illness and care. With recent developments in epigenetics, invasive but life-changing medical interventions to facilitate couples' desires to reproduce, and new regimes of biometric governance that fix (with the trappings of biological certainty) individual identities, Lawrence Cohen, Marcia Inhorn, and Margaret Lock are thrust into theorizing the effects of these bio-techno-social interventions on human experiences and local worlds. The anthropologists remain open to the possibilities that these advances may productively affirm the interlinkages of the social and biological (interlinkages that have hitherto been discounted by many bioscientific experts) and draw attention to the risk that applying technological certainty to mutable social phenomena may further naturalize social stratifications. Throughout their investigations, Cohen, Inhorn, and Lock keep in view the ways that people the world over continue to practice an "art of living socially" amid profound redefinitions of the self in context.

Mindful of Kleinman's demand for the necessity of "interference in totalizing orientations to life on the margin," Lawrence Cohen opens part III by describing the ambiguous experiences of poor transgender women in India as they encounter the nation's massive new biometric identity project known as Aadhaar (Foundation). Promising social inclusion and treatment access, technocracy here insists on "de-duplicating" identity and reordering the dynamic messiness of life. As it generates massive amounts of data, this project of "radical individuation" simultaneously produces a leakiness around gender and sexuality, as *hijras* and transgender citizens use multiple names and identities to survive in a time of "intensified affective circuits of insult and offense." Attending to "that which may resist meaning" in a community's social fabric, identity, and patterns of mortality, Cohen thus inquires into how grievability and the "nonscalable" might be intertwined. And from this ethnographic interference on the risks of "disappearance" amid new regimes of biometric governance, the anthropologist troubles the certainties of large-scale technological infrastructures and the mandates of transnational humanitarianism.

Marcia Inhorn, in turn, explores the morally ambivalent, life-making territories of in vitro fertilization (IVF) and assisted reproduction (including surrogacy) as transnational phenomena. Used to prevent demographic demise in some contexts, and in others to realize well-off couples' deep desires for offspring, these technologies are also used for sex selection and the culling of female embryos. The "global reproductive assembly line" has created what Inhorn calls "reprohubs" and a "global gynecology" made up of diverse actors from multiple countries, providing biological and technological resources, services, and family-making opportunities. These forms of reproductive care and "medical cosmopolitanism" may seem troubling as they play out unevenly across "stratifications of nation and class," yet Inhorn's "marital ethnography" and "reprotravel stories" from South Asia also "speak to the ongoing importance of local moral worlds" within these larger global trajectories and assemblages. Here, constrained physiologies, social stigma, emotionally laden aspirations, and religious sensibilities intermingle with high-end technoscience in the engineering of a possible form of "therapeutic reprieve" at all costs.

Finally, Margaret Lock invites us to track the ever mutating conceptualizations of the self that are arising through epigenetic renderings of the human-environment nexus, or "phenotypic plasticity." If twentieth-century anthropologists articulated a notion of the self as embedded in social relations and set against ideas of the modern Euro-American autonomous self, recent epigenetic findings similarly reveal the individual as an embodied, "inherently unstable" entity that demands "contextualization in time and space." Biological notions of the self as responsive, ever changing sets of interactions with social and political environments allow us to consider disease and vulnerability over a life course exposed to racism, inequality, and toxicity and to attend to intergenerational psychosocial effects resulting from colonial subjugation, for example. Such evidence of the transmission of epigenetic effects forces courts of law and health-care providers alike to reconsider "how responsibility for chronic malaise and even violence should be allocated."

Lock's essay is a tentatively optimistic one, suggesting a convergence of theories of embodiment, historical memory, and trauma from the humanities and social sciences with recent insights from the biological sciences. And though social scientists may arguably take some credit for inspiring the scope and focus of this contemporary epigenetic research, what remains to be seen is how these redefinitions of the biological self, in tandem with anthropologists' and communities' own practical solidarities and advocacy, may in turn bolster efforts toward social justice and restitution for historical wrongs—or whether they will settle into a new type of wholly biological determinism. As Kleinman and other critically minded medical anthropologists have illuminated for us, it is ultimately through the mutable domains of the institutional and the political, in law and in commitments to social welfare, that health may be made a real prospect for communities that have been marginalized by racism, colonialism, and other forms of structural and psychological trauma over generations.

A Good Death

The Promise and Threat of Biometric
Inclusion for Transgender Women in India

THE MEETING WAS HELD IN A nongovernmental organization (NGO) office above the suburban Mumbai fish market. It was 2012. I had written to the director, whom I had known for decades, to ask about a debate between his NGO (call it Sambandh) and another based in Bangalore (call it Dakshin). Both organizations promoted particular commitments to transgender health in the face of AIDS, poverty, social exclusion, and familial and state violence. They did so in the wake of the consolidation of transgender over the previous decade as a site of biopolitical governance (and abandonment) and emergent if fragile claims of rights, identities, and entitlements. The debate to which I was referring was over a new Indian national identity program known as Aadhaar ("foundation"). Aadhaar promised financial inclusion to the economically and socially marginal via the scanning and digitization of their fingerprints and irises, presumptively to rationalize the distribution of state welfare, private credit, and, in some cases, wages and consumable products. Welfare, wage, credit, and product were collapsed into an expanding figure of governable value termed *service*.[1] One's biometrics were linked to a random twelve-digit Aadhaar identification number; a facial photograph; and a series of data fields limited to name, date of birth, gender, and current address. As part of Aadhaar's promise of inclusion, the data field for gender, to be filled in at the time of scanning, was promoted as including a third, nonbinary option.

Aadhaar was administered by a massive public-private partnership called the Unique Identification Authority of India (UIDAI). In many Indian states, private corporations received contracts from UIDAI to organize infrastructure and logistics for the capture of biometric data. The Mumbai NGO had a close link to Wipro, a nationally dominant information services company that was contracted to register the population of the state of Maharashtra and its capital, Mumbai. One of the NGO's social work interns, trained at the prestigious Tata Institute of Social Sciences in Mumbai, was married to the Wipro executive responsible for the contract. With the director, the social worker organized an Aadhaar registration "camp" in September 2011 at the NGO's offices.

Dakshin's leaders were critical of this initiative, reflecting a long history of disputes between these and other AIDS-care NGOs over the moral form of care.[2] They organized a press conference in November 2011 to challenge Aadhaar as a public good for transgender persons. Their message focused not on Aadhaar's promise of inclusion but, conversely, on its threat of surveillance and the potential violence of gatekeepers controlling access to yet another punishing instrument of state identification. We are already surveilled and abused by state agencies, Dakshin's transgender clients at the press conference emphasized, detailing insult, extortion, and rape as consequences of their efforts to gain formal recognition and, thus, access to employment, housing, and state subsidies. Dakshin's leaders argued that Aadhaar threatened to intensify this violence.

I wrote to Sambandh's director to learn more about the camp. He suggested that we set up a meeting and invite interested "community leaders" when I was next in Mumbai.[3] Sambandh sponsors a *kinnar* community-based organization (CBO) that indexes governmentalized identity in an age of philanthrocapitalism. The term *kinnar* may index respectful trans- or third-gendered belonging (in variably ethnicizing ways in Hindi, Marathi, and Gujarati) with somewhat less of the abusive feel, in an age of intensified affective circuits of insult and offense, of the once far more common word *hijra*.[4] Some leaders of kinnar and transgender groups in Mumbai are known as "gurus," and their followers—variably called daughters, disciples, and dependents—are known as *chelas* or, more simply, hijras. This essay attends to discussions that happened at the meeting the director set up in 2012, which came to center on concerns about Aadhaar raised by several gurus during the 2011 camp. These concerns, temporarily interfering with the registration of persons, were *not* those enunciated at the Bangalore press conference. They opened to a different question: What is a good death, and how might the new Aadhaar ID trouble that? Against the variant stances of the NGOs—which, in framing Aadhaar's stakes as inclusion versus surveillance, mirrored broader public debate—this question was unprecedented.

Thus, in 2012 the director publicized a meeting to discuss the camp and Aadhaar more generally. I had hoped the gurus critical of Aadhaar would come, but predictably most people around the table had worked with either Sambandh or its affiliated kinnar CBO. Still, the conversation was robust around Aadhaar as an uncertain horizon. Aadhaar's presence in the world was still limited in 2012. It was only beginning to be linked to a range of health and welfare schemes. What was clear, and of prime concern, was that like other IDs, but somehow much more so, it presented particular problems with the ethics of one's name.

"What *name* would you give my brother? What would you call him? In your place?"

The demand came a fairly long time ago for this writer. It was 1988. I was a student being trained to study medicine from within and without, beginning two years of work in the Nagwa Dalit (so-called Untouchable) slum in the northern Indian city of Varanasi.

Two questions animated my early training. The first involved what Arthur Kleinman called a "category fallacy," or the ways a historically and technically located biomedical concept might, when applied generally to particular people's situations, dull attention to the *interpretation* of what matters to people, or the culturally mediated "stakes" for them, as Kleinman would suggest to us.[5] The second question concerned how the deployment of expertise in the face of human problems (e.g., in medicine, the singular attention to "disease") might defer or eliminate *acknowledgment* of the lived experience of those problems and the existential and interpersonal grounds of *care* in their face. This, too, was Kleinman's lesson. So caught up was I in naming the first question as the problem of meaning that the relation of the two questions—the limit, as well as the necessity of interpretation in the face of acknowledging that which may resist meaning—was not always apparent. I was being given the gift of interpretive anthropology; it was hard to attend, at the same time, to that anthropology's limit.

I stood outside the small house. I knew this young woman because I had interviewed and spent time with her mother, Bageshera, and Bageshera's two brothers over the previous months. The category fallacy I was hoping to address lay in how scholars of age and aging attended to distress, displacement, and the loss of a way of being in the world in late life, attended that is to a range of situations legible to them as senile dementia.[6] The three siblings were old, I was told early on, and "hot-brained," or full of angry speech: go talk to them. The low-lying lane they and their families lived on was seasonally flooded by a small river it skirted. Others in the slum tended to push me, with my unpleasant questions about things that called attention to the (inevitable) failures of caregiving, down the hill toward the poorest and palpably least resistant lane.

What name *would you give my brother?* The young woman at the bottom of the hill was referring to her younger cousin, the son of her uncle Harinath Prasad. When I walked along the lane in search of the three *burde* (old ones), this cousin was often at the threshold of his father's small house, preparing their meals. His mother had long ago died, and his sisters were married; his brother had gone to the university and held a job as a government clerk in a different city. It was winter, and he wore his shawl ladies-style as he worked, his eyes taking me in and following me. We would become friends much later, and for many years. I asked Bageshera's daughter what she meant, more or less knowing already. Her gesture took in her cousin's mien, shawl, and work. I do not remember her words, but I do remember her referring to the femaleness of it all.

What I don't trust of my recollection, although I did write those words down, was her asking me for a name. I find myself retelling the moment as if she were claiming that there was no name, as if "my place" would supplement that lack. Not long after that day on the lane, a diasporic Indo-Canadian filmmaker would make a film, *Fire*, that narrated the story of two sisters-in-law, each in different ways abandoned by a husband, who become lovers. At a pointed moment, one of the women exclaims with concern that the two lack a *word* for their love. The film's viewer is invited to imagine something like liberation through the word, the missing and universalizing *lesbian* or *gay* as an invitation to a mode of self-consciousness free of category fallacy. The moment in the film strikes a false chord. Yet this is what I remember the woman asking. To interpolate her request here places its addressee in a familiar and troubled position of authority, colluding with an anthropology that takes as its function the correct naming of the difference of others in imagined battle with a hegemonic architecture of sex. Kath Weston critically termed this style of anthropology "ethnocartography."[7] It is not, I think, what Klein-man asks for in raising the question of category fallacy—or what Bageshera's daughter was asking of me.

The experts I talked with in those years were gerontologists around the world or they were healers in Varanasi. When I wrote up the research as a book, I wrestled with whether my audience should be some of those experts and healers or anthropologists like me. The challenge put to me by Kleinman was to find a form of engagement to speak to both. Often the anthropologist reading Kleinman was the witnessing party to a provocation directed to both clinicians and ethnographers. When he turned to write extensively about caregiving, the provocation to each group was phrased as a demand for an"art" conscious of its reduction of the one cared for to an object deprived of its vitality, as if dead-in-life. To the social scientist, the call was for a return to "a *phronesis* that offers the moral and practical wisdom for the art of living socially."[8] To the fellow physician, the call was for a greater commitment, suffusing competent care: "the art of acknowledging and affirming the other as a suffering human being, imagining alternative contexts and practices of responding to calamity, and being with, conversing with, and doing for patients in desperate situations where the emphasis is on what really matters to them and their intimates."[9]

These are inevitably calls for a reorientation in time. When I was a medical student, a clinical preceptor who correctly took me for a medical anthropologist once chastised me during the presentation of a patient's "chief complaint" for including a sentence on what seemed to matter most to that patient. We do not have time for that here and now, the preceptor noted, not impatiently. Though the lesson was learned, what I find striking is a particular figure used by Kleinman to describe his mode of provocation: that of *interference*.

In the essay on caregiving I just cited, Kleinman uses interference as a way to describe contestations between caregiving and other moral demands, and elsewhere he has taken this figure further.[10] To enable the possibility of a medicine that does not position competency *against* caregiving, the productive maneuver is not complaint but interference. In a clinical training institution, inculcating competency through the cultivation of attention to a hierarchy of signs may interfere with the development of a capacity to care in the sense Kleinman terms *being-with*. The moral demands of competency may close off medicine to such care. Interference then takes several forms, from the enactment of a form of clinical practice that works otherwise to the production of a form of speech or writing that does not complain (and thus merely reinstantiate competing demands as an unending contest) but interferes in this oppositional terrain.

These days, the experts I talk with are engineers and other computer scientists, the designers of Aadhaar. Engineers have been at the forefront of UIDAI's efforts to enroll all of India's approximately 1.4 billion residents. Each set of captured and digitized biometric traces are associated with an Aadhaar number. Once one is registered, one is sent a document noting one's number and marking one's state of inclusion as a *Resident*, the term of art for someone whose biometrics are now in the UIDAI database. There is considerable variation in whether people understand Aadhaar to be the number itself (the official message UIDAI offered until 2014) or the paper document that is supposed to (but does not always) come in the mail, which is popularly referred to as the Aadhaar card.

Aadhaar's engineer founder Nandan Nilekani proposed a blueprint for a model of distribution on a national scale, framing India ontologically as a database and the government of distribution as a data problem centering on the elimination of wasteful duplicates from such a nation-as-database. In his best-seller *Imagining India* (2009), Nilekani differentiates this emergent assemblage of technology and development from the Nehruvian technocracy of his parents' generation: the latter, he argues, was suspicious of entrepreneurship and failed to deliver development's public goods. The alternative is to embrace entrepreneurial capital and through it develop a new *techne* of distribution centered on the identification and eradication of duplicate persons. Such a *techne* ensures a rationalization of distribution by eliminating efforts by both the powerful and the desperate to gain more than their allotment of a given service through the proliferation of false or duplicate identification.

Instead of a moral or legal violation, the situation of persons or coteries making such duplicate claims on a resource is subjected to an alternative mode of problematization that draws on the dominant reason of information technology (IT). Information in general degrades, subject to what since the work of Claude Shannon at mid-century has been termed *entropy*.[11] Databases, such as the list of persons meriting a distribution of service by the state, are subject to particular kinds of degradation: for one, they become riven with what in IT worlds are often termed duplicates. People who make improper claims on service are in effect *duplicating* themselves.

Duplicates happen. Despite Hegel's accusation in the lectures in *Aesthetics* that India endlessly duplicates the Idea, given its turning away (unlike China) from the "everyday life" of the World, information theory as a contemporary technics of the Idea presumes entropy as a general condition of the mutation and duplication of significance.[12] In other words, dialectic or not, no universe of discourse is free from the proliferation of copies. Any viable mode of governance must control for entropy by continually "de-duplicating" its subject population. To be developed—to succeed where the fathers have failed, to compete with China (a repeated concern for several of the UIDAI technocrats with whom I spoke)—*India must be de-duplicated.*

The understanding that a rationalization of distribution is critical to life and well-being on the social margins and that there must therefore be an audit of some kind to ensure fairness (and indeed to ensure life itself) is not limited to UIDAI's massive experiment in rendering India a database. Prior and parallel to the new technocracy have been varied other projects to audit distribution. Among the most storied has been the "social audit" tied to right-to-information legislation that enables groups of people at the village and block (group of villages) level to investigate how a public good has been distributed and to whom. Among the multiple critiques of UIDAI by scholars and activists has been the argument that people on the margin are better served by such locally responsive, scaled-down audits of distribution.

When I began to study Aadhaar, I took it as axiomatic that, to understand what the number (or ID card) was and what kind of ethics and politics would emerge in relation to it, I should ally myself with neither engineers nor critics. I satisfied neither group with this modesty: at stake for both was an urgent conception of the social as the ground for proper distribution. For activists committed to bottom-up practices such as the social audit, the social was found in a local moral world. As with the leaders and clients of Dakshin in Bangalore, the critics' experience of the world and the state led them to surmise that Aadhaar's scaling up would wildly inflate the power and lack of accountability of the state. For many engineers, on the other hand, such local knowledge was precisely the problem. The social as a figure of a just polity could emerge only if people could be freed from the drag of identity and place, no longer forced to return to a natal village or stigmatized identity to access services. Several of the engineers in California's Silicon Valley I interviewed who helped design specific features of Aadhaar were impelled by a concept they were seeking to prove: as long as identity was based on history and biography—one's caste or religion, parents' status, region or village, gender, education—the Resident would always be imprisoned within an inequitable morality. If the activists of social audit were worried about the expansion of control society under the new government of the database, for the engineers the only possible interference with the local and regional play of vested interests was a machine to unmake the historical social and reconstitute it through the radical individuation of biometrics.

Kleinman's provocation, and it is not always an easy one to bear, is to work toward a mode of interference of one's own. My experience is that Aadhaar's effects, and its politics, are not uniform and that interference works best at regional, midrange levels. This essay comes out of a conference that addressed the impact of Kleinman's work and pedagogy on scholarship located in reference to contemporary Asia; my specific charge from Kleinman was to speak in some measure to the figure of sexuality. The site of interference I take up, at Sambandh, centers on an intervention (the collaboration with Wipro to mediate transgender access to Aadhaar) focused on presumptive gender. The glide here from sexuality to gender reprises the career of Sambandh itself, which emerged as an AIDS prevention and care organization in the 1990s out of a "gay group" publishing a magazine, with its "key population" (KP), or target of public-health intervention, shifting over the subsequent decades from "gay men" to "men who have sex with men" (MSM) to a proliferating set of identity targets and then to *kothis* (legible over the 2000s as an identity of nonelite, variably female-identifying men who were not necessarily marked as transgender, hijra, or kinnar).[13] Most recently, it has shifted to transgender, encompassing people formerly indexed by the sign of the hijra and increasingly through more aspirational identifications such as the Hindi kinnar, Tamil *thirunangai*, or transgender itself.

As transgender women have emerged as the signature KP of Sambandh, its management has cultivated closer relations to kinnar, hijra, and thirunangai gurus, who are usually leaders within the local and regional form of kin and goverance known as *jamaat*.[14] The management has also promoted the creation of a transgender CBO within the envelope of Sambandh.

The continual shift in Sambandh's KP over the past two decades is not easily reduced to a demand polity of ever more marginal groups coming to make patronage claims on the NGO form. I read the shift in Sambandh's signature KP from gay to MSM to kothi to transgender as a particular response to what I call the changing forms of audit of transnational humanitarian and, specifically, infectious disease control institutions.

In the decade of the 2000s, major urban NGOs and CBOs in the Indian "MSM sector" of infectious disease control were responding to a shifting ecology of funders increasingly dominated by a few key players in global health and, in particular, by the Bill and Melinda Gates Foundation through Avahan, its Indian AIDS initiative. Avahan represented a decade-long commitment to evaluating effective HIV/AIDS prevention techniques in India; it was organized around an experiment in large-scale prevention research, with frequent audits to measure effectiveness across the major KPs. So large was the scale that the foundation's commitment radically altered the landscape of prevention research and of all the other NGO and CBO services funded through the applied research economy of the time. The monumental scale allowed Avahan to produce audits of the effectiveness of prevention practices that involved far more NGOs and CBOs than ever before. Over a decade of conversations with researchers and activists at Sambandh, I often heard of Avahan's power to alter the NGO staff's sense of the evidentiary basis for best practices through what we might term its scale of fact making. Through the massive scale of Avahan's audits of the many NGOs and CBOs it was funding, a key fact being assembled was that transgender women were a KP with troubling, worsening morbidity and mortality statistics for whom current best practices were not very effective.

It did not take the powerful fact making of Avahan for the NGO's personnel and its many kinnar clients to recognize the ongoing precariousness of transgender lives in Mumbai. But hijras were not Sambandh's KP at the outset of the Gateses' Avahan experiment. Despite the long-term presumption of official Indian state epidemiology that gay men, kothis, MSMs, and transgender women formed a single sexually deviant KP, administrators I knew at Sambandh were reluctant in the early 2000s to effect a similar collapse. They argued that hijras were tightly oriented to their jamaat hierarchy and were not likely to attend to Sambandh's health interventions. By then, a familiar account at Sambandh and some other NGOs was that of the hijra who escaped an exploitative guru through the support of an NGO as an alternative space of governance and care; still, there was a sense that CBO and jamaat were distinct moral worlds and that gurus had reason to distrust the English-speaking gay men who ran most of these NGOs.[15] In Bangalore and Chennai, NGOs had a longer record of hiring transgender researchers and outreach workers, though conflicts between gay male NGO leadership, on the one hand, and hijras and thirunangai, on the other, were not infrequent. There was a sense of a different, and explicitly more "intersectional," milieu in southern India. Differences real and imagined came again to the fore around Aadhaar in the wake of the powerful fact of transgender mortality mobilized by Avahan over a decade—thus, Dakshin's press conference. Still, despite the criticism, the Mumbai organization had gone ahead with its camp in 2011. There was a pressing sense for some I spoke with at Sambandh that Aadhaar's promise of financial inclusion for marginal people via the nation's de-duplication was worth the flak.

Aadhaar camps of varying duration are ubiquitous across urban and rural locations. The "camp" is a general biopolitical form, particularly in the post-colony, regulating and provisioning what is comprehended as a mass body.[16] If its temporary and provisional character calls to mind the literature of human-itarian exception, the exception for the health camp is normalized around particular figures of populations or locations to whom the camp allows access to care.[17] Access, in the case of the Aadhaar camp, can be denied through the same reason of localized need that subtends it. Ashish Rajadhyaksha and his colleagues have created a significant archive of short film clips, captured on mobile phones, of how people with different degrees of rights in a city or village are variably included or refused at such camps, which in urban neigh-borhoods may reflect the growing exclusion of classes of persons marked as having a diminished claim on the city.[18]

The fish sellers from the market showed up, as did other local workers. The director told me they had to get in line. "This is really for the kinnars," he said. "We made that clear." Several groups of transgender women came, along with gurus from different groups within the jamaat network. Some women had close relations with Sambandh or were part of its kinnar CBO. Others, unaffiliated, came, as well.

Few people, in 2011, had a sense of what Aadhaar would do; according to the NGO's staff and the social worker who helped Wipro administer the biometric capture, no one voiced concerns about surveillance or the police. But one concern was voiced, and forcefully. A guru got up to speak to the assembled transgender women. I was not at the camp but have heard sev-eral subsequent versions of what happened from multiple people at the 2012 meeting the director convened with me and, since then, from other people who were present. In summary, this guru told the hijras to leave; that they should not get the Aadhaar, and if they did, that they could not be buried in the *kabarstan* (graveyard).

Did hijras, then, stay or leave?

Many people stayed, I was told. But some left. What did the guru *mean*, I asked the group of Sambandh staff, transgender women, and gurus and

CBO leaders gathered at the meeting. The director said, "People are illiterate. These rumors often circulate." He proceeded to tell me about a host of other false rumors that he had heard over the years, such as how Sambandh was selling the blood of Indians it tested for HIV to America for a profit.

Another woman present, a guru herself, said that what was at stake "was the name." She asked the room: "What name will Aadhaar give you?" Elaborating for my benefit, she offered an example of a kinnar receiving her Aadhaar card. The guru contrasted this kinnar's names: a male name given soon after birth and a female name given upon entering the family of one's guru. This kinnar literally puts her *rit*, her custom, into the new family. The guru who was speaking and others present talked of their female names as "guru-given." But Aadhaar, the guru and others present worried, in its demand for a "unique" de-duplicated identity would only allow for a single name. And as access to Aadhaar was normally based on the possession of other forms of government identification, the sole name that Aadhaar would take would depend upon the name on one's existing identification.

This example was offered to me not to underscore a multiplicity in how one's several names differentially carry gender but in how these carry religion. The kinnar's birth name in the example the guru offered was that of a Hindu male. Her guru-given name was that of a Muslim female. The guru posed a question. If one's Aadhaar ID card showed a name not part of the family into which one had put one's rit—if it showed a Hindu name—could one be accepted in the kabarstan, the cemetery?

The kabarstan is here marked as a resonant feature of the moral world of Islam that becoming transgender may entail. As the anthropologist Gayatri Reddy notes, to place one's custom in a hijra family is frequently both to enter into an ethical relation to the Hindu goddess and to embrace the moral world of Islam, through conversion if one is Hindu or Christian.[19] Reddy is writing of the distinctive milieu of the city of Hyderabad. But the place of the figure of the kabarstan in what Kleinman would term the local moral world of hijras and kinnars resonates in Mumbai and elsewhere in South Asia.[20] Generally, the religious transitioning involved in putting one's rit with a guru may move in any direction: some of the guru-given names that emerged in conversation at Sambandh were signifiably Hindu. Burial also may have a Hindu context as kinnars and hijras make claims and derive authority as renunciates beyond the norms of the patriarchal family, Indeed, the recent repositioning of kinnars as essentially Hindu has involved a renewed claim on their religious authority as renunciates. But the Muslim figure of kabarstan marks the generic boundaries of an ethical life beyond specific trajectories of religious and gendered mobility, narratively and spatially fixing the burial that often concludes a hijra life.[21] Would Aadhaar, this new promised guarantee of some kind of life, disrupt that ending? Others present dismissed such concerns. Hijras, a gay man who was a researcher for an Avahan-funded project at Sambandh said, *often* change their names when they fight with gurus and place their custom with a different family. No one at the cemetery who had buried hijras before, he argued, would expect identification papers and familiar names to match.

In an elegant essay, the anthropologist Vaibhav Saria notes that, while hijras alter their names in placing their rit with a given guru—doing so repeatedly at times in the effort to create an *asli*, or authentic relation between a proper name and "the wishful construction of new identities"—the Indian state, in "its various schemes addressing poverty," is more likely to use their original male name in official identification.[22] The state's apparent reason for this has less to do with patriarchy than bureaucratic efficiency—that is, "the fact that hijras change their names." Furthermore, Saria notes, in serious criminal cases filed against hijras, such as for murder, the law is likely to include their male name as an alias. The alias not only renders criminality masculine; through the duplicate name, it also generates "a suspicion of *nakliness* [inauthenticity] that is confirmed by their criminality."[23]

Sarai's work is a powerful response to a question with which I have wrestled for many years: How can gender be made asli or nakli—that is, made real or rendered fake or duplicate?[24] What I found at the offices of Sambandh in 2012, less than a year after the camp, was that the hijras who left could not imagine a good death if they were encumbered with Aadhaar; people were developing ways, with varying rates of success, to alter the state's demand for their original male name as an unchanging reference.

At Sambandh, one kinnar guru shifted conversation away from cemeteries, to the evident relief of the director. She had, she told the room, no problem getting her Aadhaar in her female gender and guru-given name. "I travel all over India by train doing NGO work," she explained to me, "and I appreciate being treated with respect." Aadhaar affirmed who she was; it limited violence from officials and strangers; it gave her mobility. Another transgender woman, who worked as a researcher for Sambandh and was junior to the guru, looked surprised. She had tried to get the Aadhaar in her guru-given name, she said, but was required to show proof of residence and identity. All her "proof," she said, used her male name, and thus her Aadhaar has rendered her male.

While the younger kinnar was speaking the guru took out her Aadhaar to show it to me. The director encouraged the younger kinnar to do the same.

Usually in such conversations, no such hierarchical encouragement was needed: card after card would make its way onto the table as people discussed the tactics of proving themselves. "So what card did you use for proof?" the guru asked the younger kinnar. It turned out she had used a voter identification card, and this, too, was laid on the conference table. "You see," the guru offered to everyone in the room. "You need to use your PAN card." (The PAN, or permanent account number, card is an income-tax identification card.) "You see," she continued, "you can most easily get the PAN card with the name that you want. It is much harder to do that with the voter card."

At the opposite end of the slum colony in Varanasi in which Bageshera, Harinath Prasad, and their families lived was the main road through the neighborhood, and this road, in turn, led to a larger thoroughfare that went into Lanka crossing. Several women and men in the slum sold vegetables from carts at the crossing. Behind the carts was a row of shops. One of them was a tailor shop. I used to hang out there with Harinath Prasad's son, whose cousin (Bageshera's daughter) had introduced us by asking me for a name to call him by. We talked at length over the months and years, and he eventually found his way into several of my essays. As I reread them, I notice that I have given Harinath Prasad's son a different name in each. Here I retreat, uncomfortably, to how I knew him before we met. I write *son* and *he* because, in the end, these are the terms he asked me to use in the wake of other questions.

The tailor, Harinath Prasad's son told me, was his husband. The tailor was already married to someone else, and they had a son. Sometimes when the tailor was working inside or was with a customer, Harinath Prasad's son would sit on the stoop outside the shop and play with the little boy, and I would join them. "Who am I?" Harinath Prasad's son once asked the little boy. After a short pause—this game had been played before—the boy announced, "You are my uncle." "Nah," Harinath Prasad's son would chide the boy, in mock indignation. "Who am I?" he'd repeat, and the boy would repeat, "Uncle!" And this would continue. After some number of turns, the questioner appearing more vexed with each wrong answer, the little boy would capitulate. "Stepmother," he would say.

Another person in the Sambandh conference room listened as the guru detailed, in the card games one was invited by NGOs and the state to play, how to get the right name. "But you see," another person who had joined the group said, "I need my male name." She was referred to by one person there as a kothi and was dressed in men's clothes. She was involved in a court case with her brothers, she said, over family property. Though she was staying in Mumbai, her mother and her wife were living on the property. If Aadhaar reformed her legal person through the imposition of her female name, she worried, the new ID could damage the ongoing filing of papers needed to move the case along.

Over the subsequent minutes, other imperatives of living with cards asserted themselves. What emerged was a sense that the proper name, to be livable, demanded some duplication. The first speaker—the guru who, unlike others in the room, performed managing names and cards effortlessly—began to propose something like a system for which cards needed to be in which names. Discussion, and the sense of heightened stakes as Aadhaar as an instrument threatened to de-duplicate transgender life, intensified. The social work intern who had created the original camp with her husband and Sambandh's director appeared unsettled as more and more cards appeared—on the table and in the conversation—deferring the promising and well-managed future that was Aadhaar. She spoke loudly, interrupting the guru, the other women, and me. "This is not correct," she said. "You must understand that Aadhaar is not a card. It is only a number."

I presented a lecture on Aadhaar at Stanford University, at the northern end of Silicon Valley, in 2014. Stanford is an interesting site both because of the work of Jim Ferguson on how the emergent *techne* of distribution is remaking formerly productive oppositions of a critical theory and because of a new generation of anthropologists such as Ashveer Singh studying UIDAI as it is being implemented at the middle level of regional bureaucracy.[25] Universities have become critical sites of fieldwork for me, given the wide distribution of UIDAI's technocracy across a transnational reticulum of subcontracted information technology companies that establish links to universities looking to cultivate IT capital. Indeed, in my own role as an administrator of "South Asian studies" I was building donor relations with some of the same engineers that I was interested in interviewing, a particular and ever more familiar assemblage of felicity and complicity. A potential donor was in the Stanford audience. Nearby were the giant corporations. Some months before I spoke at Stanford, Facebook had begun an unpopular drive to de-duplicate its members that targeted names that appeared pseudonymous. Transgender and gender-nonbinary persons and collectives were among those who complained that such de-duplication hit at the ethical and ontogenic project of gender transition, in which the line of flight was tracked by a multiplicity of names in the database.

At the university, I laid out my question: What are the entailments and effects of de-duplication as a technocratic form, one remaking governance, securitization, welfare, and public health? An anthropologist present raised the dystopian specter of totalizing surveillance, her point echoing one of the most significant of Aadhaar's critics, legal scholar Usha Ramanathan, Ramanathan argues that as the Aadhaar program functions as a platform linking multiple data "silos" together, it enables the state and any others given access to the new database (or hacking into it) to have near-total knowledge of India's residents. Aadhaar's formal publicity has termed this linking of silos *data federation.*[26] Under a federated government of information, one's Aadhaar number might be linked to one's bank account, mobile phone account, and children's school, for example, but each of these entities would ostensibly have no access to the others through the Aadhaar platform. Ramanujan's concern was whether such federation is in fact what she and others alternatively term *data convergence*, a Big Brother total-information hybrid of state and corporation capable of new intensities of control.[27]

Behind UIDAI's push for federation is the presumption that a cause of the inefficiency or failure of the care of people at the social margin is the contemporary condition of the *silo*. Information is sequestered within silos, a proliferating set of vertically isolated entities. The future for Nilekani and his colleagues, as for surveillance capitalism more broadly, lies in "horizontalization." Aadhaar will not only return proof of identity (that you are you) to any agency that uses it to de-duplicate claimants on its services or goods, but it will also enable linkages across the different agencies that, in this political imaginary, constitute the very ground of a troublingly fragmented social.

A prominent example of the claims made for federation is the authority's promise that Aadhaar will improve India's record of tuberculosis (TB) control by treating each local clinic as a silo and linking them. The idea is not new: parallel to the development of Aadhaar has been an effort under the Revised National Tuberculosis Control Programme (RNTCP) to track TB patients digitally. But the RNTCP's branded digital scheme, Nikshay (No TB), did not have a compelling model for "scaling up." The entry of UIDAI, linking a person's access to medicine to their biometrics via Aadhaar and insuring that every time a person appeared for treatment they would proffer a fingertip to prove who they were, seemed to promise a solution to people illegible to a given clinic as someone with a history of often incomplete treatment. The idea was that every time a Resident—that is, someone whose biometrics have been captured—went to a TB clinic, he or she would constitute a *case* that, via Aadhaar de-duplication and federation, would link up to all other instances of his or her being a case, allowing a medical history to be gathered together and, ultimately, assembling a *patient*. Alone, unfederated, each of one's instances of treatment with a given practitioner was but a copy, a duplicate. To de-duplicate was to ensure that a patient did not carry—to cite again Sarai's apt phrasing—a "suspicion of *nakliness*." We can extend Roma Chatterji's figure of the file self, in which the medical file comes to stand in for the narrative and clinical continuity of the person with dementia.[28] We might speak of a *file body*—amid this hermeneutic of suspicion about whether a body on the social margin ever appears in clinic properly as itself—in which India's notable failure in TB control is comprehended as the need for authentic patienthood, to be achieved by assembling cases through a common biometric trace into a de-duplicated body. At a meeting with Nilekani, World Bank officials committed to scaling up as the critical managerial rationality for global public health appeared to ratify Aadhaar's approach as a potential way to achieve a medicine of patients at a massive scale.[29]

That one should approach such potential with circumspection—given, for example, Veena Das's current study of medical markets and the gap between knowledge and treatment—should go without saying. Das's long-term study of TB treatment in Delhi offers a precise analysis of the role of institutional neglect and what she terms *institutional incoherence* in such failures of care.[30] Most of the instances of neglect she identifies do not seem remediable by rendering individual treatment centers as silos and enacting these silos' federation.

The senior engineer (and potential donor) did not ask a question. But afterward he pulled me aside. The critical concerns of your questioners are not unfounded, he said. But one needs to understand that we wanted to design a form of identity for Indians that protected them from prejudice and vested interests. The effort was to fashion an identity that was unique in the sense that it referred to nothing but itself. "We did not," he said, "even want to have your name."[31]

In reality, he continued, they could not dispense with a name. Or an address. People needed to know they had been registered. As he narrated the chain of exigencies that piled back onto Aadhaar the varied indices of biography that the concept should have excluded, I was reminded of the tale recounted by Kirin Narayan of a *sadhu* (a holy man and renouncer) who possessed only a loincloth, the norms of decency preventing him from total renunciation. But even that iota of material possession was enough to duplicate itself treacherously: mice chewed at it when he was asleep, requiring a cat; the cat demanded other possessions to be cared for; and before you know it, the sadhu was a busy burgher encumbered by attachments to family and a large host of possessions.[32] One might term the concept of an identity without even a name as *ascetic* in its promise of a healthier social yet to come (the promised inclusion of the poor in a healthy, productive working class) radically outside of the social as it is—outside, that is, of any indices of relationship, community, history, or place. As the engineer noted, asceticism is hard to maintain, and names and forms proliferate.

I spoke to a colleague the other day, an anthropologist working on a different platform of national identification and inclusion: the Voter ID, or EPIC. She recalled a conversation with Nilekani at a soirée. The Voter ID is delivered as a card—paper or, increasingly, plastic—and like other forms of *proof*, as they are termed, it is kept as safely as precarious housing or workspace allows. In contrast to EPIC, Aadhaar was the subject of villagers' complaints: the ID card arrives as a long sheet of paper, they said, that is hard to maintain and keep safe. The anthropologist relayed this concern to Nilekani, who was then still the chairman of UIDAI. Nilekani offered a troubled look—academics tend to be critics—but answered patiently that there was a dotted line on the form that could be cut to make it the size of a card. He, of course, could have suggested that the question was misplaced; that Aadhaar is not a card, just a number. But increasingly, UIDAI had become caught between its original concept of an immaterial instrument not subject to duplication and the constant necessity to *show* the Aadhaar card to secure service, because biometric scanning—as critics had long warned—was often unfeasible. Even as some officials, such as the social worker at Sambandh, continued to stress that Aadhaar was "not a card," varied state administrations and private entities began to promise "plastic Aadhaar."[33] My colleague responded that people were reluctant to cut up a powerful document and that lamination often was not an option in villages. Nilekani's reported response was that people could simply keep the card in their wallets, and this colleague replied that most people did not have wallets.

This portrayal is of a familiar type: an encounter with an administration that seemed to be spectacularly uninformed about how people lived set against a critic making contrastive local claims. Yet this colleague's fieldwork led her to be more open than the critics to one key goal of Aadhaar: the shift toward the monetization and direct benefit transfer of welfare and away from distributions in kind. I am mindful of Kleinman's demand, as I have framed it here, of the necessity of interference in totalizing orientations to life on the margin. At this juncture, I find it as difficult to embrace Aadhaar in the hope that it will be at least as much of a rationalized ground for "making live," given the diminishing future of wage labor, as Ferguson is pressed to countenance in a very different South African milieu.[34] At the same time, though I have moved far closer to the critics than to the position say of the World Bank, I find it difficult to denounce Aadhaar as essentially a massive apparatus for the corporate extraction of wealth via the privatization of the state. Can one even write, therefore, about interference if one is uncertain as to the place of critique?

In this essay, I have attempted to open up to such a mode of interference. I have chosen to focus on the concept of the engineers as developed in something like good faith and yet as a mode of ascetic practice whose moral reason becomes undone as it enters the world. The possibility of a de-duplicated political subject *that has no name*, only randomness attached to the organic form of finger or eye to place it beyond biography and history as modes of participation that threaten duplication, may appear grandiose. But imaginaries of massive scale mark the ethical commitments of our time (and help explain the interest of the World Bank in Aadhaar). Here the effort has been to think with the way the name reattaches itself to this emergent assemblage of identification.

Naming is intensively at stake in the forms of life increasingly assembled by the scaling up of humanitarian audit and marked as transgender in India. The circulating word transgender, as with kinnar and other nominations, may at times and places offer a more respectful hailing of a gendered subject than do words such as hijra, which increasingly, if contextually, may index the memory and potential of abuse. Yet despite their "wishful" promise, names—as Saria's work engaging the ways by which hijras and others move among gurus shows—may not allow the putting aside of histories, punishing or otherwise.

At the meeting we held at Sambandh to discuss the events of the camp, it emerged that people, in living their lives, would encounter a multiplicity of institutional forms: the court, the bureaucratic office, the police station, the crowd of strangers on the train. Each of these encounters necessitated, in ways either direct or imagined, the giving of "proof" of oneself, whether to the bureaucrat, the court, or the stranger. Each of these encounters also carried a potential for violence or an opening to something else. What was clear at our meeting was that the kinds of person one must be are multiple, that one moves across such forms. Each of these encounters necessitated a different sort of proof: proof of being and inhabiting a gender and a biography appropriate to the specific potential and threat of the encounter. Proof gave one biography, gender, comportment, a name. Proof, to use the language of Jeanne Favret-Saada, "caught" one, rendered one as a given kind and history and body, and one needed to be caught in order to thrive or survive in the encounter.[35]

Yet one will need to be something else in relation to a different encounter. One must be able to duplicate oneself, to allow for a range of names to catch one as a given and fixed kind. But as the world and its institutional multiplicity gets remade within a commensurating logic of service in which the marginal subject of a distribution is always presumed to be a potential duplicate, a copy, or a counterfeit, the demand is for the scalability of proof and the possession of a single exclusive form of proof: unique. The work that proof must do in addressing the potential benefit or harm of distinct institutional encounters—what, after Anna Tsing, we might term proof's *nonscalability*—is rendered uncertain.[36]

The urgency of the future encounter with institutional form did not, for people at the 2012 meeting at Sambandh, allow for any easy submission to a de-duplicated name or gender, even as the dual scaling up—first, of urgent fact making by the Bill and Melinda Gates Foundation in the service of more inclusive AIDS prevention and care, and then of the proud fact of transgender inclusion held to by the intern and her corporate husband—appeared to necessitate a gendered solution as simple as putting a card in a wallet.

But if the meeting opened to anxiety about how a new foundation, Aadhaar, might force one to be caught by a singular form of oneself that is less livable than these allies intended, the event that preceded and shadowed the meeting—a guru's claim that Aadhaar would prevent the possibility and necessity of a good death *khabarstan mein* (in the cemetery)—is worth returning to. If one must accede to the power of scale, and the concerns of entities such as UIDAI, the Gates' foundation, and the World Bank mandate attention to scaled-up regimes of data (whether or not they can justly be framed as the foundation of a moral response to existing inequity or a violent refusal of nonscalable commitments), the fact assembled by Avahan of transgender death in the face of the comorbidities of AIDS, poverty, and transphobia makes an unexpected demand. Here, in the relayed claim of the guru, the demand is a claim over that death.

To die, and to die in an ethical manner, necessitates no less than going to court or riding on the train or negotiating an encounter with a bureaucrat—

that is, a being caught by the proof of oneself. We may debate the future of biometrics and the promises of scalability. We may side with the NGO that is trying to get access for marginal people to the one form of proof to rule them all, as we recognize that to be legible to a distribution is the ground of the biopolitics to come. We may side with the NGO that is trying to publicize how such a convergence of silos will create a condition of violent surveillance far more intolerable than the current one. But while we debate the virtues of convergent and scalable proof and the de-duplication of India, we attend, indirectly, to a guru's interference, exhorting one to leave the camp.

Harinath Prasad's son did not marry the tailor. School, marriage to a woman, a job happened. He disappeared from the slum.

Once he said to me: "If I am accepted into and join the university, then they will marry me to some girl. If not, I will stay here with the husband." His older brother had gone to college, was able to secure a government job in the state capital, Lucknow, and had gotten married. The younger brother told me that this trajectory was his aspiration, too. I wanted to ask whether something like that imagined life in Lucknow, away from his current husband, was a burden or a promise for my friend. But it seemed the wrong question somehow, and it seemed that my friend was constantly having to guide me away from wrong questions.

A few years earlier, as a younger teenager, he had been part of one of the *nautanki* (drama) troupes in the slum that performed comic skits for various lower and middle caste groups. The troupe hired women from the *mandi* (the red-light area) to dance at these performances. My friend was also a dancer, a "Boy" or *launda*. The laundas I worked with across the state border in Bihar dressed in saris and performed *launda nautch* (bawdy dancing) for men's bridal parties, labor that often included sex work with wedding guests.[37]

Harinath Prasad's younger son seldom referred to his earlier work for the nautanki troupe as a launda, save to say that several "uncles" in the slum had organized it. The one time I tried to bring up what was expected of him as a dancer and singer he deflected the question, and I was in that moment reminded of his schoolmaster father and his sense of propriety. I often thought of Harinath Prasad at such moments, and in this essay I have given my friend a name—one of many that he bore, in this case through his father. I have called him a son. Perhaps I did so because I worked with Harinath Prasad for a long time before I got to know his son; perhaps I did so because there is some form of filiation I cannot escape, particularly in an essay that would honor filiation—here, my own. Perhaps as I was introduced to my friend as the child who cooked and cared for his father, introduced with the words "What would you call him? In your place?" So instead of offering a proper name, I turn the question back.

We talked, over the years, my friend and I, not of dance or uncles but of his current husband and his maybe future wife. He would go to the university like his brother. However, there emerged some problem around his admission: he was not, he would sometimes say, like his brother. We started having these conversations about the future some months after that day at the tailor's shop playing with the little boy. Back on that day, a few minutes after the game of naming as stepmother, our conversation was interrupted. A policeman from the *thana*, the station across the road, came outside and looked toward us. He gestured slightly with his head, and my friend excused himself and went into the station. I knew the thana, or assumed I did, from accounts with the old people of the Nagwa Dalit slum I used to interview. They told me about being beaten as proxies for adult children accused of theft while doing domestic work at the wealthy homes that surrounded the slum. I tried to involve the boy in other name games but was not sure which name to use. About ten minutes later, Harinath Prasad's son emerged from the thana and returned to us. I was about to ask him what the policeman wanted, but his look silenced me. It seemed to me that something important depended on my not asking.

Sometime later, during a visit to my boyfriend and me at my rented room, Harinath Prasad's son was excluded from an inside joke (if my memory is correct). He began to sing a song from the Hindi film *Pehchan*: "Bas yehi apradh, main har bahar karta hun, aadmi hun aadmi se pyar karta hun" (Only this one fault, I commit every time; I am a man, and I love Man). It is a song in the theme of *insaniyat* (humanity), a word much bandied about, about a man whose only crime is that he loves other men, which, the song's context implies, refers less to homosexuality than to a dangerous humanism. Still, the double entendre was there. Or was it? I had learned not to ask.

Harinath Prasad's son did get into college. He did get married, and he left the slum. He lives near his brother in Lucknow. I have not seen him since his marriage. I recently got his phone number in Lucknow from a neighbor in the slum. He does not answer my calls.

I wrestle with how to think about *disappearance*. There is the disappearance of the guru and the hijras who followed her from the Aadhaar camp; from the sphere of influence of Sambandh's director; and, as it turned out, from being captured by this ethnography, save as secondhand news. There is the disappearance of the nonscalable from the world mandated by the concept of the engineers and the scaling-up imperatives of the World Bank. There is the disappearance of my friend from the slum and from his tailor and his stepson and from the police.

My motivation to attend to disappearance comes in part from the work of Chris Roebuck.[38] In addressing the lives of economically and racially marginalized transgender women in the Tenderloin district of San Francisco in the context of AIDS and its governance, Roebuck turns to Judith Butler's question of grievability, of the form of life that cannot be mourned.[39] Roebuck's work is an effort to use language to acknowledge a marginalized form of life as it acknowledges itself—as beautiful, as all too human, as entirely of its structurally violent conditions yet, profoundly, *beside* them.[40]

There is a counterpoint, in my reading of Roebuck's work, to the question of death as grievable in the figure of a disappearance. People *disappear* from the Tenderloin, from its spaces of recognition and sociality and care. They disappear due to death and from physical attacks; they disappear given the structural violence of United States immigration policy. They disappear in ways that cannot be accounted for. This is often the thing about disappearance. They may also *disappear into the future*. A familiar story circulates about those who escaped the Tenderloin for the suburbs, for a marriage to men of relative means who would care for them. Disappearance holds uncertainty. The future cannot be discounted, entirely.

What is it to claim a good death? How might grievability and the nonscalable be intertwined? One may attend to life under big data as promising, if you believe what the engineers do when they point out to the social scientists: *you and your social have failed*. One may attend to life under big data as monstrous, and examples of monstrous effects are legion. And one may ask: Why was it, at a given moment, that Aadhaar, amid the scaled-up fact of a community's mortality, seemed to trouble less the question of a good life (at stake for the activists on all sides of the Aadhaar question) than that of a good death?

The guru, despite the earnestness of the inclusionary form of Aadhaar, left the camp. I am left with little. There are debates among NGOs. There is a series of internet sites promising the secret, ritual truth of how hijras die. There are the many scholarly panels and conferences on Aadhaar and big data in which I participate. But I am no happier with my own, intermediate position than I am with the certainties on all sides that wall me in. Perhaps I have been instructed by a friend—what would you call him?—that interference may at times involve learning how to stop asking the wrong questions.

Notes

I am grateful to Veena Das and Arthur Kleinman for comments on the original version of this essay and to Anjali Arondekar and Thomas Blom Hansen for comments on its second airing; to Vivek Kumar for the generous gift of access enabling this research; to my former students Tara Gonsalves, Chris Hanssmann, Shakthi Nataraj, Eric Plemons, Chris Roebuck, and Gowri Vijayakumar and to Gayatri Reddy and Vaibhav Saria for their ongoing work on the biopolitics and necropolitics of transgender survival and grievability; and to Ashok Row Kavi and Ashveer Singh for conversations that jump-started this project. I am mindful of the long and ongoing history of gay men and others speaking for transgender people. Though my effort here is to do otherwise, the events I narrate with their focus on the good death come uncomfortably close to an all-too-familiar rendering of transgender as fatally abject. The University of California, Berkeley, where this essay was written, sits on the territory of *xučyun* (Huichin), the ancestral and unceded land of the Chochenyo-speaking Ohlone people, the successors of the sovereign Verona Band of Alameda County. I recognize that my work in this essay has benefitted from the use and occupation of this land.

1 | Cohen, "The Social De-duplicated."

2 | Cohen, "The Kothi Wars."

3 | I render conversations that rely on audiotape or on extensive notes written one to several hours later, or both, and place all such mediated speech, mine and by others, within quotation marks.

4 | Since the first version of this essay was written, kinnar has come for some upper-caste and high-profile Hindu transgender and gay activists to take on an additional if contested cultural valence, as an explicitly caste Hindu form of ethical life, one set against hijra as a presumptively Muslim form of ethical life. This emergent religious and communal differentiation is also coded in class terms, with kinnar marking middle-class aspiration and participation in the formal sector of capital and hijra marking the criminalized and informal social margin whether Muslim or low caste. See Bhattacharya, "The Transgender Nation and Its Margins"; Biswas, "The Iconography of Hindu(ized) Hijras; Dutta, Hossain, and Pamment, "Representing the Hijras of South Asia"; Upadyay, "Hindu Nation and Its Queers"; and on the social marginality, informality, and pleasures of a hijra form of life that kinnar may refuse, see Saria, *Hijras, Lovers, Brothers*. The NGO Sambandh has been a notable site where the Hinduization of transgender has been both enacted and contested.

5 | Kleinman, "Depression, Somatization and the 'New Cross-Cultural Psychiatry.'"

6 | Cohen, *No Aging in India*.

7 | Weston, "Lesbian/Gay Studies in the House of Anthropology."

8 | Wilkinson and Kleinman, *A Passion for Society*, 163.

9 | Kleinman, "Catastrophe and Caregiving," 23.

10 | Dalstrom, *Arthur Kleinman on Caregiving.*

11 | Shannon, "Prediction and Entropy of Printed English."

12 | Hegel and Knox, *Aesthetics, Volume 1*, 335.

13 | See Cohen, "The Kothi Wars."

14 | In framing hijra and kinnar structures of relatedness and hierarchy under the umbrella term of *jamaat*, one of several figures for both local and regional transgender association and governance, I follow the work of Shakthi Nataraj. Nataraj attends to the two collective forms at stake in the political and ethical lives of urban thirunangai (the respectful and preferred Tamil term among communities often referred to in national media and academic writing as hijras) in Chennai, the CBO or NGO on the one hand and the *jamaat* on the other, where *jamaat* comes to index the organization of lineage, ritual and sexual labor, and bodily transformation among thirunangai. Nataraj shows the dense and contested interplay of *jamaat* and NGO/CBO norms and forms in the agonisms and solidarities of everyday ethics. See Nataraj, "Trans-formations."

15 | I cannot overestimate the importance of Shakthi Nataraj's work in attending to when and how CBO or NGO versus *jamaat* distinctions come to matter. This essay is written in the wake of one's teachers; it is no less formed in the wake of one's students.

16 | Cohen, "Accusations of Illiteracy and the Medicine of the Organ," 125–26.

17 | Redfield, "Doctors, Borders, and Life in Crisis."

18 | Rajadhyaksha, *In the Wake of Aadhaar.*

19 | Reddy, *With Respect to Sex.*

20 | See Kleinman, "Local Worlds of Suffering" and "The Delegitimation and Relegitimation of Local Worlds," in which "the moral" becomes a critical problem-space to reframe disciplinary engagement with the local. The moral here is a significant departure from the cultural. In his teaching, Kleinman often spoke of the importance of attending to "what's at stake" for people (see Kleinman and Kleinman, "Suffering and Its Professional Transformation"), a formulation that he would develop further through the figure of the moral. The importance of the stakes and the moral as a theme over Kleinman's career belies the sufficiency (if not the utility) of critique of the *clinical* medical anthropology with which he was associated by the presumptively contrastive position of a *critical* medical anthropology. The moral was never, that is, merely the interpretive and normative force of a semiotic and apolitical rendering of culture or society, or a refusal of the ideological and phantasmatic structuring of experience. It is, however, a strong refusal of the reduction of experience to a statement of its ideological and phantasmatic conditions in Kleinman's return again and again to localized stakes. Its critical distinctiveness from the ethical as concept is that the moral is not only the iterative and necessary performance of the good, of healing and care, but the ground as well of harm and hurt. Herein, in this terrifying proxim-

ity of care and harm (and on this theme see Garcia, *The Pastoral* Clinic) lies the critical salience and pathos of a world with stakes. Kabarstan, in the moment around which this essay circles, anchors the material and performative ground of a good death but it also marks the often tight embrace of care and harm on the social and gendered margins (as powerfully rendered in Saria, *Hijras, Lovers, Brothers*). For a literary preoccupation with the density of kabarstan in hijra worlds, see Roy, *The Ministry of Utmost Happiness*.

21 | I would make no claim about the normative ritual of death among kinnar, hijra, and other transgender women in Mumbai. The point is that the interference at the camp was remembered as speech about a graveyard and access to it and that discussion of that speech some months later opened up to a more general set of questions about the alleged power of Aadhaar to fix the name. It might be fair to state that, when they die, people are variably cremated or buried, and that both the named religion of one's guru and intimates and the particular ties with one's natal (and often affinal) kin may matter in the kind of death one makes. There is something like an industry of disclosure in the face of the "secret" practice of hijras, including an imperative to speak of death (notably in Jaffrey, *The Invisibles*). After the 2012 meeting, I kept encountering variants of such disclosure in the form of internet blogs and soft journalism: see Maask, *Myths Surrounding Hijra Community*; Thakur, "A Eunuch's Journey"; Thorat, "17 Things You Didn't Know about Hijras." Each of these authors describes both Hindu and Muslim ceremonies as normative forms of death among hijras, though only one of them (Maask) is at pains to show that these forms of death are neither secret nor religiously non-normative. The others are invested in disclosing non-normative, esoteric forms. To trouble such investment, Maask here cites "Humaira, another hijra we interviewed," who notes, pointedly, "When there is only one Quran and only one way of burying the Muslims, why would we have a different burial? Our burial is similar to the burials of any male or female Muslim and it takes place in the morning, evening, anytime." The coordinates of such a death, as Humaira claims it, are inclusive within an Islamic moral world.

22 | Saria, "To Be Some Other Name."

23 | Saria, "To Be Some Other Name," 7.

24 | Cohen, "The Pleasures of Castration."

25 | Ferguson, *Give a Man a Fish*.

26 | See Cohen, "The Nation, De-duplicated" and Cohen "The Social De-duplicated."

27 | Ramanathan, "A Unique Identity Bill."

28 | Chatterji, "An Ethnography of Dementia."

29 | World Bank, "India's Massive I.D. Program Exemplifies 'Science of Delivery.'" The World Bank's enthusiastic commitment to the Aadhaar program has been troubled for the apparent misuse of financial data in making claims for the program, see Venkatanarayanan, "The Curious Case of the World Bank and Aadhaar Savings."

30 | Das, *Affliction*, 47–54.
31 | Cohen, "The Social De-duplicated."
32 | Narayan, *Storytellers, Saints, and Scoundrels.*
33 | Cohen, "The Nation, De-duplicated."
34 | Ferguson, *Give a Man a Fish*. "Making live or letting die," as opposed to "making die or letting live," is the classic conceptual distinction between biopower and sovereignty developed in Foucault, "The History of Sexuality."
35 | Favret-Saada, *Deadly Words.*
36 | Tsing, "On Nonscalability."
37 | Cohen, "Science, Politics, and Dancing Boys."
38 | Roebuck, "*Workin' It.*"
39 | Butler, *Frames of War.*
40 | See Stevenson, *Life beside Itself,* which elaborates this figure of beside.

Medical Cosmopolitanism in Moral Worlds

Aspirations and Stratifications in Global Quests for Conception

INFERTILITY, OR THE INABILITY TO CONCEIVE a desired child, is one of the world's most neglected reproductive health problems.[1] As many as 186 million people—both men and women—suffer from infertility worldwide.[2] However, most have no access to in vitro fertilization (IVF), the assisted reproductive technology (ART) that was designed to overcome infertility and that has been available in the Global North for more than forty years. Unfortunately, in a world still stratified by political, economic, and social inequalities, it is the countries of the Global South that have the least access to ARTs, even though they have the highest rates of infertility.[3] Even in the Global North, ARTs may be available, but they may remain inaccessible for the majority of infertile people due to the technologies' high costs and various legal barriers to access. As a result of these reproductive inequalities, couples in both the Global North and the Global South may look beyond their national borders for infertility care, engaging in transnational "quests for conception."[4] Indeed, such transnational quests are a growing global phenomenon, with thousands of infertile couples moving around the globe in attempts to "make a baby" and make parents of themselves in the process.[5]

Nearly thirty years ago—when ARTs were still relatively new to the world and twenty-first-century quests for conception had yet to be set in motion—Arthur Kleinman published an article that was perhaps one of the most influential in the history of medical anthropology. It was titled, "Local Worlds of Suffering: An Interpersonal Focus for Ethnographies of Illness Experience," and its message was repeated in his later books, including *Writing at the Margin: Discourse between Anthropology and Medicine* and *What Really Matters: Living a Moral Life amidst Uncertainty and Danger.*[6] In his initial essay, Kleinman urged medical anthropologists to attend to what he called *local worlds*—"recognizable as a particular form of life, a local way of being human."[7] Furthermore, Kleinman emphasized that these local worlds are *moral worlds*, "for what precedes, constitutes, expresses, and follows from our actions in interpersonal flows of experience are particular local patterns of recreating *what is most at stake* for us, what we most fear, what we most aspire to, what we are most threatened by, what we most desire to cross over to for safety, and what we jointly take to be the purpose, or the ultimate meaning, of our living and dying."[8]

In *What Really Matters*, Kleinman went on to adumbrate the importance of *aspiration* in local moral worlds. As he explained: "Living a life embraces positive and negative conditions, and indeed is a story of how they come together. Enlightenment about genuine reality should not demoralize us; it gives meaning to our small triumphs and daily pleasures. The fact that selves and worlds can be reworked in response to hazard and insecurity, and that they are worth remaking, in spite of their limits, is what makes aspiration so important."[9]

However, as a physician-anthropologist who had spent much of his research career in Asia, particularly in Taiwan and the People's Republic of China, Kleinman was also keenly aware of the ways in which human aspirations could be hampered and curtailed by "cultural, political, economic, institutional, and social relational sources and consequences."[10] Indeed, in much of his oeuvre, Kleinman focused on *social suffering*, or the ways in which lives can be radically altered by political dangers, economic uncertainties, social misfortunes, and the individual experience of illness.[11]

A signature of Kleinman's scholarship was thus his insistence on the importance of human *experience* within these local moral worlds. "Experience," he said, "should be seen as a flow, a medium moving between and within persons that is the condition for, as well as the achievement of, actions and transactions."[12] Kleinman urged medical anthropologists to describe the flow of interpersonal experience in local moral worlds to understand "the deep interiority of the experience of suffering."[13] To do so, Kleinman famously called on medical anthropologists to collect *illness narratives*—or a "view from up close in the words of the participants that captures the microcontext of experience."[14] However, Kleinman also emphasized the need for contextualization—"a view from afar that relates this highly focused perspective to the larger-scale political, socioeconomic, and cultural forces that impinge on the local world."[15]

In this chapter on twenty-first-century transnational quests for conception, I intend to demonstrate the ongoing conceptual force of these key themes from Kleinman's work. Transnational reproductive travel, or what I call *reprotravel*, is a world fueled by human aspiration—in this case, to make a coveted "test-tube baby."[16] But it is also deeply riven by global stratifications of nation and class. Although reprotravel is often characterized as either "North-North" or "North-South" in nature (e.g., Euro-Americans traveling to neighboring countries or to countries in South and Southeast Asia), in this chapter I show that reprotravel entails "South-South" movements as well, with couples of different economic strata and nation-states making valiant quests across continents and international borders in search of ARTs. In particular, I focus on quests for conception within Asia, the region of Kleinman's own ethnographic engagements. As I show, modern-day reprotravel connects China, India, and the Arab Gulf, a form of *inter-Asian* transnationalism that merges culturally and politically distinct nation-states in new circuits of reproductive mobility and transaction.

To demonstrate these inter-Asian connections, I include in this chapter two detailed *reprotravel stories*, in which infertile couples from South Asia—one Hindu, one Muslim—narrate their painful journeys to and from India and China to the emerging global city of Dubai, United Arab Emirates. There, I met infertile couples from around the world who had traveled to the UAE to receive care at a highly sought-after global IVF clinic.[17] Some of the reprotravel stories I collected there were from women alone; others were from men. But most were from infertile couples who spoke with me together in a rather uncommon form of *marital ethnography*. As with illness narratives more generally, these men and women shared the painful details of their infertility diagnoses and the social situations that eventually drove them to seek care across international borders. These reprotravel stories shed light on the ways in which economic stratifications and divergent religious sensibilities profoundly shape the trajectories and outcomes of infertile couples' reproductive quests. But more generally, they speak to the ongoing importance of local moral worlds within larger global trajectories and assemblages.

Indeed, toward the end of this chapter I place these stories in a global perspective by introducing a conceptual vocabulary with which to describe this twenty-first-century reprotravel phenomenon. The making of babies across international borders necessitates new ways of thinking about globalization and transnational mobility. Thus, I offer a *reprolexicon* to characterize global reprotravel in the twenty-first century.[18]

Reprotravel to Cosmopolitan Dubai

As an anthropologist of reproduction in the Middle East, my research on reprotravel began in Egypt, moved to Lebanon, and ended up taking me to the United Arab Emirates, where the city of Dubai has branded itself as a medical tourism destination.[19] Dubai itself is a border city—situated strategically between the Middle East and Asia. Given its location on the eastern side of the Arabian Peninsula, Dubai shares the Middle Eastern cultural dispositions of its Arab Gulf neighbors. However, Dubai is geographically located in western Asia and is connected across the Indian Ocean to South Asia. In demographic terms, Dubai is, in fact, South Asian: more than half of its residents hail from India, with many of them viewing Dubai as India's westernmost city.[20]

Dubai is also the Middle East's only global city.[21] To wit, of all the cities in the Middle East, Dubai is the only one to have cultivated a reputation as a high-tech, global hub for medical treatment and consumption. As a result, Dubai is now considered one of eight destinations for medical tourism within Asia.[22] Within the Middle East as a whole, Dubai is home to the region's only "medi-city." Called Dubai Healthcare City, this medi-city is registered as one of thirty-six tax-exempt "free zones" in the UAE, a list that also includes Dubai Silicon Oasis, Dubai Internet City, Dubai International Academic City, and Dubai Knowledge Park. Dubai Healthcare City—which was initially developed with input from a Harvard University team—is said to include more than one hundred and twenty medical facilities and more than four thousand health-care professionals.[23] Despite some setbacks associated with the economic downturn of 2008–2009, the medi-city has nonetheless become a destination point for medical travelers from around the world. It has also served to stanch the flow out of the region of wealthy Gulf Arab patients, who in prior years would have traveled abroad for medical treatment to places such as Bangkok.[24]

Given its growing reputation as a destination for high-tech medicine, Dubai is also emerging as a global *reprohub* to which infertile couples from at least five continents travel for assisted conception. The UAE in general, and Dubai more specifically, boasts a booming IVF sector. Thus, it was there, in 2007, that I carried out my ethnographic fieldwork at a busy global IVF clinic called Conceive, located strategically on the border of Dubai and its neighboring emirate of Sharjah.

For me as a medical anthropologist, Conceive provided an object lesson in globalization. Muslim patients from Pakistan met with Hindu physicians from India, were cared for by Catholic nurses from the Philippines, had their embryos handled by Greek Orthodox and Palestinian embryologists, and received follow-up care from East African and Arab clinicians, most of them Muslim. Conceive was the brainchild of Dr. Pankaj Shrivastav, the clinic's physician director, who was widely revered as the "father of IVF in the UAE" and whose patients referred to him as "Dr. Pankaj." Born in India and educated in the United Kingdom, Dr. Pankaj could be thought of as part of the generation of European-trained gynecologists who began taking the art of assisted conception to other countries around the globe.

Now nearly two decades old, Conceive is a stunning example of a cosmopolitan clinic. With more than twenty staff members hailing from the Middle East, Africa, South and Southeast Asia, and Western Europe, Conceive practices a kind of global gynecology, making infertile patients from abroad feel comfortable with its IVF services and its multicultural patient care, which is delivered in English, as well as in Arabic, Hindi, Urdu, Tagalog, and several other languages. In the Middle East as a whole, the practice of global gynecology in a cosmopolitan clinic is unusual, perhaps even unique. Most clinics and hospitals in other Arab countries (such as Egypt and Lebanon, where I have also worked) are staffed by local Arab physicians, who treat mostly Arab IVF patients. However, during the course of my research at Conceive I was able to track the comings and goings of a diverse group of nearly 220 reprotravelers from exactly fifty nations. Many of these reprotravelers were Arab, but most were not. Indeed, the vast majority of patients coming to Conceive were from Asia—primarily India and Pakistan, but also Southeast Asia, including the Philippines and Malaysia.

The explicit attempt by both patients and staff at Conceive to overcome multiple differences—to be open to, and tolerant of, medical care delivered across geographic, ethnic, linguistic, religious, political, economic, gender, and cultural boundaries—provides a case study of twenty-first-century medical cosmopolitanism, a feature of health-care delivery in a small, but growing, number of global hub cities, the majority of which are located in Asia.

What do I mean by *medical cosmopolitanism*? This term has two distinct but related meanings. First, it entails the concept of *cosmopolitan medicine*, a term introduced by the physician-anthropologist Frederick Dunn in the early medical anthropological volume *Asian Medical Systems: A Comparative Study*, edited by Charles Leslie.[25] Cosmopolitan medicine was meant to signify the production of Western-based biomedicine and its rapid global ascendancy. Dunn favored the term *cosmopolitan* for its associated meaning of "cosmopolitanism." As Dunn noted: "A dictionary definition of 'cosmopolitan' conveys the ideas of 'worldwide rather than limited or provincial in scope or bearing; involving persons in all or many parts of the world.'"[26] Dunn described cosmopolitan medicine as "global, largely urban," involving processes of professionalization and specialization among "secondary elites." He cautioned that cosmopolitan medicine might have a "profound impact" in non-Western settings, responding with biologically based solutions and technologies, such as IVF, when most global health problems were, at their root, political and economic in nature.

Over time, and under the influence of the theories of Michel Foucault, the term *cosmopolitan medicine* gave way to *biomedicine*, a reflection of the centrality of Foucauldian "biopolitics" in Western thought, as well as the increasing importance of the "bio" in the life sciences and biotechnology industries.[27] Today, the term *biomedicine* is used almost exclusively by scholars to signify Western biotechnologically based medicine. However, I would argue that Dunn's earlier notion of cosmopolitan medicine signals the "global" in a way that the Foucauldian term *biomedicine* does not. What concerned Dunn— much more than Foucault—was the globalization and eventual hegemony of Western medicine around the world, concerns that were truly prescient. Four decades later, Western-invented, high-tech, urban-based curative medicine— Dunn's definition of cosmopolitan medicine—has, in fact, spread far and wide, including to the Middle East and Asia.

As I would argue, the UAE—and particularly the city of Dubai—manifests the second distinct feature of medical cosmopolitanism that I want to emphasize. Namely, the UAE is the Middle East's most cosmopolitan nation, and international tourism is now the main engine of the country's economy, especially in the city of Dubai. The cosmopolitan nature of this tourist city undergirds the lure of Dubai for medical travelers, who can gain easy access to hotel accommodations and generally receive month-long visitors' visas, extendable for up to three months, before they are required to leave the country.

Given the well-developed tourist infrastructure and the relatively lax criteria for getting a visa, it is not surprising that Dubai is among the top ten most visited cities in the world, along with Bangkok, London, Paris, Singapore, and New York City.[28]

Travelers to this gleaming global city tend to be connected by a certain shared outlook on life—a cosmopolitan disposition—that leads them to a place such as Dubai. Indeed, in my study of reprotravelers from fifty nations, most were attracted to Dubai for its cosmopolitan reputation. In general, these reprotravelers were highly educated, transnationally sophisticated, dual-career couples who had traveled to Dubai for IVF care in a comfortable, cosmopolitan milieu. Thus, I came to think of these reprotraveling couples as *global mobiles* who were attracted to Dubai because of its reputation as a medically cosmopolitan reprohub.

Global Mobiles: Gandhali and Paavan

Such was the case with Indian couple Gandhali and Paavan, whom I met in Conceive's ultrasound scanning area. There they explained to me that they had traveled from China to overcome their infertility problem. Both twenty-eight years old and married for seven years, Gandhali and Paavan were a college-educated, highly successful Indian couple who had married for love—Gandhali moving from Mumbai after marriage to join Paavan and his family in Dubai's affluent Sindhi merchant community. After marriage, Gandhali, who had a bachelor's degree in communication studies, opened an advertising agency based in Dubai. Paavan, meanwhile, started a successful import-export business with China, and four years after their marriage, the couple decided to relocate to Guangzhou, the capital of Guangdong Province, to expand the business. In this respect, Gandhali and Paavan were representative of many of the young, dual-career Indian couples in my study. Highly educated and professionally ambitious with entrepreneurial aspirations, these middle- to upper-middle-class Indian couples were global mobiles, traveling frequently to take advantage of family ties, business connections, and entrepreneurial opportunities in the growing global hub cities across South, East, and Southeast Asia.

Gandhali and Paavan had homes in three Asian cities: their main residence in a foreigners' high-rise apartment complex in Guangzhou; an unoccupied house that they owned in Mumbai; and an apartment in Dubai where they had lived at the beginning of their marriage and where they stayed when they returned to Dubai for business, family visits, and, now, infertility treatments.

Their infertility had come as a great surprise. Assuming that they were young and fertile, and more interested in building businesses than a family, Gandhali and Paavan had used condoms for the first four years of marriage. But when they stopped using contraception, Gandhali did not become pregnant. Puzzled, the couple considered seeking a diagnosis at the American hospital in Guangzhou, a city of nearly fourteen million people. Although Gandhali believed that she might find a fertility specialist at that hospital, Paavan was highly skeptical about the general quality of medicine in China. In a vibrant couple's interview—filled with animated dialogue—they explained their treatment decision making in this way:

GANDHALI: We don't trust medicine there [in China].

PAAVAN: We've never heard bad things about it, but there is the language barrier.

GANDHALI: I got a cold, and my maid got a syringe. I don't want to take any medicine for a cold.

PAAVAN: And a lot of Chinese still rely on herbal medicines. Even urban, educated people still prefer traditional to Western medicine. Their mentality is completely different.

GANDHALI: So we decided that we needed to come here or go to India.

PAAVAN: The thing with India is, we've never lived in India—or, rather, I've never lived there, and I'm not very comfortable there. We have a house in Bombay, but we would have to get it cleaned and settled in before we could use it. I can't take fifteen to twenty days out in India. There's not good access to the internet as frequently, and I haven't really lived there.

GANDHALI: Just as important, here we have family. The clinic here does the same thing as in India, but there [it] is much cheaper. It's 10 percent of the cost.

PAAVAN: The quality of Indian clinics is very good, but it's not 10 percent.

GANDHALI: Here, it's 25,000 dirhams [$7,146] to do IVF. Over there, it's maximum 100,000 rupees [$1,385].

PAAVAN: So that's maybe 8,000 dirhams [$2,286], one-third of the cost.

GANDHALI: Plus, a few people we know got some treatment from Dr. Pankaj. One couple in our building here has twins from Dr. Pankaj. So that kind of motivated us to have trust.

MARCIA: They told you that their twins were from IVF?

PAAVAN: We don't know the full story. Indian couples with fertil-
            ity problems don't really discuss much. It's more like,
            "My mother found out from someone." It's through the
            grapevine.

Based on these perceptions of IVF in the three countries, Gandhali and
Paavan decided to travel from China to Conceive. At Conceive, Paavan undertook his first semen analysis and learned that his sperm count was lower
than one million (a count of fifteen million is diagnostic of male infertility).
Paavan, who was only twenty-six at the time, was devastated:

PAAVAN: They said our only option is ICSI [intracytoplasmic sperm
            injection, the variant of IVF used to overcome male infer-
            tility]. I was affected pretty badly by the news. . . . Really, it
            just hits you. Your confidence level goes down. I was very
            bad for maybe four to five months after that, feeling de-
            pressed. And in India, there's lots of alternative medicine
            there. My parents are kind of into that. So for maybe six
            to seven months, I was doing—I don't know exactly what
            I was taking: some tablets, some weird concoctions that
            came from India. But I went for a semen test again, and
            it was the same thing . . . ever since it's been the same. I've
            got sperm, but the numbers are really low, the motility is
            pretty low, and the sperm quality overall is D+.

MARCIA: But you know that ICSI was designed for these kinds of
            problems?

PAAVAN: Yes, ICSI—we've read a lot about it, as well, on the inter-
            net, and the doctors explained what happens with ICSI.
            But what really affected me is that if . . . ICSI wasn't there,
            there would have been no option for me. But then again,
            I've been thinking a lot recently. I'm not really a believer
            in God per se. But nature doesn't intend for me to be a
            father. So I don't know how right this is, morally speak-
            ing, to do ICSI. I feel like I'm doing this because of a lot of
            pressure from my family, my friends, and my wife. I would
            have preferred, left to my own decision, to adopt or maybe
            use a sperm donor. I've been told the possibility that if we
            have a boy with ICSI, the same problem will be carried into

him, as well. Actually, my right testicle is 50 percent of the normal size, and the doctor told me that this could happen to my son. And since ICSI is fairly new, I heard that there could be abnormalities in the child; ICSI is relatively new, so very little is known about that. So, you know, what concerns me is the whole question, philosophically, it's bothering me a little bit, that "nature doesn't want me to have [a child]."

Paavan was not the only man in my study who was worried about siring an "abnormal child" through ICSI. As Dr. Pankaj often warned patients with severe male-factor infertility problems, ICSI could, in fact, perpetuate genetically based male infertility problems into the next generation of male offspring. In some cases, Dr. Pankaj recommended to couples that they transfer only female embryos if they wanted to avoid such outcomes. Paavan found the ethical implications of passing on male infertility to any future son deeply troubling. Yet Gandhali's desire to become a mother outweighed her concerns:

GANDHALI: I don't actually believe this. I've heard nothing really about the health of children from ICSI. Frankly, all my friends are getting pregnant, one by one, except me. I just want to get pregnant. I want *his* child, so I don't want to use a sperm donor, even if it's available over here.

PAAVAN: I don't think it is, although we've never looked into it seriously.

GANDHALI: We'll do the ICSI, no matter what. Believe me, as soon as you get married, the pressure is on—immediately. My mom—

PAAVAN: Her parents, my parents.

GANDHALI: The uncles, the aunts.

PAAVAN: And nowadays, any relative we meet, any relative we meet after a long time, the first question is: "When are you going to get good news?" Anywhere we go, in China, in Dubai, in India. My friends who married in the last three to four years are very much after me, too. They're starting to get pregnant.

GANDHALI: Now I wish I would have done ICSI several years ago. We would have had a baby by now. The thing is, my friends are having kids before me, even if they got married after me. It's the "social eye" that looks at you.

PAAVAN: Every couple that becomes pregnant, there's that much more pressure on us. What especially bothered me is that my grandfather had never said anything. But in the last five to six months, even he's asked.

GANDHALI: In India where he lives, women are completely pressured.

PAAVAN: But even more so in the UAE, I think. It's worse here among our local friends [Emiratis]. It's the first question they've asked us from the time of our marriage. This is how it starts: "Are you married?" "Do you have kids?" "No! Why?" That's the way it is with locals, or any Arab for that matter. There is *so much stigma* attached to this. Even with my best friends, I *never* talk to them about this.

GANDHALI: You can't talk to anyone.

PAAVAN: I'm *very* close to my sister, and I never told her, and she just found out.

MARCIA: How?

PAAVAN: Through my mother.

GANDHALI [*turning to Marcia*]: No, *I* told his sister that. *I* told her.

PAAVAN [*surprised*]: You did? Why?

GANDHALI: Maybe I was depressed. I just told her. I don't know.

MARCIA: How did she respond?

PAAVAN: Actually, she was very pissed at me. She lives in the United States, and she was feeling cut off from the family. She wanted me to tell her this directly.

GANDHALI: But he didn't want me to tell anybody except "the moms."

MARCIA: Why just the moms?

GANDHALI: We are attached to our moms more than our fathers.

PAAVAN: I *should* tell my mother. She will want to know what's wrong. And she suggested coming here. It's the same with your mother.

GANDHALI: Since the first year, it's been, "Why haven't you had babies? Tests should be done." Every day, the whole year.

When we found out, I told her, and she was upset for a day or two. But then she began pushing us to start treatment, and we kept delaying it. -

PAAVAN: Initially, it was alternative medicines we tried. That was the initial thing. But afterward, we decided to give it a break. We took a vacation.

GANDHALI: And we settled in China.

Although relocating to China was like taking the lid off an infertility pressure cooker for Gandhali and Paavan, the move was also culturally jarring. The young couple felt "cut off from the cultural mainstream" in a country where *Newsweek*, *Time*, CNN, BBC, and Wikipedia were still blocked by the government. Unable to speak Chinese fluently, Gandhali and Paavan also found their ability to enjoy life in China quite limited. Gandhali admitted that she spent most of her time at Starbucks, which was conveniently located next to their apartment complex. "It's just coffee, massages, and eating," Gandhali complained. Most important from a fertility perspective, "overindulging" in various "vices" in China had caused her to gain weight—five to six kilograms (about twelve pounds)—which had triggered a new diagnosis of polycystic ovary syndrome (PCOS), a condition related to diabetes that leads to female infertility:

GANDHALI: Dr. Pankaj told me to reduce my weight the first time I came for treatment.... In China, I used to drink a lot. We all used to drink. And after that, my insulin was up pretty high. When I came back to start treatment, he put me on Metformin [a diabetes medication] and told me to come back after I lost five to six kilograms. There's a lot of eating and drinking there. I've stopped drinking completely, because it's not OK at all. Sindhis aren't supposed to drink. Our parents didn't know that I drink. And just the week before, I told his mother, when she asked me where we went, I told her, "We went out to a pub." "A pub! So, what—you all drink alcohol? You drink whiskey or what?" You see, you can't drink or smoke in front of Sindhi parents. There are very few who are open-minded about that.

PAAVAN: And they're vegetarians, our families. Even though Sindhis are not strict vegetarians, they hardly ever eat meat.

But you *can't* be a vegetarian in China. To be a vegetarian, I couldn't eat. They say in Cantonese: "Anything with a back facing the sun can be eaten."

GANDHALI: And he started smoking because of depression.

PAAVAN: That has to do with China.

GANDHALI: After every little bit, he runs out to smoke.

PAAVAN: That started with China, really. A lot of men smoke there. *A lot.* When you're conducting business, you almost feel to get closer and to make a deal you *must* smoke and drink. In the office, it's mostly smoking. But in lots of cases, you go to a function and the boss comes with cigarettes packaged as a gift, and it's rude to say no. I used to smoke in college, but I was able to stop pretty quickly, so I can cut down any time.

GANDHALI: Knowing the treatment, you shouldn't be smoking! I can't take smoking. I hate the smell.

Given that smoking can negatively affect ICSI outcomes, Gandhali was probably right to admonish Paavan about his smoking. I, too, told the couple that smoking is generally bad for male reproductive health. I asked Gandhali and Paavan if they planned to return to "smoky China" at the completion of their ICSI cycle:

GANDHALI: As soon as I get pregnant.

PAAVAN: I'm going back next week.

GANDHALI: Thanks for telling me. I didn't know that.

PAAVAN: I have to go back. I have work waiting for me there.

Despite the couple's bickering, it was clear that Gandhali and Paavan loved each other very much and viewed their childlessness as a shared struggle. Because they were such a loquacious and forthcoming young couple, I decided to ask them at the end of the interview: "How's your marriage holding up?" Gandhali answered for both of them: "Now, since the treatment started, he's been more depressed. He's been a little aloof because of the treatment. And because of the [hormonal] medicine, I'm getting a little finicky, picking some fights without reason. In the first few days, I was crying all day. But every time we travel for treatment, we're getting closer. We're young, and it's like we're growing up together."

Poor Migrants: Fatima and Mahmoud

Cosmopolitan elites, such as Gandhali and Paavan, were not the only repro-travelers finding their way to Conceive. Very poor infertile couples consti-tuted about 5–10 percent of the clinic's patient population. Most of these poor couples had come to the UAE as migrants from India, Pakistan, and the Philippines. At Conceive, I met some of these impoverished migrant couples who were hoping to make a test-tube baby. Their presence was in-dicative of three oft-ignored global realities. First, poor people want children just as much as elites do. Second, poor infertile couples may have enduring, committed relationships in the face of intractable infertility problems. And third, poor couples may be willing to go to extraordinary measures to ac-cess IVF, engaging in catastrophic expenditure and risking destitution in the process.

Fatima and Mahmoud, who hailed from Kerala, India, were one such couple. As soon as I met them, I realized that they were religiously pious Mus-lims: Mahmoud wore an Islamic skullcap over his balding scalp and sported a calloused prayer spot on his forehead above his sparkling green eyes; Fatima was dressed completely in black, covering herself with an *abaya* (a long black women's cloak) and facial veil so that only her eyes—behind heavy glasses—could be seen. The couple was very poor. Mahmoud made only 3,000 dirhams a month (about $857) as an office clerical assistant, with half of his salary going to rent their small apartment in Abu Dhabi, where they had lived for six of their eight years of marriage.

Fatima had spent most of the previous six years in that apartment, ventur-ing out primarily for doctor's appointments. Unfortunately, she suffered from a painful condition called endometriosis, caused by the excess proliferation and sloughing of endometrial tissue into the pelvic cavity. Fatima needed laparoscopic surgery to remove the excess tissue and relieve the unremitting pelvic pain, so she traveled with Mahmoud during his one-month annual leave back to Kerala, where they were hoping to obtain the surgery for one-fifth of what it would cost them in the Emirates. However, once in India Fatima's case was determined to be severe. Her surgeon ended up removing Fatima's right fallopian tube and ovary.

Demoralized by the outcome, Fatima returned with Mahmoud to Abu Dhabi, where they were referred by a kindly female gynecologist to a govern-ment IVF clinic in Al Ain, a remote desert city in the Emirates. There they were overjoyed to hear that IVF would be completely free to them. They ac-cepted their place on the one- to two-year waiting list, believing that they were being tested by God for their faith and persistence. A full two years passed before an appointment was finally made. By this time, however, the Emirati government had changed its IVF public financing scheme to reserve state-subsidized IVF for Emirati citizens. This news came as a great blow to Fatima and Mahmoud. As Mahmoud lamented, "You know, we waited for two years like that—*two whole years*—before they started calling us for the initial checkups. But now, they tell us, you have to pay the full cost if you're an expat. That would be around 12,000 dirhams for IVF, excluding the medicine, or 20,000 dirhams [$5,717] altogether."

Feeling priced out of the high-end private IVF sector in the Emirates, Mahmoud and Fatima traveled back to India on Mahmoud's next annual leave, checking on a "well-known" hospital in Karnataka. There they were told that IVF was still in the "planning stages" and that they would have to wait another one to two years before a clinic would be opened. Fatima, meanwhile, was diagnosed with a cyst on her remaining ovary. The cyst had to be removed with a second laparoscopic surgery, and Fatima was instructed to return in another year once an IVF clinic had been established in Karnataka.

When they returned to Abu Dhabi, Fatima became pregnant, but the pregnancy turned out to be an emergency ectopic (tubal) pregnancy, which was removed by medication. The same cycle—returning to India, being told that they had to wait for an IVF clinic to be opened, undergoing laparoscopic cyst removal, then becoming pregnant with an emergency ectopic—happened once again, although this time in their home state of Kerala. "After that, I was *so* depressed," Mahmoud explained, for he had come to realize that India's purported IVF clinic boom had not at the time reached the southern states, which he, Fatima, and the majority of Indians living in the Emirates considered their real home.

After returning to the UAE from Kerala, Mahmoud and Fatima learned about Conceive, with its Indian clinical director. As pious Muslims, Fatima and Mahmoud would have preferred a female Muslim physician. But they decided that the "quality of a doctor"—not the doctor's nationality, gender, or religion—were what really mattered to them in making a test-tube baby. Furthermore, once they met Dr. Pankaj, they were pleased with his demeanor and clinical competence. In fact, Dr. Pankaj was the first physician to diagnose Fatima's PCOS and insulin resistance (the same infertility-related conditions suffered by Paavan), which needed to be treated before she could safely embark on a cycle of IVF. Dr. Pankaj also determined that Mahmoud's sperm profile had been deteriorating over time, a finding that Mahmoud himself attributed to "all of the tension."

When I met Fatima and Mahmoud at the clinic, they had just undertaken their first IVF cycle, and they laughed while telling me that it had taken them five full years to finally access this reproductive technology. Luckily for them, Fatima became pregnant on the first IVF cycle, which they attributed to the "great job" being done by Dr. Pankaj and his clinical staff. Nonetheless, as Indian Muslims they did not plan to tell anyone about undertaking IVF at Conceive with a Hindu physician. As Mahmoud explained, "IVF is not accepted in our community. Actually, some people believe that what we're doing is against God's wishes. We don't believe this, but some people do. They don't agree with IVF." Mahmoud also stressed the need for absolute secrecy to prevent "family interference." Nonetheless, he had been forced to borrow money from his relatives, telling them only that Fatima was "receiving treatment." He explained:

> For six years, I've been spending all my money on this. I don't have anything left. I've spent *a lot* of money over five to six years. So I took [out] a loan from my father and his relatives. They're helping, but I'll pay them back. It is my wish to pay for this from my own pocket. But it is *very* difficult to save for this. I brought her here only for this—to have a baby—nothing else. And a loan was necessary for that. And I've traveled a lot for this—two countries, two emirates!

Now $6,000 in debt to family members—an amount that would take them years to pay back—Mahmoud and Fatima were nonetheless ecstatic. Returning from the first ultrasound scan of her pregnancy, Fatima had the final word, which truly summarized their shared sentiments. "We were coming here from Abu Dhabi *very tense*," she said. "But we reached here, and we became *very happy*."

A Reprolexicon

In these reprotravel stories of two Indian couples—who literally crossed Asia in search of assisted conception—we can open a window into local moral worlds. As we have seen, these moral worlds are replete with powerful reproductive aspirations amid intense physical pain and emotional suffering. They invoke not only profound religious uncertainties, but also an implicit faith in the power of biomedicine to solve problems of both a human and physical nature. These moral worlds are saturated with social stigma and the resulting loss of privacy and personhood, but the social consequences are eased by the edifying effects of love, care, and conjugal support. We see, too, how families may rally when loved ones are sick, but how economic disparities may temper these forms of family aid and charity. Finally, these reprotravel stories reveal the widespread cultural chasms in the delivery of health care from one nation to another and how reprotravel to distant destinations may thus represent a logical form of therapeutic reprieve.

To understand these moral complexities and vital logistics, it is necessary to frame these issues conceptually in a way that widens the discussion from "the local to the global."[29] To do so, I offer here a reprolexicon: five key tropes that help to characterize the phenomenon of reprotravel on a global scale.[30] Some of this reprolexicon is unabashedly derivative, inspired by the work of globalization theorists within anthropology. However, other terms are original, designed to capture the dynamics, directionality, subjectivities, and affect associated with twenty-first-century reprotravel. I begin at the meta-level and end at the micro-level of human experience, where the animating force of reprotravelers' stories gives life to this conceptual vocabulary.

GLOBAL REPRODUCTIVE ASSEMBLAGE

In their well-known collection *Global Assemblages: Technology, Politics, and Ethics as Anthropological Problems*, Aihwa Ong and Stephen Collier build on Foucault's and Gilles Deleuze's analysis of "assemblage" to propose the concept of the "global assemblage," or a "contingent ensemble of diverse practices and things that is divided along the axes of territoriality and deterritorialization."[31] The range of phenomena that best reveal such global assemblages are, according to Ong and Collier, "technoscience, circuits of licit and illicit exchange, systems of administration or governance, and regimes of ethics or values."[32]

Twenty-first-century reprotravel could be conceived of, quite readily, as a *global reproductive assemblage*. This global reproductive assemblage involves the global diffusion of IVF and its underlying technoscience; international circuits of traveling people and, increasingly, their body parts; systems of administration that involve the medical and tourism industries; increasing regulatory governance on the part of both nations and professional bodies; and growing ethical concerns about various forms of licit and illicit exchange, including unprecedented evasion of the law across national and international borders. Indeed, as a kind of metaconcept, the global reproductive assemblage brings together these many diverse elements operating on a global scale, which make IVF and its associated mobilities a distinct form of global travel in the twenty-first century.

Before the concept of global assemblages was introduced into academic discourse, the anthropologist Arjun Appadurai had already put forth his influential notion of "scapes."[33] In the mid-1990s, he outlined a "global cultural economy" in which global movements operate through five pathways. According to Appadurai, globalization is characterized by the movement of ethnoscapes (or people), technoscapes (or technology), financescapes (or capital), mediascapes (or images), and ideoscapes (or ideas and ideologies), which now follow increasingly complex trajectories, moving at different speeds across the globe.

Using Appadurai's language of scapes, I would argue that global reprotravel involves a *reproscape*—a kind of metascape that combines numerous dimensions of globalization and global flows. This reproscape entails a discernible geography traversed by global flows of reproductive actors, technologies, body parts, money, and reproductive imaginaries. In spatial terms, these global flows are also moving in particular directions, which may become quite regularized over time. For example, egg donors and recipients now head to Spain and Eastern Europe, while those who need donor sperm rely on Denmark and California.

The Middle Eastern reproscape also entails a distinct geography traversed by global flows of reproductive actors, technologies, and their body parts. For example, Dubai is at the center of a reproscape in which couples are heading into the UAE from Western Europe, South Asia, East and West Africa, and other parts of the Middle East. This reproscape is both spatial and dynamic, involving geography and movement. Whereas the global reproductive assemblage entails a coming together of diverse IVF elements, the notion of a reproscape is more dynamic, entailing movements of many kinds.

However, these movements are not unfettered. The adjective *stratified* might be added to the term *reproscape* to describe the inequalities, disjunctures, and obstacles that inhibit and even prevent flows of people, technology, and other forms across uneven global terrains. To take but one example, elites from the Horn of Africa may come to Dubai to undergo a single cycle of IVF. But the vast majority of infertile sub-Saharan African couples, from places such as Somalia and Djibouti, will never take part in such reproflows to Dubai.[34] In other words, the stratified reproscape in which reprotravel takes place is an uneven terrain, since some individuals, some communities, and some nations have achieved greater access to the fruits of reproductive globalization than others.

Furthermore, this reproscape is highly gendered, a feature of globalization that was not the focus of Appadurai's original work on global scapes. For example, reproductive technologies such as IVF are enacted on women's and men's bodies in highly differentiated ways. Furthermore, the global reproscape entails new forms of gendered reproductive labor among reproductive "assistants," most of whom are women, who undergo risky forms of hormonal stimulation, egg harvesting, pregnancy, and labor. These variable measures of reproductive value are clear indicators of the stratified reproscape in which some reproductive bodies are valued more than others.[35]

REPROFLOWS

The concept of *reproflows* brings these bodies and body parts back into the discussion of IVF as a global form. If a reproscape entails the geography and directionality of reproductive movements in space and time, then within each reproscape there are specific types of flows that are entirely unique to the world of IVF. On one level, reproflows involve the movement of many kinds of human actors. These include the IVF scientists, physicians, embryologists, and other kinds of IVF technicians who travel to and from sites of training, international conferences, and medical trade shows and to the countries and clinics where they provide their services. Among these reproductive actors are embryo couriers, who cross international borders carrying their precious cargos in carefully sealed cryopreservation tanks. Reproflows also involve the thousands upon thousands—perhaps millions—of men and women now flowing across national and international borders in their search for IVF technologies and related forms of reproductive assistance. Reproflows also include the reproductive assistants, including traveling gamete donors and surrogates, who may be flown across international borders in increasingly regularized circuits of reproductive exchange.

On another level, reproflows also engage nonhuman actors, which are crucial elements in the global reproscape. Reproflows involve the movement of IVF technologies from the sites where they were developed (e.g., England in the case of IVF) to many other countries around the world, flows that are made possible through processes of manufacture (in countries such as the United States and Italy) and global dispersion via medical trade shows and pharmaceutical representatives. Reproflows also involve many kinds of reproductive entities and substances, including the embryos passed from country to country through the work of embryo couriers; the frozen sperm samples, ready for use in donor insemination, that are posted through various international delivery services; and the reproductive hormones, or the costly medications used to stimulate women's ovaries into oocyte hyperproduction.

Finally, in the domain of reproductive physiology, reproflows speak to the quintessentially fluid nature of men's and women's bodies and to the biological movements of conception that take place every minute in IVF clinics and laboratories around the world. For example, reproflows entail the flow of semen into plastic cups in IVF clinic bathrooms, as men are asked to masturbate themselves to ejaculation or to be masturbated by their wives. Reproflows include the flow of oocytes suctioned from women's ovaries and flushed from pipettes into waiting petri dishes in IVF laboratories, where they are handled and inspected by embryologists. And reproflows involve the flow of menstrual blood when conception is not achieved during a failed IVF cycle.

REPRODUCTIVE CONSTRAINTS

Biologically based *reproductive constraints* of many kinds continue to plague the embodied world of IVF—making IVF fail more often than not, thus seriously demoralizing those who have traveled to use it. In the world of assisted reproduction, bodily flows are often blocked, hindered, or rendered inert. For example, reproductive hormones are injected without stimulating the maturation of eggs. Semen is ejaculated without yielding viable spermatozoa. Eggs are fertilized with sperm but do not become human embryos. Embryos are transferred into wombs but are not implanted in uterine walls. Pregnancy tests are positive but lead to negative outcomes, such as stillbirths and miscarriages.

Biological obstacles are not the only deterrent to IVF successes. Indeed, there are numerous other arenas of constraint—structural, sociocultural, ideological, and practical obstacles and apprehensions—that may deter IVF seekers from accessing assisted reproductive technologies within their home countries.[36] On a global level, the two most fundamental arenas of constraint are probably economic and legal. That is, IVF seekers may not be able to afford these services in their home countries, given the global average of $3,500 for a single IVF cycle (the cost ranges from $1,200 per cycle in Iran and Pakistan to $12,500 per cycle in the United States).[37] Furthermore, IVF seekers may be barred from accessing IVF in their home countries by various legal prohibitions, which are most prominent in parts of Western Europe.[38] However, it is important to emphasize that economics and law are not the only arenas of reproductive constraint. Instead, a complex set of factors militates against access to IVF, thus setting in motion reprotravel across national and international borders.

These arenas of reproductive constraint can be grouped into four broad categories: (1) resource considerations, including the high costs of IVF, lack of expertise and equipment, resource shortages, and waiting lists either for IVF itself or for donor gametes; (2) legal and religious prohibitions, including religious bans, national laws, and the denial of treatment to certain categories of people; (3) quality and safety concerns, involving poor-quality care, unsafe practices, and low success rates; and (4) sociocultural issues, revolving around medical confidentiality, cultural and linguistic barriers, and lack of supportive services. In general, reprotravelers often say that they are "forced" to travel from home countries to access IVF services that are safe, effective, legal, and affordable.

REPROTRAVEL STORIES

Finally, as a medical anthropologist of reproduction, I have thought a great deal about infertile couples such as Gandhali and Paavan and Fatima and Mahmoud, who have traveled great distances, often at considerable expense to their bodies and their wallets, to conceive a longed-for child. It is these aspirations for parenthood—or the yearning to become parents of children who are wanted, needed, and cherished—that undergird the global movements of all reprotravelers. Such aspirations for parenthood and desires to bear children are found among both men and women in a world in which nearly 95 percent of all adults still express the desire to have children at some point in their reproductive lives.[39]

For reprotravelers such as Gandhali and Paavan and Fatima and Mahmoud, in their global quests for conception in places such as Dubai, it is the search for new life—a child, who can make a woman into a mother and a man into a father—that is most at stake in local moral worlds. Although we may critique the globalization of IVF on many levels—as a neoliberal, capitalist global reproductive assemblage; as a stratified reproscape of global inequalities; as an exploitative, gendered form of reproductive labor; and as a high-end reproductive technology that is often ineffective, as well as physically taxing—ethnographic encounters with the infertile render visible both the pain and the desire found in human aspirations for parenthood. For Indian couples such as Gandhali and Paavan and Fatima and Mahmoud—but also for most infertile couples, from many parts of the world—reprotravel is undertaken for two important reasons: first, because infertility is a profound source of human suffering, leading to local moral worlds replete with desperation and despair; and second, because IVF is often the only way to overcome this suffering, thereby leading to the great joy that only an IVF baby can bring.

In the end, then, as a medical anthropologist deeply inspired by Arthur Kleinman's call to document both the suffering and aspiration in people's local moral worlds, I want to emphasize how reproductive aspirations comprise a vital part of human experience; how infertility can thus be understood as a profound form of human suffering; how desires to overcome this suffering are at the core of infertile couples' quests for conception; and how the births of beloved test-tube babies constitute the ultimate joy of couples' tortuous IVF quests. In the twenty-first century, reprotravel across national and international borders can thus be seen as an understandable and legitimate response to infertility, the magnitude of which cannot be underestimated—in Asia and beyond.

Notes

I thank Arthur Kleinman for his ongoing intellectual inspiration and caring support as a colleague and mentor. I also thank João Biehl and Vincanne Adams for their fine editorship of this volume and Ken Wissoker of Duke University Press for publishing so many important volumes in medical anthropology. This chapter is adapted from *Cosmopolitan Conceptions:* IVF *Sojourns in Global Dubai* (Duke University Press, 2015), based on a study I undertook in 2007 in the UAE. I thank all of those at Conceive who made the study possible, especially Dr. Pankaj Shrivastav and the many reprotravelers who sought his exceptional care. The study was generously supported by the US Department of Education's Fulbright-Hays Faculty Research Abroad Program and the Cultural Anthropology Program of the US National Science Foundation.

1 | Inhorn and Patrizio, "Infertility around the Globe."
2 | Rutstein and Shah, *Infecundity, Infertility, and Childlessness in Developing Countries.*
3 | Inhorn and Patrizio, "Infertility around the Globe."
4 | Inhorn, *Quest for Conception.*
5 | Inhorn, *Cosmopolitan Conceptions*; Thompson, *Making Parents.*
6 | Kleinman, "Local Worlds of Suffering"; Kleinman, *What Really Matters*; Kleinman, *Writing at the Margin.*
7 | Kleinman, "Local Worlds of Suffering," 129.
8 | Kleinman, "Local Worlds of Suffering," 129.
9 | Kleinman, *What Really Matters*, 14.
10 | Kleinman, "Local Worlds of Suffering," 128. See also Kleinman, *Patients and Healers in the Context of Culture*; Kleinman and Kleinman, "The Transformation of Everyday Social Experience"; Kleinman et al., *Deep China.*

11 | Kleinman, *What Really Matters.*

12 | Kleinman, "Local Worlds of Suffering," 128.

13 | Kleinman, "Local Worlds of Suffering," 129.

14 | Kleinman, "Local Worlds of Suffering," 131. See also Kleinman, *The Illness Narratives.*

15 | Kleinman, "Local Worlds of Suffering," 131.

16 | Inhorn, *Cosmopolitan Conceptions.*

17 | Inhorn, *Cosmopolitan Conceptions.*

18 | A fuller version of this reprolexicon, along with twenty-three additional reprotravel stories, are in Inhorn, *Cosmopolitan Conceptions.*

19 | Inhorn, *Cosmopolitan Conceptions*; Inhorn, *Local Babies, Global Science*; Inhorn, *The New Arab Man*; Inhorn, *Quest for Conception.*

20 | Vora, *Impossible Citizens.*

21 | Sassen, *The Global City.*

22 | Horowitz and Rosensweig, "Medical Tourism."

23 | Ismail, "Dubai Healthcare City to Compete for Foreign Patients."

24 | Whittaker, "'Outsourced' Patients and Their Companions."

25 | Dunn, "Traditional Asian Medicine and Cosmopolitan Medicine as Adaptive Systems"; Leslie, *Asian Medical Systems.*

26 | Dunn, "Traditional Asian Medicine and Cosmopolitan Medicine as Adaptive Systems," 135.

27 | Clarke et al., *Biomedicalization*; Foucault, *The Birth of the Clinic.*

28 | As reported in Morton, "The Ten Most Popular Cities of 2019."

29 | Inhorn, *Local Babies, Global Science.*

30 | Inhorn, *Cosmopolitan Conceptions.*

31 | Deleuze, *Foucault*; Ong and Collier, *Global Assemblages*, 338.

32 | Ong and Collier, *Global Assemblages*, 4.

33 | Appadurai, *Modernity at Large.*

34 | Inhorn and Patrizio, "Infertility around the Globe."

35 | Colen, "Like a Mother to Them."

36 | Inhorn, *Local Babies, Global Science.*

37 | Chambers, "The Economic Impact of Assisted Reproductive Technology"; Collins, "An International Survey of the Health Economics of IVF and ICSI."

38 | Pennings, "International Evolution of Legislation and Guidelines in Medically Assisted Reproduction."

39 | Boivin, "International Estimates of Infertility Prevalence and Treatment-Seeking."

Environments and Mutable Selves

THE IDEA OF "SELF" IS SELF-EVIDENT, or so it seems. Of course, we worry at times that we are not true to our self, or that self is out of sorts, but for the most part we assume that self subsists quietly in our subconscious. This essay highlights varying conceptualizations of self in time and space and shows how, as supposed processes of embodiment are revised and interpreted in light of current scientific findings, the material self that is emerging is proving to be a moveable, shifting, context-dependent entity.

Environments and Mutable Selves opens by briefly summarizing key themes in the work of the anthropologists Marcel Mauss and Franz Boas that presage a displacement of the autonomous self. A discussion then follows of the Japanese concept of *jibun*, glossed in English as "self." Jibun has been extensively debated and written about for more than 150 years by scholars both inside and outside Japan. This concept is explicitly located at the nexus of shifting social relationships; hence, self and the social are by definition interactive and not readily separable entities. However, for well over a century the idea of an autonomous self has been present in Japan as a self-consciously imported entity put to strategic use at times in business, politics, the writing of literature, and daily life. Explication of jibun in this essay serves to decenter a persistent assumption that the autonomous Euro/American self is the norm for modernity everywhere. Many readers will already be acquainted with the anthropological literature produced over the past fifty years about concepts and practices associated with self and emotions the world over.[1] This research uniformly stimulates reflexive examination of the autonomous, decontextualized self as a historically and culturally constructed, ideologically grounded entity, and the Japanese example set out later is just one illustrative example among many possible alternatives that causes us to do so.

Findings from the bourgeoning world of behavioral epigenetics are then introduced. The discipline of epigenetics, first consolidated more than half a century ago, has been renewed over the past two decades as a lively molecularized science, to which the concept of environment is central. Epigenetics can be glossed as "over or above genetics." More specifically, it refers to heritable changes in gene expression that do not involve changes to underlying DNA sequences, and practitioners in this rapidly expanding field explicitly claim that they have uncovered molecular links between "nature" and "nurture."

This research makes clear that molecular pathways active throughout life result in an inextricable entanglement of environment and body/mind. Contemporary molecular biology suggests, then, that self is not sealed off or embodied in mind; nor is it produced solely by means of language and moral exchanges. Self is an elusive, unstable entity. Iterations of context-dependent selves is a useful way to think about this concept.

People and Environments

When Mauss discusses the idea of self—of *moi*—and its relationship to person, he notes: "Each one of us finds it natural, clearly determined in the depths of consciousness, completely furnished with fundaments of the morality that flows from it."[2] Mauss demands a historical consideration of self but also undertakes a comparative examination of this concept. With reference to published materials on the Zuni and other Pueblos more generally—to the Haida and Kwakiutl of the Canadian northwest to various Australian indigenous groups—Mauss argues that the idea of person or individual among these peoples is thoroughly embedded in and inseparable from social life. He then makes clear the transformations that "person" undergoes over the centuries in Europe, culminating in the modern self, an entity that he identifies as having a "psychological consciousness"—that is, an individuated awareness of self. The idea of self is not innate, as we suppose, Mauss insists, but, rather, "originated and slowly developed over many centuries and through numerous vicissitudes, so that even today it is still imprecise, delicate and fragile, one requiring further elaboration."[3]

When Mauss delivered the Huxley Memorial Lecture in 1938, in which he set out his ideas about self in public for the first time, he concluded with the comment: "Who knows . . . whether this 'category,' which all of us here believe to be well founded, will always be recognized as such?"[4] He argued that anthropology, sociology, and history teach us to perceive how human thought "moves on." We know, of course, that Mauss himself moved on from the dominant thinking of his day when he elaborated extensively on "techniques of the body" and the manner in which they are learned: his was a major advance in restoring the suppressed idea that nature and nurture are inseparable, in marked contrast to the thinking of his uncle Émile Durkheim, Alfred Kroeber, and others, who deliberately sundered society from biology.[5]

In retrospect, it is apparent that the majority of social and cultural anthropologists did not welcome Mauss's theorizing. On the contrary, with the consolidation of the discipline of genetics, and the gradual formation of deterministic neo-Darwinism over the course of the twentieth century, a separation of the social and biological sciences became ever more marked. What is more, a widespread popular assumption (not necessarily shared by all anthropologists) is that the essence of "self" is to be found in the genes alone, leaving "nurture"—culture, learned behavior, social life—as the icing on the cake. Ironically, mapping the human genome resulted in some major surprises (as discussed later), with the result that, despite continuing remarkable advances in genomic knowledge, the assumption that genes alone determine the origin and unfolding of human life has been nudged to one side.

Boas, writing earlier than Mauss, argued that adult phenotypes are dependent on environmental exposures during human development. Boas capitalized on the insights of the eminent Danish scientist Wilhelm Johannsen, who first posited the genotype-phenotype distinction in 1908 when he intimated that life events and environmental exposures are literally embodied, with lasting consequences for health and illness, possibly over ensuing generations. Boas's prescient insights, set out in the first decade of the twentieth century, are largely ignored by cultural anthropologists today and are unknown by the majority of geneticists.

Boas's research involved the measurement of the cephalic indexes of several thousand immigrants and their children living in New York. The findings revealed that the brain sizes of immigrant children differed from those of their parents, surprising Boas and forcing him to conclude that the head shapes of immigrants converge to a common type as a result of similar environmental pressures. He wrote: "We are necessarily led to grant . . . the great plasticity of the mental make-up of human types."[6] Boas was equally at pains to emphasize that the organization of the brain is basically the same for all mankind: "There can be no doubt that, in the main, the mental characteristics of man are the same all over the world," but he readily acknowledges a "diversity produced by the variety of contents of the mind as found in various social and geographical environments."[7]

Behavioral epigeneticists are today dealing with rapidly proliferating research findings at the molecular level that mesh with Boas's postulates. Their methods are designed to produce findings that situate research subjects in context from the moment of conception—in environments macro and micro—making the very possibility of autonomous selves untenable. Body boundaries are envisioned as permeable, malleable, and changeable over time; any thought of an innate, hardwired self cannot be sustained. Nor can the idea of autonomous bodies independent of context. Boas can plausibly be thought of as a proto-epigenesist.

Relational Selves: The Japanese Instance

The word *jibun*, translated into English as "self," implies that this concept cannot be separate from the social realm. Literally, *jibun* means "self part," implying that individuals are inevitably embedded in human relationships, groupings, and communities at large. Ruth Benedict's classic *The Chrysanthemum and the Sword*, based on interviews with Japanese living in the United States who were interned during World War II, is a study of so-called personality patterns in which Benedict concluded that Japan is best characterized as a "culture of shame."[8] External sanctions imposed on children as they grow up result in feelings of shame, Benedict argued, as opposed to what she understood as a more mature way of coping with imposed controls by means of internalized guilt. Benedict's research has been criticized over the years, with good justification, but it nevertheless stimulated a large body of research on mother-infant behavior in Japan carried out by both anthropologists and psychoanalytically oriented researchers. Robert Smith, an anthropologist who conducted ethnographic research in Japan over many decades, concluded when commenting on the Japanese self: "There is no fixed center . . . from which the individual asserts a noncontingent existence."[9] And the general conclusion drawn repeatedly about early child-rearing has been that Japanese babies are encouraged to be oriented toward others and interdependent from the day they are born, whereas American babies are, from the outset, taught to be independent.[10]

The classic movie made by Margaret Mead titled *Four Families* (1960) features differences in human relationships in a selected Japanese, Indian, French, and Canadian family as each goes about daily life. The contrasts in the care of the families' youngest members are striking. Viewers are shown how, in the Japanese family, the baby is held closely, often by grandma, in the deep, hot *ofuro* (bath), and sleeping on *tatami* (mat) is communal. In contrast, in the Canadian family, from Manitoba, the infant is held over a kitchen sink and roughly sponged and then is wrapped up warmly for the night and put to sleep in his own room, where the light is turned out and the door is shut— leaving the baby "to develop his character," as Mead put it. Punishment of small children in Japan today continues, for some, to be separation from the family; the child is made to stand outside the house, rain or shine, until he or she is brought back in to apologize. A recent example of this treatment went viral when a Japanese boy was forced out of his family's car that then took off, leaving the boy by the roadside.[11] In North America and the United Kingdom, by contrast, a common threat is to send a child to her room if she does not behave properly, although a moment's thought makes clear, given that the so many children have computers in their rooms and carry cell phones from a young age, that such disciplinary measures are no doubt severely compromised.

Marked linguistic distinctions between inside (*ura*) and outside (*omote*) have been written about extensively by both the anthropologist Takie Lebra and the psychoanalyst Takeo Doi.[12] Both discuss extensively how, in theory, Japanese are expected to keep certain aspects of self inside—notably, many emotional feelings—while the outward expression of self is formalized and follows expected patterns of exchange and behavior. Doi's first book in English, *The Anatomy of Dependence* (1971), was an effort to explain the Japanese concept of self that results from the intense relationships between babies and their mothers. His second book, *The Anatomy of the Self*, is subtitled, "The Individual versus Society." This book first came out in Japanese titled simply *Omote to Ura* (Outside and Inside) and is an explicit effort to explicate the relationship among language, mind, and behavior in Japan, in which some commonalities can be detected with the West. It is an effort to make the strange familiar to curb the exoticism associated until recently with Japan.

The edited volume *Narrating the Self* makes clear that novelists in Japan were struggling throughout the early twentieth century with the concept of self.[13] The genre of the so-called I-Novel, published between the 1920s and 1960s, reveals an enormous gulf between the form the novel took in Japan and Europe at this time. I-Novels are written in the first person singular (hence, the genre's name) and attempt to portray the struggle to attain a modern internalized self. This genre is completely at odds with what was being written in European novels of the day, in which fictional characters were developed with great care.

As early as the mid-1970s, several authors began to critique the very assumption of an inherent dichotomy between an internalized and a relational self. Thomas Rohlen, for one, made clear that the practice in Japan of building one's spirit—*seishin*—is an expression of individuality. Such activities include Zen meditation, the martial arts, practice of the tea ceremony, and calligraphy. Among modern corporations, endurance walks and military boot camp experiences are carried out to teach fortitude, cooperation, self-confidence, and other qualities thought to contribute to the workplace and, hence, indirectly to society at large.[14] Dorinne Kondo criticized the research on self in Japan by arguing that approaches tend to emphasize "static, essentialized, global traits disconnected from power relations in society." She suggested that a more critical approach would ask "to what extent general 'essences' of selfhood can be distilled out from the particular contexts in which they took place."[15] Kondo argues that, rather than creating arguments that suggest a smooth totality, ambiguities and contradictions should be brought to the fore, as should struggles about power, hierarchy, and discipline. Her research among people working as artisans led her to conclude that multiple selves and identities are inevitable and that fragility of identity is often apparent.[16]

The question of alienation in contemporary Japan has repeatedly emerged in research since the 1970s, whether in schools, in the factory, among so-called salarymen, or among housewives.[17] One housewife I interviewed voluntarily said that she had "no self" because she felt that her life was taken up entirely by looking after other people. The refusal of many Japanese adolescents to go to school in recent decades is an example of profound social alienation. In some instances, major psychiatric disorders are evident, and medical care is needed. But by far the majority of "school refusers" are articulate about the reasons for their behavior. Many complain about overmanipulation by their families; teasing by peers; stresses associated with the competitive education system in Japan; and hours spent commuting on trains. Teachers, parents, and neighbors informally diagnose these young people as having "school refusal syndrome." A good number remain relatively isolated in their homes for months on end, frequently in bed much of that time, their desperate parents unable to bring the crisis to an end. When medical help is sought, often with reluctance because of embarrassment, family therapy with the child's teacher present is usually suggested, although the father is frequently absent due to work obligations.[18]

Since the late 1990s another condition has been recognized in Japan: hikikomori (withdrawal), characterized as a profound lack of interaction with other people. A very large number of affected individuals (the exact number is impossible to estimate) shut themselves away in their parents' homes, refusing to leave for months or even years on end, usually eating alone and frequently passing their time using electronic devices. Hikikomori affects individuals ranging in age from teenagers to the late thirties, the majority of them young men. Several noted Japanese psychiatrists insist that this phenomenon is primarily a social matter, and one or two social commentators have gone as far as to assert that affected individuals are healthy but are forced to live in a society that makes unhealthy demands on them. Efforts to deal with the problem are largely by means of support groups attended by anguished parents usually unaccompanied by the affected individuals. Japanese media has dubbed these and other efforts to deal with the phenomenon the "hikikomori industry."

Based on ethnographic work, the anthropologist Amy Borovoy concludes that the origins of this condition are multiple, but "the fact that these various dilemmas lead to the shared outcome of shutting oneself away at home is remarkable."[19] A number of people with hikikomori start out as school refusers who may have undergone bullying or ostracism at a young age, but others retreat later in life, after failing to find satisfactory work after graduating from college or university. Borovoy and others note that, at times, severe psychiatric disorder is evident involving violent outbreaks, obsessive-compulsive disorder, and hallucinations. Hikikomori lays bare what Borovoy suggests should be understood as the "darker side" of a commitment to equality. She documents how, in the Japanese mental health-care system, great lengths are taken not to diagnose individuals with mental health problems to avoid the consequences of labeling someone as different and damaged. Borovoy also makes clear the extent to which mainstreaming is normative in Japan so that all children will be exposed to the same education and, hence, in theory, have equal opportunities. She uncovers "holding areas"—so-called step classrooms, prolonged sick leave, and mothers available at home to tend solicitously to their children—that protect affected people until they can be persuaded to reenter everyday life. Ultimately, everything is done to stop the removal of young people from school, social life, and the workforce.

Extreme feelings of alienation can, of course, lead to suicide. In Japan, suicide has long been classified into several types, depending on the context in which it takes place. One form, *kakugo no jisatsu* (suicide of resolve), is understood as an act of "free will." This type of suicide has been "estheticized" for centuries and continues to be so today in popular culture, in the media, and even among many psychiatrists. Formerly, this type of suicide was associated with the samurai class, but also included are people who believe that they have become a burden to family or society, such as the elderly or those who have failed others in a profound way. Suicide rates in Japan (among the ten countries in the world with the highest suicide rates) have remained at about thirty thousand per year for more than a decade, and approximately one hundred persons a day commit suicide.

Junko Kitanaka argues that Japanese psychiatrists sometimes exhibit deep ambivalence about the medicalization of suicidal patients, and the majority recognize suicide of resolve as in some way "worthy." Psychiatrists strive to achieve a "minimum of shared understanding with patients about the biological nature of 'mental illness,'" but at the same time, they deliberately avoid what is thought of as existential discussions and do not actively explore psychological aspects of the patient's distress. Kitanaka argues that psychiatrists can be complicit in reproducing cultural assumptions about suicide when they reinforce a moral hierarchy in which some suicides are estheticized as courageous while others, although they may be sad and moving, are nevertheless thought of as mundane and pathological.[20] It is striking that this psychiatric practice shows marked overlaps in the practice that takes place in many of the clinics in Japan run by East Asian medical practitioners.[21] In both situations, although narratives about the intolerable life situations of patients are usually listened to with great sympathy, medical practitioners do not think that the suffering of individual patients should be "psychologized" or individualized. Nor do they make recommendations for changes in the everyday lives of patients. Rather, the task is to ease "real" bodily pain to give patients sufficient resolve to participate again in everyday life. Furthermore, Kitanaka makes clear how the management of depression in Japan is gendered, with much less attention, until recently, being given to women than to men, who are assumed to be justly suffering due to an insupportable workload.

When writing about the elderly in Japan, John Traphagan notes that, because social engagement is understood as the morally right thing to do, the thought of losing oneself to dementia is particularly abhorrent. "Self-building" is actively promoted by the government in Japan, and ubiquitous pamphlets charge residents to persist in the task of self-improvement. One document put out by a Center for Lifelong Learning in Kanegasaki, in Iwate Prefecture, states that the center is "for the purpose of residents to carry on an abundant and bright life, an institution where one can be healthy through study, learning, sports, and recreation."[22] Creating and sustaining a purpose in life (*ikigai*) that involves self-cultivation, interaction with others, and physical activity is integral to maintaining health and avoiding dementia. When successful, the government has, in effect, demonstrated fiscal responsibility by avoiding expenditure for housing the elderly.

The question arises as to where jibun is located, and a brief discussion about the ubiquitous terms *ki (ch'i)* and *kokoro (xin)* provides some clarification. These words have been in use in everyday life for hundreds of years in both China and Japan and are referents for body states, emotions, and human behavior. Ki is also a fundamental postulate used in East Asian medicine, a concept somewhat akin to the Greek concept of *pneuma*. It exists both exterior and interior to the body and is profoundly implicated in sustaining health and emotional well-being. Many people think of ki as a concept without any material reality, but nevertheless mastery of ki is central to smooth human relations. *Kokoro* has a broad range of meanings—heart, mind, spirit, vitality, sincerity, care, will, intention, and yet others; it has a corporeal quality associating it with the heart, but a different term is used for the anatomical heart, and *kokoro* is more diffuse. One should "cultivate" or polish kokoro through many of the activities associated with seishin (described earlier). Such language usage ensures that mind is not separated from body and that the mind/body is never sealed off from the exterior world. Jibun, oneself, flows though body boundaries, and ki and kokoro are concepts freighted with a moral discourse that enables jibun to participate appropriately in daily life.

In recent decades, as literature, movies, art, and a body of social-science research about Japan so clearly show, anomie and alienation are readily apparent. The social self must surely be on the wane; however, cultivation of self is equally evident among many people of all ages.[23]

Environments and Selves

An explicit assumption that "self" is embedded in a larger social milieu from which individuals at times retreat and withdraw has been well documented by anthropologists the world over. However, the physical body has rarely been explicitly included in anthropological analyses. The soma remains, in effect, black-boxed, and discussion is focused primarily on linguistic analyses.

We have recently entered an era in which the lasting effects of environments on the human body from the moment of conception are beginning to be documented, making it necessary to think about self from a new perspective. Over the past decades, analyses of "self and non-self" have become an urgent matter in connection with immunology, blood transfusions, organ transplants, and human reproduction. The development and application of these technologies have made it clear that the embodied self must be understood fundamentally as both biologically and subjectively experienced: without the application of biological knowledge, these technologies result in disastrous illness and death or fail in their objective to create new life. But anthropological research in connection with transfusions, transplants, and the new reproductive technologies has shown how, when successful, individuals very often report that their selves are fundamentally transformed in mind and body.[24] Epigenetic research makes clear how nurture and nature are deeply entangled throughout life, with enormous consequences for human development, the embodiment of self, and health and illness.

Conrad Hal Waddington is regarded as the founding father of epigenetics. Born in 1905, Waddington eventually came to be regarded by some scientists as a revolutionary. The *Encyclopedia Britannica* describes him as an embryologist, geneticist, and philosopher of science. He acquainted himself with paleontology while teaching at Cambridge University and eventually became known as the founder of systems biology. Waddington explicitly derived the term *epigenetics* from the Aristotelian word *epigenesis*:

> Some centuries ago, biologists held what are called "preformationist" theories of development. They believed that all the characters of the adult were present in the newly fertilized egg but packed into such a small space that they could not be properly distinguished with the instruments then available. If we merely consider each gene as a determinant for some definite character in the adult (as when we speak loosely of the "gene for blue eyes, or for fair hair"), then the modern theory may appear to be merely a new-fangled version of the old idea. But ... embryologists ... have reached quite a different picture[:] ... the theory known as epigenesis, which claims that the characters of the adult do not exist already in the newly fertilized germ, but ... arise gradually through a series of causal interactions between the comparatively simple elements of which the egg is initially composed. There can be no doubt ... that this epigenetic point of view is correct.[25]

Waddington initially argued that the field of epigenetics should be confined to demonstrating causal interactions between genes and their products that result in the phenotype (physical traits). His position was influenced by the dawning realization of several researchers that embryological development must involve networks of interactions among genes that form a complex integrated system and that the completely bifurcated subjects of genetics and embryology should be better integrated, although many embryologists feared that their field would be overtaken by genetics if such a move took place. Waddington expressly made "development" central to his arguments because of its double meaning: the growth of individuals *and* evolutionary change.

He insisted that genes are responsible only for guiding "the mechanics of development" and that phenotypes result from ongoing interactions among cellular environments and genotypes. He was emphatic that no single gene functions solely to bring about one or more phenotype and, further, that synchronic processes in the intracellular environment and among genes greatly modify linear unidirectional accounts of developmental processes and evolutionary change. These arguments are today subsumed under the much used concept of "phenotypic plasticity"—that is, the ability of an organism to create the phenotype most advantageous in response to environmental changes.

Embryonic "pluripotent stem cells" become differentiated during development so that they acquire specific functions—such as, for example, liver or brain cells in the various tissues and organs of the body—a characteristic first made clear by Waddington. Furthermore, he recognized "critical periods" during individual development that are universally accepted today. Waddington upended the dominant thinking of his time—namely, that genes are the source of life and determine development—when he insisted that genes must be activated and deactivated by complex intracellular processes.

Working in the same era as Waddington, the physician-philosopher Georges Canguilhem, active in the French Resistance, argued for recognition of the concept of the "milieu." Emphasizing the biological relationship between "the living and its milieu," Canguilhem insisted that the "individuality of the living does not stop at its ectodermic borders any more than it begins at the cell."[26] The research and writing of both Canguilhem and Richard Lewontin is at one with that of Waddington, but, significantly, they both extend the idea of environment *beyond the body* into the world at large.[27] Lewontin states: "Organisms have skin, but their total environments do not. It is by no means clear how to delineate the effective environment of an organism."[28] For these commentators, "nurture" is inseparable from "nature." This recognition of the extent to which the material body is permeable demands a revision of received wisdom about self and about self and others.

Molecular Epigenetics and the Reactive Genome

Waddington's work was overlooked for three decades, and several scientists claimed that it had no worth, but it was eventually revitalized to become the foundational approach of molecular epigenetics. In the interim, the human genome had been mapped, a project that contributed greatly to undermining an era of hard-line genetic determinism. The dethroning of the deterministic gene started even before the Human Genome Project (HGP) commenced when, in 1968, it was found that large amounts of DNA sequences are repetitive. Following the HGP, the idea that genes determine life unraveled, in large part as a result of what the map revealed.

It was formerly assumed that the genome is composed entirely of genes that code for proteins, although certain scientists had long suspected that this could not be the case. The HGP revealed that genes that code for proteins make up only about 1.2 percent of the genome and are unevenly distributed on chromosomes, clustering at particular sites. Furthermore, among these genes many code for more than one protein; sometimes they code for many. Humans have approximately twenty thousand genes, not one hundred thousand, as had been predicted. Numerous plants have many more genes than do humans, and the diminutive worm *C. elegans* has about the same number as we do. The size of a genome bears no relationship to its complexity, and the genome is not equivalent to the organism, "The role of the genome has been turned on its head," Evelyn Fox Keller argues, "transforming it from an executive suite of directional instructions to an exquisitely sensitive ... system that enables cells to regulate gene expression in response to their immediate environment."[29]

When scientists found that large segments of the genome were not functional, they disparagingly labeled this matter "junk" and set it to one side. But an article by Wayt Gibbs published in *Scientific American* in 2003 stated: "New evidence ... contradicts conventional notions that genes ... are the sole mainspring of heredity and the complete blueprint for all life. Much as dark matter influences the fate of galaxies, dark parts of the genome exert control over the development and the distinctive traits of all organisms, from bacteria to humans.... [S]ome scientists now suspect that much of what makes one person, and one species, different from the next are variations in the gems hidden within our 'junk' DNA."[30]

It is now well established that the activities of non-coding RNA (ncRNA) constitute the most comprehensive regulatory systems in complex organisms. These activities function to create the "architecture" of organisms, without which chaos would reign. To this end, ncRNA profoundly affects the timing of processes that occur during development, including stem cell maintenance, cell proliferation, apoptosis (programmed cell death), the occurrence of cancer, and other complex ailments. It has been shown recently that the epigenetic regulation of chromatin structure is of crucial importance in these processes.

Among other things, this emerging knowledge makes clear that the task of the genome is to respond to environments that we are currently altering at a phenomenal rate, and the central dogma on which molecular genetics was founded has been exploded. Today the majority of biologists, whatever their specialty, accept that cellular differentiation is governed by something akin to what Waddington described as the epigenetic landscape, a complex panorama of networks and feed-forward loops that determine whether or not stem cells go into a lineage. A large number also agree that environments interact directly with individual genomes, bringing about epigenetic changes. Many such changes are reversible, while others apparently are not. The biologist Scott Gilbert summarizes the position taken by researchers who continue the Waddington tradition this way: "Organisms have evolved [a reactive genome] to let environmental factors play major roles in phenotype determination. . . . [T]he environment is instructive."[31]

Steven Rose, a professor of neurobiology, argued two decades ago, while countering genetic reductionism, that we must be concerned above all with the dynamics of life—that is, with process and the continuous interchange between organisms and their environments. Our "lifelines," he argued, constituted by life processes, generate our sense of self.[32] Rose insisted that we are defined by our histories at least as much as we are by our molecular constituents and individual histories composed of lived experience in environments, natural and social. Over the years, biomedical reductionism has also been critiqued by researchers investigating the history of concepts of disease.[33] In addition to this, numerous other medical anthropologists, philosophers, and individuals in social medicine have contributed to a vibrant literature that counters reductionism.

In summary thus far, genomic medicine furnishes, in effect, decontextualized information. In contrast, epigenetics has the potential to create a field that is complementary to medical anthropology, social, and historical medicine and create at the molecular level dynamic, fluid images of self, recognized as inherently unstable, that demand contextualization in time and space. One thriving subfield of particular interest when considering the self is environmental epigenetics, in which researchers track the transmission of signals originating externally to the body to the body interior, and vice versa. In other words, genes are activated (switched on) and, when appropriate, deactivated (switched off) by means of complex processes. These signals incite trains of molecular activity that modify DNA expression, at times with lifelong effects on behavior, health, and illness. Animal studies show that such modifications can be transmitted intergenerationally, and increasingly research suggests that this may also be the case in humans. Thus, not only is genetic determinism challenged. So is the assumption of an autonomous self from which the moral order flows.

Epigenetic researchers are usually careful to point out that we have yet to fully identify the mechanisms that transmit signals emanating from social environments that result in DNA changes. To date, DNA methylation, among several epigenetic mechanisms that control gene expression, has received the most attention. Methylation is a highly conserved process found widely in both animal and plant worlds that permits any given genome to code for diversely stable phenotypes. The process, stimulated by enzyme activity, is one in which a methyl group consisting of one carbon atom bonded to three hydrogen atoms is attached to cytosine or adenine DNA nucleotides, thus blocking the transcription of genes. This permits differentiation of embryonic stem cells into specific cells and tissues. Such changes are usually permanent and unidirectional, take place in utero and in the early postpartum years, and continue throughout the life span.

Environmental epigeneticists posit that DNA methylation and related mechanisms have a second, very important function: these processes do not take place solely as a result of endogenous stimuli, but are also responses to environmental signals external to the body that modulate patterns of cellular activity *directly*, without the involvement of genes. An iconic, oft-cited research project made use of a model of maternal deprivation created in rats by removing young pups from their mothers, thus curtailing maternal licking and grooming during critical developmental periods. This deprivation altered the expression of genes that regulate behavioral and endocrine responses to stress, as well as hippocampal synaptic development. These changes could be reversed if pups were returned in a matter of days to their mothers. Furthermore, when the birth mother was a poor nurturer, placement of her pups with a surrogate mother who licked and groomed them enabled the pups to flourish.[34] Crucially, it was shown that pups or foster pups left to mature with low-licking mothers not only exhibited a chronically increased stress response but also passed this behavior on to their own pups. Hence, variations in maternal behavior result in biological pathways that lead to significantly different infant phenotypes that can persist into adulthood.

A substantial body of research has now accrued supporting a position that forces internal and external to the body, in addition to genes, contribute to the phenotype of the next generation, and possibly of several generations. Work with single-celled organisms, nematodes, rodents, and primates has demonstrated transgenerational epigenetic effects. When it comes to humans, vociferous arguments take place among researchers as to whether or not such transmission occurs. Marcus Pembrey and Lars Olov Bygren carried out research in Överkarlix, an isolated Swedish municipality near the Arctic Circle, examining the historical records of three generations of births and deaths, as well as annual harvest records. They found strong correlations between epigenetic changes in eggs and sperm in grandparents that resulted from famine, along with the occurrence, years later, of diabetes in their children and grandchildren. They argue that these findings are proof of transgenerational epigenetic effects.[35] Not everyone is fully convinced.[36] Nevertheless, it is clear that epigenetic changes influence cell memories for at least one generation, and perhaps more.

Epigenetics and the Life Course

It has been demonstrated repeatedly that prenatal exposure to "maternal stress, anxiety, and depression" have lasting effects on infant development that are associated with the appearance of psychopathology later in life. A review of 176 articles based on findings from both animal and, to a lesser extent, human research notes that "the in utero environment is regulated by placental function and there is emerging evidence that the placenta is highly susceptible to maternal distress and is a target of epigenetic dysregulation."[37] The mental health community draws on the concept of emotional dysregulation to refer to what is commonly known as mood swings. Psychiatrists have long associated such swings with early psychological trauma, including child abuse or neglect, chronic maltreatment in institutions, and brain injury; they have also been linked to deficits in the frontal cortices of the brain. Now, increasingly robust evidence indicates that epigenetic effects are involved in such dysregulations. Furthermore, as is well known, a large body of research suggests that postnatal maternal care can induce further emotional disruptions.

Antenatal depression and anxiety symptoms exhibited by mothers are picked out for particular attention as states contribute to an in utero environment that brings about dysregulation. In other words, in this type of research, the environment is effectively scaled down to molecular activity inside a single organ of the body: the uterus and its fetal contents. Certain research has also shown that fathers' sperm can contribute to dysregulation.[38] Such findings are based primarily on correlations, although researchers are beginning to map segments of the pathways whereby environmentally induced epigenetic marks appear to be associated with behavioral outcomes pre- and postnatally.[39]

In an article published in *BioSocieties*, Ilina Singh comments on a warning sent out to members by the American Academy of Pediatrics in 2011 cautioning about the harm caused to children by "toxic stress." Singh interprets this warning as a move toward further monitoring of families—notably, pregnant women and young mothers, who, she suggests, are likely to be targeted for observation, their behavior subjected to surveillance designed to avoid fetal and infant stress. Medical and social support for young childbearing women is to be lauded, but, as Singh states, the possibility is that newly revamped home visits to pregnant women, such as those being carried out through a partnership of nurses and family practitioners in New York, might well become, in effect, "womb visits." The poverty and often violent living conditions of many mothers-to-be may be virtually ignored, and attention may light almost exclusively on the pregnant belly and its dysregulated contents.[40] Research findings from the Mapping of the Human Brain project are providing remarkable insights into the singularity and complexity of genes that appear to put a fetus at risk for autism following birth, and it appears that epigenetic changes in utero are implicated. As research such as this progresses, the womb and its environments will be monitored yet more closely.[41]

One of the most cited studies in which the fetal environment has become an object of study is in connection with pregnant women affected by the so-called Dutch Hunger Winter. This research has been followed up over two ensuing generations. Thirty thousand people died from starvation as a result of a food embargo imposed by the Germans in World War II that brought about a complete breakdown of local food supplies, adding to the misery of an already harsh winter. Birth records collected since that time have shown that children born to women who were pregnant during the famine not only had low birth weights but also exhibited a disproportionally high range of developmental and adult disorders later in life, including diabetes, coronary heart disease, and breast and other cancers.[42] Furthermore, it has been shown that the second generation, even though prosperous and well-nourished themselves, produced low birth-weight children who inherited similar health problems, which are thought to be founded on epigenetic effects. Moreover, exposure to severe food deprivation during the first trimester of pregnancy showed a substantial increase in hospitalized schizophrenia for women once they became adults, but not for men. The Dutch Hunger study is often cited as a sound example of intergenerational transmission of epigenetic effects. These findings suggest that highly traumatic experiences affect not only physical well-being but also the sense of self and identity of affected individuals.

In addition to the effects of malnutrition on fetal development, a large literature has accrued since the 1990s showing a strong relationship between "childhood maltreatment" and negative mental health outcomes, ranging from aggressive and violent behavior to suicide. Investigations are beginning to expose the pathways of implicated epigenetic processes regarded as crucial mediators of the biological embedding of childhood maltreatment. The conclusion drawn from this research is that the "epigenome is responsive to developmental, physiological and environmental cues."[43]

Inevitably, researching human molestation is fraught with difficulties owing to ethical issues, and abuse is not amenable to measurement. But over the years, research has become more sophisticated. Rats and humans have a similar stress mechanism; to measure the effect of epigenetics on the human brain, researchers targeted the NR3C1 gene, which had previously been studied in rats. One experiment used thirty-six autopsied human brains, of which twelve came from individuals who had died by suicide and had experienced childhood abuse; twelve came from individuals who had committed suicide and had not been subject to abuse; and another twelve were those of "normal" controls.[44] The results showed that abuse resulted in DNA methylation patterns that, in turn, altered the functioning of the NR3C1 gene such that the glands that secrete stress hormones stayed constantly alert in abused individuals, making them susceptible to anxiety, depression, and possibly suicide.

These findings are presumed to substantiate a molecular mechanism whereby nature and nurture meld as one. In this particular case, childhood adversity is associated with sustained modifications in DNA methylation across the genome, among which are epigenetic alterations in neurons of the hippocampus that may well interfere with processes of neuroplasticity—that is, the ability to use multiple potential pathways in the brain. The researchers acknowledge that the sample is small and that such research cannot be thoroughly validated. The absence of a control group that experienced early life abuse and did not die by suicide is another shortcoming. Furthermore, the abuse that the subjects experienced was informally reported as exceptionally severe. It has recently been established that behaviorally induced methylation changes are not limited to brain tissue: changes can be detected in white blood T-cells that correlate with the brain tissue changes. This is good news for researchers, who can now use blood samples procured from living subjects rather than be confined to donated brains.

Obviously, fetal malaise and that experienced by young children is at times caused directly by the behavior of parents and stepparents. Such behavior is frequently aggravated by the socioeconomic status of the family and may be exacerbated by substance abuse. However, it is clear that history, politics, social environments, racism, chronic discrimination, war, and other major social disruptions must be given consideration equal to, or perhaps greater than, that of immediate family circumstances when attempting to account for these epigenetic effects. Such research raises challenging questions about the distribution of responsibility for ill health over time and space among individuals, families, communities, bureaucrats, politicians, capitalists, and others. Causation is complex, but outcomes involving serious mental health problems are striking and clearly impact not only health but also the sense of self and identity as subjectively experienced by individuals over their life course, reinforced in part by people around them.

Epidemiological research in the United States, for example, has shown that the disproportionate burden of abnormalities, disease, and mortality borne by African Americans, compared with whites, is associated with low birth weight, which, in turn, is substantially linked to the subjective experience of racism. This research implicates changes in gene expression resulting in epigenetic changes as a major contributor to the problem.[45] And the moniker the Glasgow effect is used to describe Europe's sickest city, in which epigenetic markers have been shown to contribute to dramatic class differences in disease incidence and life expectancy.[46] Nancy Kreiger and George Davey Smith stress that it is essential to examine the "literal" effects of the embodiment of racism, inequality, and discrimination. In addition to this, it should go without saying that narrative accounts of the self as subjectively experienced are indispensable. In sum, discrimination of various kinds, coupled with poverty, affect neurodevelopment from the time in utero on, and toxic environments seriously compound the situation. When addressing the problems of poverty, emphasis is often given to providing schooling that will enable children to overcome their difficult start in life. Epigenetic findings make clear that the effects of poverty are such that a great deal more than schooling must be attended to if babies born into poverty are to flourish.

Colonization and Historical Trauma

Canada is home to roughly 1.2 million individuals who endorsed the category "Aboriginal" in the 2006 Canadian census. The majority of these people live in communities that continue to contend with the devastating legacy of settler colonialism, among them entrenched poverty and invidious discrimination manifested in so-called mental health problems of many kinds. They include substance dependence, depression, violence, and extraordinarily high rates of suicide, especially among young people, estimated in some Inuit communities to be six times the rate in other parts of Canada.[47]

Mental health professionals and individuals living in First Nations communities have consistently associated these high rates of pathology with the experiences of colonization that commenced five centuries ago. A concept of "historical trauma" has been adopted to call attention to the collective, cumulative, and intergenerational psychosocial effects that resulted from past colonial subjugation and persist in abated form to the present day.[48] With colonization, population densities increased, considerably facilitating the rapid spread of disease, and the mortality rate from infectious disease was extraordinarily high. The Haida Nation, with whom Boas worked for some time, went from an estimated population of twenty thousand prior to 1770 to fewer than six hundred by the end of the nineteenth century.[49] The full effects of population decimation are rarely fully appreciated: given the climate and an economy based on hunting, the ability of those that survived to procure food was in effect destroyed; hence, individuals "with the dubious good fortune of living through the initial sickness" died of hunger.[50]

Extensive efforts to "whiten" Indians commenced in the nineteenth century through the establishment of residential schools. Young children were rounded up and sent great distances from their homes to be housed in institutions where they were not permitted to speak their own languages or participate in anything regarded as cultural practice.[51] Today, the residential schools, the last of which were closed only in the 1990s, are regarded among First Nations and Inuit communities as the primary source of their current malaise. It recently came to light as part of the ongoing Truth and Reconciliation Commission of Canada that repeated sexual abuse took place in these schools, one of which was characterized by an investigating Supreme Court justice as practicing "institutionalized paedophilia."[52] Systematic nutritional medical experimentation was also practiced on some of the students, resulting in malnutrition in many and death for many more. Tuberculosis was rampant, and few attempts were made to curb it. In one notorious school, the death rate of children was apparently 75 percent in the first sixteen years of its operation.[53] The majority of individuals who grew up in these conditions, now middle aged and older, have until very recently been unwilling to ruminate about their younger lives, but many freely admit to being unable to adequately parent their own children.

Despite major changes for the better in recent years, racism and discrimination continue to be blatantly evident against First Nations. Shocking poverty persists on many reservations, a number of which have no running water. Toxic contamination is frequently present. Schools on reservations are poorly provided for compared with schools elsewhere in Canada. The education gap has increased in recent years between First Nations children and other Canadians, and alcohol and drug abuse and violence against women and children is extraordinarily high.[54]

Not all reservations exhibit high rates of illness and suicide. Some survivors report that they enjoyed school, and others became devout Christians—a conversion that apparently assisted in their survival. Clearly, accounts of differences among First Nations are of the utmost importance when attempting to account for malaise. Second, ongoing land claim settlements have improved the lot of some First Nation communities, but settlements have not been made with the majority of communities. And third, the establishment of healing programs and suicide prevention gatherings conducted by First Nations themselves that make use of indigenous healing practices together with biomedicine exist in certain communities and receive some government support. Such changes are regarded as a positive form of empowerment by many First Nations leaders, but they are not yet broadly entrenched.[55]

Although First Nations received a formal apology from the prime minister of Canada two years ago, the budgets of twelve government-funded programs for First Nations have been cut, and nine are now closed.[56] Rates of suicide, substance abuse, and disappearance and death of young First Nation women continue to be extraordinarily high.[57] If the concept of historical trauma is to be taken seriously, then a great deal more than an apology and a reconciliation commission are needed to counter the crudely racist attempts to obliterate the Indian—the effects of which are being played out among third and fourth postcolonial generations.

It is not yet known whether intergenerational transmission of DNA modifications has contributed to this situation, although this seems highly likely, but demonstration of epigenetic changes obviously are not required to verify the extent and depth of this ongoing abuse that a number of survivors of residential schools and their offspring describe as genocide.[58] Accounts of trenchant memories about past and present experiences, both individual and among families, are indispensable in attempting to understand the extent of experienced trauma. But evidence of intergenerational transmission of epigenetic marks can make such accounts all the more significant in courts of law and among health-care providers and force a reconsideration of how responsibility for chronic malaise and even violence should be allocated.

Conclusion

Anthropological apprehensions of the self are found throughout the ethnographic archive, reminding us that neither the concept nor its experiential demands has ever been settled. Assumptions of a culturally and socially constituted autonomous self that were a hallmark of early anthropological research quickly proved to be inadequate as various sites revealed that a relational self may be normative, exemplified in the case of Japan. These recognitions early on challenged a medical anthropology that relied on cultural wholes, as well as biomedical idioms of pathology that cohered around a stable notion of the self, and ultimately enabled anthropologists to become provocateurs in the world of medicine. But we have gone long beyond that.

Today, as anthropologists engage in new ways with the biomedical sciences, similar interruptions can be seen. As genetic assumptions about autonomous selves have, in the era of epigenetics, given way to relational biologies, social and biological scientists work together to decipher how material and social environments and exposures are scripted into heritability by way of changes in methylation. These shifts in knowledge have kept pace with a shift in politics, giving new life to the recognition that matters such as socioeconomic precarity, violence, and political disenfranchisement can be accounted for, not just through anthropological archives, but also as part of the biological record. I think of these interruptions as forms of interference in the arc of promise of medical anthropology and as continuations of the effort to rethink how and what our work produces, not just in ethnographic sites, but also in the political worlds where our findings increasingly have impact.

Notes

1 | Including, notably and among others, Das, *Life and Worlds*; Desjarlais, *Body and Emotion*; Heelas and Lock, *Indigenous Psychologies*; Lebra, *Japanese Patterns of Behavior*; Lutz, *Unnatural Emotions*; Rosaldo, "The Shame of Headhunters and the Autonomy of Self."

2 | Mauss, "Une catégorie de l'esprit humaine," n.p.

3 | Mauss, "Une catégorie de l'esprit humaine," n.p.

4 | Mauss, "Une catégorie de l'esprit humaine," n.p.

5 | Lock, "Comprehending the Body in the Era of the Epigenome"; Meloni, "How Biology Became Social."

6 | Boas, *The Mind of Primitive Man*, 64–65.

7 | Boas, *The Mind of Primitive Man*, 104.

8 | Benedict, *The Chrysanthemum and the Sword*.

9 | Smith, *Japanese Society*, 81.

10 | Caudill, "Tiny Dramas."

11 | "Boy Missing in Japanese Forest after Parents Kicked Him out of Car as Punishment."

12 | See Doi, *The Anatomy of Self*; Lebra, *Japanese Patterns of Behavior*.

13 | Suzuki, *Narrating the Self*.

14 | Rohlen, *For Harmony and Strength*.

15 | Kondo, *Crafting Selves*, 41.

16 | See also Lock, *Encounters with Aging*.

17 | Clark, *The Japanese Company*; Imamura, *Urban Japanese Housewives*; Rohlen, *Japan's High Schools*; Rosenberger, "Productivity, Sexuality, and Ideologies of Menopausal Problems in Japan"; Vogel, *Japan's New Middle Class*; Vogel, "Professional Housewives."

18 | Lock, "A Nation at Risk."

19 | Borovoy, "Japan's Hidden Youths."

20 | Kitanaka, *Depression in Japan*.

21 | Lock, *East Asian Medicine in Urban Japan*.

22 | Cited in Traphagan, "Being a Good Rôjin," 275.

23 | Garon, *Molding Japanese Minds*.

24 | Crowley-Matoka, *Domesticating Organ Transplant*; Lock, *Twice Dead*; Sharp, *Strange Harvest*.

25 | Waddington, *The Strategy of the Genes*, 156.

26 | Canguilhem, *Knowledge of Life*, 111.

27 | Lewontin, "It's Even Less in Your Genes."

28 | Lewontin, "It's Even Less in Your Genes," 23.

29 | Keller, "From Gene Action to Reactive Genomes," 2425.

30 | Gibbs, "The Unseen Genome," 48.

31 | Gilbert, "The Reactive Genome," 92.

32 | Rose, *Lifelines*.

33 | See, e.g., Cohen, *No Aging in India*; Hacking, *Re-writing the Soul*; Young, *The Harmony of Illusions*.

34 | Meaney et al., "Early Environmental Regulation of Forebrain Glucocorticoid Receptor Gene Expression."

35 | Pembrey et al., "Network in Epigenetic Epidemiology."

36 | Champagne, "Epigenetic Mechanisms and the Transgenerational Effects of Maternal Care."

37 | Monk et al., "Linking Prenatal Maternal Adversity to Developmental Outcomes in Infants," 1361.

38 | Siklenka et al., "Disruption of Histone Methylation in Developing Sperm Impairs Offspring Health Transgenerationally."

39 | Monk et al., "Linking Prenatal Maternal Adversity to Developmental Outcomes in Infants."

40 | Singh, "Human Development, Nature and Nurture."

41 | Semeniuk, "The Hunt for Humanity."

42 | Heijmans et al., "Persistent Epigenetic Differences Associated with Prenatal Exposure to Famine in Humans."

43 | Lutz and Turecki, "DNA Methylation and Childhood Maltreatment."

44 | McGowan et al., "Epigenetic Regulation of the Glucocorticoid Receptor in Human Brain Associates with Childhood Abuse."

45 | Kreiger and Davey Smith, "'Bodies Count' and Body Counts."

46 | Ash, "Why Is Glasgow the UK's Sickest City?"

47 | Kral, "Postcolonial Suicide among Inuit in Arctic Canada."

48 | Niezen, *Truth and Indignation*.

49 | Laas, *Journal of the Haida Nation*.

50 | Daschuk, *Clearing the Plains*, 12.

51 | Carr, *Bearing Witness*.

52 | Carr, *Bearing Witness*, 19.

53 | Carr, *Bearing Witness*; Niezen, *Truth and Indignation*.

54 | Friesen, "Widening Education Gap Leaves Aboriginal Canadians Further Behind."

55 | Niezen, *Truth and Indignation*.

56 | Bennett, "The Budget and First Nations."

57 | Leblanc, "List of Missing, Killed Aboriginal Women Involves 1,200 Cases."

58 | Niezen, *Truth and Indignation*.

Tracing Arts *of* Living (Or, Anthropologies *after* Hope Has Departed)

HOW DOES CARE CONTINUE IN AFTERMATHS—of ethnographic encounters, of hope and death?

In part IV, Robert Desjarlais, João Biehl, and Jean Comaroff explore people's ongoing relations with caregivers, interlocutors, and kin in the wake of ends of various sorts, together brainstorming a new anthropological commitment to the figure of the human in the wake of the Anthropocene. Desjarlais and Biehl explore the radical unpredictability of social relations and the ways subjects leave behind traces that transcend and exceed bounded encounters and lives and that ethnographic storytelling animates time and again. Meanwhile, Comaroff builds from these attunements to insist on anthropology's capacity to care for human and nonhuman lifeworlds and to produce meaning at the edge of environmental calamity.

Arthur Kleinman's work has persistently drawn on his extended relationships with individual ethnographic subjects and their stories. Biehl and Desjarlais take inspiration from this temporality and mode of ethnographic encounter in exploring the many domains of social life that coalesce in the experience of illness, suffering, mourning, and care—the domestic, the religious, the ritual, the political, the economic, the psychological, the historical—and that, in turn, are also changed and shaped by an illness.

Throughout part IV, Desjarlais, Biehl, and Comaroff consider how care— the heart and soul of Kleinman's *oeuvre*—continues to bind in ways that transcend individual lives: the spectral presences of the dead that animate households, families, and social worlds, inspiring deepened meditations and prompting newly forged relations, friendships, commitments and ongoing obligations.[1] As stories, these ethnographic presences continue and shape the world in unexpected ways.

Following this line of inquiry, in his essay Desjarlais explores the wisdom about the art of living in "a dying world" elicited from his ethnographic openness to Buddhist funeral rites and his inquiry into the attachments of the living to the dead and the dead to the living. Might it be, Desjarlais piercingly asks, "that to anthropologize is to learn how to die?" Drawing on decades of fieldwork with Hyolmo people and zooming in on their meditative rites and provisional becomings in the face of death, Desjarlais suggests that through a rhythm of *poiesis*—the art of bringing something into being that hitherto did not exist—the Hyolmo enable the dead and the living to move back and forth into and out of one another's presence, as senses, attachments, and selves are creatively made and unmade. That is, the Hyolmo consider the generativity of a person's life as due to both his or her "forg[ing] a path, a line, or a trajectory in the world" and to that person's work to make the conditions of dying an "active, conscious project in life." When so much appears to be in demise today, we, too, are called to an ethics of care and to "a certain kind of demise writing, in which one writes within an intensity of dissolution," Desjarlais adds, "within the arc of a creative, uncertain, open-ended dying." Such an anthropology *in the mode of dying* may enable a humbler openness to the forms of life, presence, and care that persist in one's wake.

Biehl's essay chronicles the unexpected encounters that followed the death of his primary interlocutor Catarina, the main character of the book *Vita*. As life goes on, the "ethnographic sensorium" becomes a nexus for the reconnection of various members of the family who had dispersed alongside Catarina's abandonment as mad and intractable—a reassembling that, after she was left to die, Catarina had sought through her own storytelling and writing. Here, the *ethnographic open* allows "image-survivals" to travel, setting "surprising and unforeseeable processes in motion" that, in turn, become alternative figures of ethical and political thought and of futurity. When one reanchors the ethnographic project through wonder and bonds of accountability, the simplistic binaries of interlocutor versus collaborator, research subject versus friend, story versus theory are creatively blurred. Experimental and radically unpredictable, Biehl notes, ethnographic subjects thus "imprint our own doing, thinking, writing and imaging with the multiple and the unfinished"—persistent traces of care.

While social scientists have taken up the challenge of responding to the threat of abrupt climate change and the failed promise of a humanist agenda by trying to think beyond the human, Jean Comaroff's chapter builds on Desjarlais's and Biehl's meditations on care to offer a series of critical provocations. Anthropology's history of engagements with peoples' "labile entanglements with other beings and forces, animate and intimate, social and material," in relation not just to human conceptualizations but also the material conditions of life itself might be engaged by anthropologists calling for ontological and multispecies turns. Comaroff calls for renewed rigor in ethnographic commitments to the way that lives and worlds (human and nonhuman alike) are, and have always been seen as, crafted, inhabited, and forged through relational priorities and powers.

Humbly aware of our species' limits and interdependencies, we must not cede the ground of the real, the ethical, and the politico-economic to "postpolitical, posthuman forces, from biodeterminism to technoeconomic rationality," Comaroff warns. Opting for a radical humanism in our worlds on the edge, then, is not necessarily a return to casual anthropocentrism but a principled "commitment to care, to interfere, and to make the very best of borrowed time."

In an afterword, Arthur Kleinman reflects on the *Arc of Interference* chapters in relation to the moral and emotional transformations that underlay his evolving commitments as an ethnographer and caregiver, especially vis-à-vis the influences of his late wife and lifelong collaborator, Joan Kleinman. "The soul of care" lies in its irreducible sociality, efforts at presence, and persistent moral obligations. Care, in other words, is as much a set of practices aimed at improving the well-being of others and alleviating their suffering as it is an art of existence that enhances the meaning, fulfillment, and even pleasure of day-to-day life for all involved. The caregiving process, Kleinman points out, "continues even after death in the caring for memories" that become integral to the fabrics and forces that keep "individuals, families, communities, and even societies going." Caregiving and studying care thus offer "a way of critically getting at life itself"—an interference that remains uncaptured by prior determinisms and conventional ways of knowing.

Note

1 | Kleinman, *The Soul of Care*, 236.

Anthropology in a Mode of Dying

One writes here in a tone of care and appreciation for the work of a mentor, for the rich arc of a scholarly life, for a person's singularly innovative engagement with ideas. One writes in the terrain of keen insights on illness, medicine, healing, social suffering, psychiatry, medical anthropology, care, and morality sharpened, refashioned, and generously shared through years of research, writing, and teaching, such that those ideas take on new forms in a series of lives while always carrying the vital trace of the scholar-teacher who made possible the work that emerges. I write, as well, within the awareness of a fragile world, of forms of life and death at risk of perishing. Through this I seek, alongside others, altogether faintly, to find arts of life that might carry us further in life, even if this art of living relates intimately to an art of dying.

"TO PHILOSOPHIZE IS TO LEARN HOW TO DIE," or so wrote Cicero, echoing a sentiment that is axiomatic to ancient philosophy and recurrent from Plato on. As Simon Critchley explains the abiding idea, "The main task of philosophy, in this view, is to prepare us for death, to provide a kind of training for death, the cultivation of an attitude towards our finitude that faces—and faces down—the terror of annihilation without offering promises of an afterlife."[1]

Might it also be that to anthropologize is to learn how to die? And would the means and lessons of that education be distinct from those common to philosophical reasoning? That is, can a careful attentiveness to how others die, near and far, to ways of living and dying in human communities, to the all-too-human responses to a loss, to the politics of death and annihilation, to the profound and ubiquitous method of rituals, to the affective force of images, to the stark depths of grief, to the spectral play of memory, to a sense of vitalities echoing on—can all of this enable one to cultivate an expansive grasp of the actualities of death? Can an anthropology of death and dying teach one how to die, and thus how to live?

Such considerations might be particularly relevant in the contemporary world, where so many systems of life appear to be on the demise, from environmental decline to the waning of the polar ice caps and rising waters, the extinction of numerous species, and the severe diminishment of resources in the Anthropocene; from the collapse of political systems to conditions of poverty and existential precarity and political apprehension; from epidemics to epidemic carcinogenesis and the looming termination of many forms of life, as well as devastating spectacles of violence, destruction, and massive displacement. It's also the case that many now die in technologically mediated ways, where the idea of "death with dignity" often comes into question. What does it mean to live and die today? What forms of thought and writing might be best attuned to ways of living and dying in a world powerfully tied to environmental, sociopolitical, and existential change—as well as processes of sudden or gradual demise? How might we learn how to live well within a world so often marked by scenes of dissolution? Perhaps a certain kind of *demise writing* is called for, at times—a writing of and in disaster, a fragmentary writing, in frailty, uncertainty, of making and unmaking, a ruin of words that carries the potential for creative change, emergent life, and subtle shifts in knowing, becoming, relating.

These questions have been on my mind while I have been completing a body of research and writing that attends to themes of life and loss among Hyolmo people.[2] Hyolmo people are an ethnically Tibetan Buddhist people from the Hyolmo region of Nepal whose ancestors moved from Tibet to settle in the Hyolmo region of north-central Nepal, and who have recently found homes in the Kathmandu Valley and in places as far-flung as Japan, Great Britain, and the United States. I have been conducting ethnographic research with Hyolmo people for some twenty-five years now, both in Nepal and in the United States.[3]

I would like to draw from these sustained dialogic engagements to speak to questions of life, mortality, and afterlife as known by Hyolmo people. My work in this area has been driven by two abiding questions: What can the processes associated with living, dying, and death tell us about how certain features of human existence—such as consciousness, memory, desire, and bodiliness—are enacted and dissolved through a range of social, ritual, and communicative practices? And what might all this tell us about the figure of the human within the span of life?

While much of my thought ties into the fact of death in the Hyolmo world, the words involved point to something more heartening than death alone, for they speak to the creative, generative dimensions of Hyolmo efforts in the world. In general, human endeavors carry this creative capacity. Something profoundly generative and reverberative courses through Hyolmo lives and deaths. Life itself is generative, even within the burned-out shadow of death. And yet there is also another story to tell, for the vital dimensions of life stand in tension with moments of dying and legacies of death within the world.

Poiesis in Living and Dying

Hyolmo Buddhists are often concerned with a good death, one that helps them to achieve liberation or a good rebirth. Undertaking a quiet apprenticeship on the matter, they often adopt a number of techniques that help them to die well, from preparing for their deaths to giving a last testament in their final days and forging a calm and peaceful state of mind in the hours of their demise. Family and friends often help in these endeavors. They try to calm and support the fading loved one; they help him to sever his attachments to his life, exchange final words and glances, and accompany him in the process of dying, up to the "mouth" of death itself. As Hyolmo people know it, after a person dies, his consciousness departs from his body and enters into a phantasmagoric liminal realm between one life and the next, known as the *bardo*. This "between" can last up to forty-nine days after the death—until, basically, the consciousness moves into a new life form and is subsequently reborn in that life or it achieves nirvana altogether and steps out of the samsaric cycle of worldly, karmic existence. While in the bardo between, the consciousness is bereft of a tangible body. That spectral subject lacks the capacity for personal action, while needing to find the right route to a good rebirth.[4] He or she must therefore depend on the aid of the living, who must perform a number of rituals on his or her behalf.

"The dead are attached to the living, and the living are attached to the dead," goes one Hyolmo saying. The task of the living is to cut off the deceased from their world, to diminish their attachment to that world, to the point of a zero-degree desire. They must render the deceased no longer a living, fully human, flesh-and-body person. If the funeral rites go well, the personhood of the deceased fades in time. His persona becomes increasingly nameless, apersonal, and distant from the world of the living. Family members sponsor and participate in these rituals in a spirit of care and responsibility while often attending to wounding grief that diminishes, but never fully expires, in time.

The living and the recently dead are thus engaged in delicate technologies of cessation and transformation. Dying calls for an active patterning of self and other, as do the funerary rites. An element of *poiesis* courses through Hyolmo responses to death. There is a creative making, a generative fashioning of sense and consciousness, that serves to aid the deceased's plight while tending to the ache of grief and longing.

Poiesis implies a begetting, a fabrication and bringing forth, of some new form or reality; something that was not present is made present. The concept first took form in Greek philosophy, most significantly in the writings of Plato and Aristotle. It has subsequently been adopted by modern philosophers such as Martin Heidegger and Hannah Arendt, as well as by some anthropologists.[5] Taken from the Greek *poiein* (to act, to do, or to make) and related to the words *poetics* and *poetry*, the term *poiesis* has come to designate any making or doing beyond purely practical efforts. Poiesis is involved in the crafting of poems and in the art of shipbuilding.

Ideas of poiesis skirt dichotomies problematically common to Western thought, such as art and deed, virtuality and actuality, and idea and matter.[6] Imaginative visualizations are as much a matter of poiesis as religious statues. Such begetting is central to procedures of dying, death, and mourning in Hyolmo communities. Consciousness is transformed, ceremonies are performed, substitute bodies are made and unmade, and memories are revised—all in ways that entail techniques of fabricating, bringing forth, and transmutation.

A strong inclination toward creative fashioning recurs in many domains of life in Hyolmo communities, from the inventive industriousness often displayed by individuals and families to the "skilled means" employed by Buddhist adepts and the diligent attempts to generate positive karmic merit for oneself and others. The focus on self-transformation central to Tibetan Buddhist religious practices similarly involves motifs of overt and active fashioning.[7]

While ideas and doings of poiesis are central to many Hyolmo lives, they involve only one particular rendering of something at work in the lives of peoples throughout the world. Poiesis is found in the strivings of all peoples—and, perhaps, of all life-forms more generally. Poiesis is there in the urge we have to make something of our lives, both individually and collectively. The concept ties into Spinoza's idea that "each thing, as far as it can by its own power, strives to persevere in its being," and it has resonance with Gilles Deleuze's philosophy of becoming. It echoes Kathleen Stewart's considerations of "cultural poesis," which she richly locates in "the generativity of emergent things." It relates to Tim Ingold's inquiries into "making" and the "form-giving" principles of creation. And it parallels a theme in Michael D. Jackson's writings on the generative capacities of human beings.[8] We are always going beyond what is given to us, in one way or another. The capacity for generating is built into us. Poiesis is found in moments of joy and suffering, and of life and death.

Poiesis is evident in the ways people fashion something out of the elements of their lives, even if those elements are bone bare, at times. The catch to all this, however, is that those weavings often run up against the weavings of others similarly intent on making something of their lives. We all know of moments of counter-poiesis; one person's strivings cross creations with another's. Or, more harshly, our efforts hit up against the world at large, blind and inert to human strivings. A "coefficient of resistance" is forever involved in any human strivings in life, to use a Sartrean term.[9] We create and fashion, most often, within situations of struggle, denial, want, and the wastages of time. There is a recurrent tension between what people aspire to in their lives and the forces that shape and constrain those lives.

Poiesis can assume many forms. Among them are inclinations, in no particular or purely distinct or finite order:

> To make new things, more or less concrete or virtual
> To alter or fashion the appearances of the world
> To shape or change the consciousness of someone or something
> To construct memories
> To change the form of someone or something
> To teach something significant or lasting
> To create relations between forces in the world
> To alter the ways in which relations take form or proceed
> To forge a path, a line, or a trajectory in the world
> To bring forth something previously dormant, hidden, or
>   germinating
> To play with the forms and formations of life

To unmake something; to dissolve something or take it apart

To withhold from acting in the world

Each of these efforts plays a central role in how Hyolmo peoples go about their lives, as well as how they tend to moments of death and loss. Rituals are performed. Consciousnesses are fashioned and refashioned. Selves are made.

And selves are unmade. The procedures of dying and death often entail a poiesis of cessation, in the seemingly paradoxical sense that a dying self endeavors to dissolve its self. There is often a gentle art to dying. Dying often emerges as an active, conscious project in life, as an action to be undertaken. A person strives, often with the help of others, to create the conditions whereby she can contribute to the creative subtraction of her place within, and longing for, the world. Many strive to craft appropriate states of mind while dying. They try to dissolve their attachments to the world, visualize the forms of Buddhist deities, and contemplate the impermanent nature of all life. Through these efforts, a person can maintain some control over the dying process and be conscious of his or her passing.

Mourners, in turn, try to facilitate these endeavors on behalf of lost loved ones while trying to abate their own attachments to them. Much of the dying process and the cremation and funeral rites orbit around an intricate making of unmaking, a calm forging of undoing, dissolving, and stillness. Attachments are diminished; sensory engagements are extinguished; and the now gone one is resolved of his worldly existence. In many respects, these efforts fit well with the intent of Buddhist teachings and practices, which work toward the idea of relinquishing ego, attachments, sensory dependencies, and the sense of a solid and unchanging self in the world. Dissolving, taking away, releasing, removing until all is emptiness, until the self itself is stilled: these hard-gained endeavors apply both to Buddhist practices and Hyolmo methods of dying and post-life transformations.

In thinking of how people engage constructively in the world, we need to entertain Buddhist ideas of "taking away" and consequential "nondoing" as much as we do Western philosophical ideas of poiesis as entailing a directly active "bringing forth." Stable ideas of active and passive break down here. At the same time, the poiesis here implies a *provisional* making and fashioning, one couched in the virtuality and impermanence of its own constructedness.

Given that people usually do not engage in these efforts on their own, it's clear that much of the "bringing forth" that takes place in situations of dying and death, as in those of life, have a decidedly *social* cast to them. We're speaking, most often, of a kind of *co-poiesis*, of a collaborative fashioning and unfashioning of self and other, as well as of a *poiesis on behalf of another*. What people often bring forth, or dissolve, is on behalf of others. This is particularly crucial after a person dies, as the dead can accomplish little on their own. They must rely on the living to do this. The ritual assistance is a welcome responsibility, as the living long to act in ways that can benefit lost loved ones. These efforts at assisted cessation trip up prevalent ideas of agency in Western social and political thought, which often paint "personal agency" as being a question of actions undertaken by individuals, often while under the constraining weight of political forces. Individual action in the world is usually not from one hand only. And yet we can also envision a scene where one hand strives to erase another, or itself.

The designs most in circuit here involve social and ritual practices whose effects are to transform people or situations in some way. What are being changed are perceptions, karmic statuses, moods and longings, forms of attachment, sensual and social relations, and ways of knowing and being in the world. Each step of the way, as people die, mourn, and console, forms of consciousness are invoked, memories are revised, senses are engaged and disengaged, and selves are named and unnamed in an evolving charge of relations. The realities and virtualities generated in these moments are in line with a world familiar with tantric energies and transformative intensities. They proceed without any single author or known agent. They have powerful effects in and on life, and beyond it.

There is a singularity to many deaths. Something in the way the details of a death unfold make them stand apart from the typicality of cultural discourses and representations or any general story one might want to tell about how women and men die. Dying unsettles the same, the familiar, the expected— much as life does, when it comes down to it. It's also true that death is cultural, that dying and cessation take on particular forms in distinct social and historical settings. Most Hyolmo people desire to die in their homes, among loved ones. The dying should be at ease, surrounded by family members, relatives, and friends, without fear or longing, prepared to die. While many say it's best to die while sleeping, with an absence of awareness, others, especially those familiar with Buddhist principles, find it's important to die while awake and conscious of one's death. In that way, a person can say goodbye to loved ones in good terms and embrace new situations to come.

Others are not so fortunate. Hospitals present bad places in which to die. For most Hyolmo people, they are an unpleasant scene of medical instruments, tubes, infections, contagions, unfamiliar protocols, and operations that go well or poorly. They can be costly in the long run and far from home.

It's difficult for many family members to stay with a hospitalized person for long stretches of time, leading to a situation wherein a person might die alone or with only one or two acquaintances nearby. "When we see on television a person dying in a hospital alone," one man told me, "we say that it's a very bad death. 'What bad karma,' we say. 'Not even a chance to say goodbye.'"

Hospitals are known as spiritually impure places. The fact that many different people, including many who might be spiritually impure, have died within their confines, perhaps in the same bed that "one's own" would be assigned, make them a place of impurity (*dhip*). Such "death impurity" can further harm and weaken a person, as well as contaminate her body or consciousness if she does die. For this reason, many resist being taken to a hospital if it looks like they might die there.

In recent years, a few people living in the United States who have been gravely injured have been cared for in hospitals. They have been kept alive, while in comas, with the aid of life-support systems, attended to by family members. "That is very sad," a friend said in speaking of these situations while conversing with me in his home in Kathmandu one evening. "If a person like this had died by now, he would have already come back [been reborn]. That kind of thing is difficult for everyone. If something like this happens in Nepal, the person would die soon after getting injured. They don't have those kinds of machines here."

Unable to die, a person is stuck between lives. The tempo of a good death is obstructed. The person is also situated between two technologies of death: the Buddhist practices he and his family might know well and the biomedical procedures of a big city hospital. Once those procedures embrace an unconscious body they establish a situation often found today in American hospitals: "a prolonged hovering at the threshold between life and death," as the anthropologist Sharon Kaufman has observed. "Instead of death," Kaufman notes, "the hospital opens up an indefinite period of waiting during which patients do not cross that threshold until it is decided when it is *time* for them to die."[10] Like others in hospitals sustained through ventilators and additional life-support systems, the person enters a "zone of indistinction"—biologically alive, though only because he is "sustained by biomedical technology, and without signs of unique, purposeful life."[11]

Situations such as these throw Hyolmo families up against forms of the "new death" that is taking hold in many societies.[12] These emergent, technologically mediated ways of dying configure death as occurring not as it will appear "naturally" but "delayed, managed, and timed."[13] The medical technologies continue to such an interminable point that they beg the question, painfully felt, of whether or not a person whose body is sustained in such a way is still vitally alive. The gamut of biomedical interventions applied in hospital settings to prevent a person from dying often stand in stark contrast to forms of dying in the Hyolmo region, where there is more a sense of calm, compassionate, and patient attending to a person's cessation than any kind of radical efforts to forbid the death from happening. There is caring comfort in the face of death, but there is also a sense of quiet restraint and "practices of nondoing."[14] This sentiment can be compared to the combative zeal that medical practitioners in Europe and the United States often have in trying to preserve a life.

Ritual Poiesis

The generative dimensions of Hyolmo lives and deaths are as much in evidence in the funeral rites that follow a death as they are in the life that preceded those rites. The funeral rites, which are usually performed in the first seven weeks after the death, similarly involve ritual and sensorial means to transform situations, consciousnesses, relations, and the phenomenal grounds of people's lives. One aspect of the rites that is worth noting here is that a series of tangible images of the deceased serve to simulate the deceased's identity as it changes through time. Each of these images is first invoked, then taken away by being either burned or dismantled.

In the hours and days immediate to a death, the body is prepared for the cremation and visualized as a deity. It is then cremated in an elaborate ceremony of dissolution and ritual sacrifice.

Once the cremation is completed, a *malsa* (resting place) is made and set up in the home of the deceased. Composed of the former clothes of the dead person, this resting place serves as a way station whereby the consciousness of the deceased can remain in its former home. The malsa is later dismantled, and the clothes are discarded.

During the first main funeral rite after the death and cremation, a *jhang par* (name card) is used. This piece of paper often holds the printed figure of a human being on one of its sides and prayers on the other. The name of the dead person is written in an appropriate place in these prayers. At the crux of the ritual proceedings, a lama summons the consciousness of the deceased, then transfers it into the name card. The lama burns the print just as he "elevates" the consciousness to the Pure Land of Amitābha. The consciousness is elevated, lifted up, and transported to a purer, more enlightened realm, just as the name card, and the figure and identity inscribed within it, is dissolved into flames.

During the final funeral rite, commonly held in the seventh week after the death, a life-size effigy of the deceased is often made. Built out of the clothes of the dead person and adorned with a sheer white cloth of a face, it is set up in the place of the funeral proceedings. People tend to treat the effigy as a simulacrum of the deceased, and they often relate to it as though the dead person's consciousness is inhabiting that lifelike form. A name card is again produced and again set to flames to a flurry of dramatic music. At this moment, the effigy is dismantled into a pile of loose clothing.

The effigy's sudden dissolution serves as an object lesson in the methods of life, death, and impermanence. The presence-then-absence of the effigy nods, again, to the constructed, relational, and empty nature of all reality. The act of "dismantling the effigy" reflects a second cremation: the deceased's body is eliminated once again. Gone in a matter of seconds, it is torn asunder, disaggregated.

In effect, then, images of the deceased are made, then destroyed, time and again throughout the funeral rites. While it's difficult to say for sure why this is the case, it's evident that the making and unmaking of corpse images models the flow and ebb of life, as known by Hyolmo Buddhists and, perhaps, Buddhist peoples more generally. Composite forms arise, exist, and cease to exist. Something once constructed is soon deconstructed. People are made, then unmade. A series of minor, fleeting rebirths and sudden, dramatic re-deaths occur throughout the funeral rites. Apparently, there is a need to enact the death of a person, time and again.

Once the name card is burned for the last time, people tend not to speak the name of the dead person again in daily life. "The dead have no need for names," I have often been told. Indeed, the funeral rites as a whole trip a process of *effacement*, in which the deceased person's "name" and "face" are gradually but decisively dissolved. The body is soon covered up in a white cloth. The body is cremated. No body remains after that. The effigy carries a pure-white face. The name card, bearing the figure of a human being, is burned, after which the deceased no longer has a proper "name." Bones, ashes, and the cinders of the name card are taken and molded into generic figurines known as *tsha-tsha*, which are placed in "pure places" far removed from the traffic of everyday life. No names are inscribed on these figurines, resulting, in time, in an air of collective anonymity to the dead.

The identity of the deceased undergoes a comprehensive transmutation. What occurs is a ritually geared movement from more personalized and concrete physical representations of the deceased to more depersonalized, abstract, and collective ones. Step by ritual step, image after image, the deceased comes to be signaled in more remote, subtle, nameless, and unworldly terms. Other transitions arise, as well. The dangerous impurity and coarseness generated by the corpse alters into the purity and transcendent otherworldliness associated with figurines and relics. Corpses, effigies, and name cards are but fleeting images; the qualities central to figurines, relics, and shrines point to objects that can last for years, generations even. In this dizzying swirl of cessation and continuity, representations of the deceased skirt from the world of the living and the dying, from painful cycles of samsara and suffering, to realms removed from this world, gesturing toward the timeless and the painless.

The imagery advanced by the funeral rites serves as an object lesson in the ways of life. It teaches both the living and the dead that living forms exist, then cease to exit. The funeral rites offer a weeks-long meditation on what Hyolmo people call *chhiwa mitakpa* (death and impermanence). Form slides into emptiness, and emptiness into form. The recurrent, successive body images model the life-and-death process in a temporally abrupt, accelerated form: arising, abiding, ceasing. Something is assembled, then disassembled. "The great lesson of Buddhism," the scholar John Strong points out, "is not that of impermanence, if, by impermanence is simply meant 'nothing lasts forever.' It is rather that of process—that things, beings, buddhas come into existence due to certain causes and go out of existence due to certain causes."[15] The funeral rites convey just this lesson. A Buddhist philosophy of life and death is conveyed, but through ritual practice, rather than explicit statement or textual exegesis. Traces of a person are here, then gone, present and absent afresh, in a cycle of rebirth and re-death. Form flows into formlessness, then tides back to form and formlessness again, with neither of these ever fully complete.

An Archipelago of Care

The living work on death. They turn it. They carefully rework the nature of relations. They establish new connections when a life ends. Similar to the ways in which "neurogenesis" can occur after a stroke, in which stem cells in the adult brain multiply and send "immature neurons" to areas of damage, there is a kind of "vitagenesis" at work in people's lives in the wake of death, in which new strands of life emerge in forms both actual and virtual.

Death is often taken to be the absolute other of life. Yet it can also be said that the words *life* and *death* mark situations more complicated than that binary arrangement alone. Being alive is clearly different from not being alive; there is a "difference of kind" between the two, not simply a difference of degree.[16] Yet the ever changing flow of life and death, presence and absence, includes varying intensities and thresholds of existence, the circling of memories plush with life, moments at once actual and virtual, ghosts as real as people and people as vacant as ghosts. The end of one set of bonds leads to new strands of connection. Cessation itself is a kind of becoming. A life implies the imminent remove of that life, while the loss of a life brings a wealth of memories, feelings, and reverberations. There can be a richness to loss, much as there can be a paucity to life, making for nondualistic vitalities quick to alter. Moments of dying are found in moments of living, and vice versa.

My work with Hyolmo people has led me to appreciate better the intricate weave between life and death. I cannot say whether or not I have learned how to die—this will be revealed some future day, I suppose. But all of this anthropologizing of death in Nepal has led, I believe, to a keener take on life, territories of death included. I have come to perceive life in ways at once unnerving and exhilarating, as consisting of so many "fields of apparitions," to use the Buddhist phrasing. I now take the elements of life to be spun out of such fields of apparition, ever changing, ever shifting, juiced with remarkable energy, tied to others, vexed at times, haunted, luminous, subject to countless forms and dissolutions.

When I began this research on dying and death among Hyolmo people, I saw in death endings only, a terminus of life and relation. It's now clear that new connections take form, in vast swirls of continuity. Mourners find new ways to relate. They rethread linkages with the strands available to them. Rituals fill in the blankness. An abiding theme in many a life is the knack for crafting new conditions and relations within life. Life itself is generative, transitive, echoic. And yet so often, as well, people face continued hardships, and there is a fine, shaky line between despair and renewal.

Care is a pervasive element of Hyolmo lives and deaths—much as it is for human lives in general, as Arthur Kleinman has so poignantly conveyed in recent writings.[17] In considering Hyolmo engagements with the dying and the funeral rites that take effect after a person dies, especially in light of Kleinman's compelling writings on the significance of caregiving in human existence, it becomes clear that care is an integral aspect of responses to frailty, old age, dying, and post-life formations among Hyolmo people. Helping others to prepare for a good death; visiting the sick and dying at their homes; giving support to worried and grief-stricken family members and making them not feel so alone; providing gentle, calming care in the hours of a death in tender, unassuming ways; gathering family members to the site of a dying life; listening and heeding a dying person's last will; trying to make the death a calm and comfortable one; carefully "transferring" the consciousness out of the body after a person dies; preparing a body for cremation and then "eliminating" the corpse through transformative rituals; compassionately dissolving the identity and material existence of the lost person through a series of funeral rites that work to transform the existence of a recently deceased person and enable the possibility of spiritual liberation or a rebirth in an advantageous new life form; caring for the memory of the deceased: with all of this, Hyolmo engagements with dying and death imply, through time, a virtual archipelago of care, in which island-like acts of compassionate care appear in so many moments of everyday life and rituals of post-life transformation.

Hyolmo people approach death with an ethics of care. That sense of care is an extension of the consideration that Hyolmo people frequently pay to others throughout their lives, whether it is helping others when they are sick or in need or building a house. It is especially pronounced when another is in a condition of dying. People visit the home of a dying person, attend to her needs, satisfy desires, comfort her. Friends and family are usually present when another is dying, and they try to make that person's passing less painful and less solitary. Dying well requires the help of others; a person can't go it alone.

The philosopher Emmanuel Levinas has posited that one of the ethical obligations of human beings is to not "leave the other alone in the face of death."[18] Levinas contends that the sociality of people, based on the presence of the inescapable "face of the other," implies the obligation not to remain indifferent to the death of another, "even if responsibility then amounts only to responding, in this impotent confrontation to the death of the other, 'here I am.'"[19] We can all identify, if we're honest about it, with the occasional urge to get away from the sick and the dying, to walk away from the misery of others, if only because attending to that misery and all the crap that comes with it can be an unpleasant and thankless task. But something usually brings us back or keeps us there among those in need, responsive to their needs, before and after they die. We answer, usually, if we can, when we're called. Hyolmo communities know well this ethical responsibility and the moral breach implied when it is not heeded. "Here we are, beside you, now and later," families and neighbors appear to be saying through their actions. "We can't prevent your death. But we can make it a less painful and less lonely one."

This creative, energetic poeisis of care for the dying and the dead—and the bereaved—is open-ended. There is no finite end point in time or relation. The care seeps within the strands of relationality of everyday life; it diffuses into emptiness. While those who care for the dead are "present" in many ways, through a series of ordinary and ritual acts of care—to draw from Kleinman's important observation that care so often involves "being present" in the lives of others—those who are cared for are tangibly absent.[20] In many respects, care after a death for a recently deceased person becomes rather spectral in nature: the living caring for an absent loved one, unsure how certain gestures of care might reach that absent figure, and without receiving response or acknowledgment that the care has reached its intended subject or is effective. This spectral care is an ultimate form of care, for it occurs without response, without any certain knowledge or tangible awareness that the care reaches somewhere or someone absent.

In time, through recurrent ritual practices that are rather "memorial" in nature, people care for distant ancestors, who become increasingly absent from the lives of the living, anonymous, vague, and remote. Yet people continue to care for those distant elders, as that is what is called for. Much the same moral orientation is found within Kleinman's writings on care: care is what is called for in the lives of humans and in the anthropological study of those lives, even if such care is complicated and morally vexed at times and rather diffuse, open-ended, and spectral in nature. An anthropology of care gets at fundamental, ethically immanent aspects of human existence.

Demise Writing

My thoughts turn to narratives of dying, particularly those that I collected while conducting fieldwork in Nepal in the early 2000s. The accounts that people related to me—loose *récits*, really, culled from memory, with little explicit social or moral commentary—were matter-of-fact in their language and emotional tone and sometimes point-blank, graphic even, in their terms. To give one account:

> One of my uncles died. It was from cancer. Maybe it wasn't from cancer—actually he was suffering from TB. Was it TB, or cancer?—It's difficult to say. The sons brought him to the hospital and he was admitted there, but in the end he died at the age of sixty, due to TB.
>
> While he was dying, for him it was the most difficult death. Here and there he was hanging on, what to do? *Āiya-āmā*, so uncomfortable. For some eight, nine hours, he was very uncomfortable, the villagers had filled his house, after being so uncomfortable, he couldn't die, the breath

couldn't leave. There were so many expressions of pain [*āiya-āmā*], of being seared [*ātau āmā*], leaping, jumping in a disordered way he died. In this way he died, this man.

Writing about dying is unsettling. If thoughts of death are unnerving, then stories of dying are doubly so. Dying tears at the self. Dying tears at the world. Tending to the actual ends of people ruptures any secure sense we might gain by thinking about death as either a null point in existence or a self-contained category of thought or experience. The abstract purity of death, as an idea or ideal in the world, stands in contrast to the jittery, open-ended tracks of dying. The wrenching sharpness of dying is forever wounding, forever cutting into the flesh of life and the cold stillness of death. "It is though there is, in death, something stronger than death: dying itself—the intensity of dying," as Maurice Blanchot conveys it. For Blanchot, death is "power and even potency—and thereby limited." Dying, in contrast, is "absence of power" (*non-pouvoir*).[21] "Interrupting the present, always a crossing of the threshold, excluding all term or end, providing neither release nor shelter," Blanchot writes. "In death, it is possible to find illusory refuge. . . . Dying is the fleeting movement that draws into flight indefinitely: impossible and intensively."[22]

While I was writing *Subject to Death*, accounts of dying made up the ethnographic terrain that affected me the most (the grief of friends and acquaintances came a close second). Only after reading Blanchot's words have I been able to gain sense of why this might be so. Dying pulls indefinitely. It draws us away from any easy models of life and death and situates us in moments of pain and non-closure and a terrible, unending openness.

For Blanchot, who is in implicit conversation with Hegel and Heidegger, among others, the philosopher's concept of death implies a potential mastery and assuredness in which a person can search for authenticity in death and, potentially, become master of himself. Death is of a clear formation; within time, it appears relatively changeless. It offers an illusory refuge and holds the possibility of transcendence. Dying, in contrast, is passive, impersonal, endless, limited, strangely other. In depicting death and dying in such terms, Blanchot is not speaking solely of these forms of cessation. He is also trying to get at a certain, dissonant ontology of existence, one that attends to a "strange, insectlike buzzing in the margins."[23] At the same time, Blanchot seeks to express an orientation, through writing, that attends to the incessant dying, weakness, passivity, and dissolution that shadows many situations in life. Dying, for Blanchot (*le mourir*) is, in contrast to death (*la mort*), something beyond subjective or temporal horizon, beyond clear-cut meaning and conceptualization, beyond power or possibility. Dying is on a par with the disastrous, the collapse of existence, the end of a world and a self's relation to it, ruptures in perception and time, and the liquidation of stable meaning and knowledge. Writing should attend to the inassimilable force of such disasters while working in correlation with the dissolutions involved. Blanchot advocated that one write not simply to destroy, conserve, or transmit but "in the thrall of the impossible real, that share of disaster wherein every reality, safe and sound, sinks."[24] This is, in part, what he meant by the phrase "writing of the disaster" (*l'écriture du désastre*), the title of one of his later books.

To think the way one dies: without purpose, without power, without unity, and precisely, without "the way."[25]

What would be involved if one were to think, anthropologically, within an interval of dying—to write, that is, from a fractured space of weakness and of nonmastery, without power, without unity or determination, without potency and domination, without the strength of a clear "way"?

This writing would entail a modality that approaches the singularity of the extreme, an "un-story" that bears ruptures, effacement, exposure, excess. Such writing would rest on fragile, awkward discourses that are torn, incapable, feverish, violent; where hallucinations are as real and unstable as white blood cell counts; where the writing transpires within an intermediate between, implying not just ethnography but a "phantasmography," in which the phenomenal and the phantasmal are deeply intertwined.[26] This thinking and dying would require an "exigency of strangeness."[27] It would proceed in relation to alterity, an otherness that exceeds our grasp; dying is always other. This modality of knowing would know faintly of nonknowing, a deprivation of sure truths and clear foresight. Such writing would attend to the many little deaths and grand deaths encountered in life. It would reflect and inhabit a "wounded space, the hurt of the dying"; an unceasing, passive, neutral dying; "broken reserve, a deep cut in the possibility of any cut at all."[28]

The writing would attend to the materialities and vitalities of life, the matter of bodies and technologies, without rending this all into a formal, interpreted whole. It would heed "the danger that the disaster acquire meaning instead of body."[29] The writing would suggest a perilous threshold between being and nonbeing, "an exhaustion of appearance," wherein the subject becomes absence, where words imply less a subject with a subjectivity than a "subjectivity without any subject," with no fixed and stable subject position or truth in perspective.[30] The name wears away, and words as such would "cease to be arms: means of action, means of salvation."[31] Words would assume, rather, an air of dissolution, subtraction, passivity. There is being and becoming, yes; but there is also dying, disarray, and the receding absence of will, presence, and power.

Living these days carries a fair share of dying, and our modalities of perception and writing should reflect this. We should locate ways to write about what it means to live in a dying world. We also need creative and thoughtful apprehensions of this process—we need a poeisis, a creative, generative engagement that entails the undoing of certain modes of thought and forms of power, knowledge, and capability, which, while seemingly true and powerful, can work to undermine certain systems of life. We need to care for absence, and those who are absent, and anticipate further losses; we need to care, creatively, for dissolution and creative transformation. We also need to strike out what is injurious to life and death. There is value in relinquishing certain presumptions and ways of thinking and being. To continue on in life, we need to learn to die in some ways. We need to fall apart and take on new forms of emergent life. We need to find ways to live with less; to accept limited agency and finite possibilities; to know weakness and uncertainty; and to comprehend the complicated, interwoven processes involved in change, disassembling, and renewal. A contemporary art of living requires an art of dying. The call on us is to approach an orientation similar, perhaps, to the transformative *making of unmaking* that Hyolmo Buddhists know within the span of their lives. This orientation also implies one of care; care for the living and the dying; a care for dissolution and transformation; care and appreciation for changing forms of life and death; care for the future, for the past and present; care for wrecked life and continued life; compassionate care for others; spectral care for those absent or faintly present; frail, uncertain care for what is not there or no longer there.

"When all is said," wrote Blanchot, "what remains to be said is the disaster. Ruin of words, demise writing, faintness faintly murmuring."[32]

In this time of the disastrous, when so much appears to be in demise, it may be that what is most called for, anthropologically, is a certain kind of demise writing in which one writes within an intensity of dissolution. This implies a poeisis of frailty and weakness within the arc of a creative, uncertain, open-ended dying. If to anthropologize can be to learn how to die, then by writing in a mode of dying we might learn how to live, and thus care more in life, for life as well as for death and for dying remnants of life, in a changing, possibly dying world. Through moments of creative living—and dying—new forms of life might emerge.

Notes

Special thanks to Arthur Kleinman for inviting me to contribute this chapter to the present volume and to Vincanne Adams and João Biehl for their perceptive reflections on an earlier version of the chapter.

1 | Critchley, *The Book of Dead Philosophers*, xv–xvi.
2 | Desjarlais, *Subject to Death*.
3 | See, e.g., Desjarlais, *Body and Emotion*; Desjarlais, *Sensory Biographies*; Desjarlais, *Subject to Death*.
4 | I take the term *spectral subject* from Boulter, *Beckett*.
5 | See, e.g., Arendt, *The Human Condition*; Heidegger, *The Question Concerning Technology, and Other Essays*; Lambek, *A Reader in the Anthropology of Religion*; Stewart, "Cultural Poesis."
6 | On this see, Lambek, *A Reader in the Anthropology of Religion*, 15–16.
7 | See, e.g., Gyatso, "The Ins and Outs of Self-transformation."
8 | See, e.g., Deleuze, *Difference and Repetition*; Ingold, *Making*; Ingold, "The Textility of Making"; Jackson, *Life within Limits*; Spinoza, *The Collected Works of Spinoza*; Stewart, "Cultural Poesis."
9 | Sartre, *Search for a Method*, xii.
10 | Kaufman, *And a Time to Die*, 4.
11 | Kaufman, *And a Time to Die*, 98.
12 | Lock, "Inventing a New Death and Making It Believable."
13 | Green, *Beyond the Good Death*, 47.
14 | Sedgwick, *Touching Feeling*, 175.
15 | Strong, *Relics of the Buddha*, 6.
16 | To use terms from Deleuze, *Difference and Repetition*, 4.
17 | See, e.g., Kleinman, "Caregiving"; Kleinman, "Forum." See also Kleinman's afterword in this volume.
18 | Levinas, *Entre Nous*, 112.
19 | Levinas, *Entre Nous*, 128.
20 | See Kleinman's afterword in this volume.
21 | Blanchot, *The Writing of the Disaster*, 47, translation modified. I follow here the modified translation in Hill, *Maurice Blanchot and Fragmentary Writing*, 303.
22 | Blanchot, *The Writing of the Disaster*, 47, translation modified. I follow here the modified translation of Hill, *Maurice Blanchot and Fragmentary Writing*, 303.
23 | Blanchot, *The Work of Fire*, 333.
24 | Blanchot, *The Writing of the Disaster*, 38.
25 | Blanchot, *The Writing of the Disaster*, 39.
26 | Desjarlais, *The Blind Man*.
27 | Blanchot, *The Infinite Conversation*, 129.
28 | Blanchot, *The Writing of the Disaster*, 8, 30.
29 | Blanchot, *The Writing of the Disaster*, 41.
30 | Blanchot, *The Writing of the Disaster*, 30.
31 | Blanchot, *The Writing of the Disaster*, 11.
32 | Blanchot, *The Writing of the Disaster*, 33.

Ethnographic Open

Portals

There is always a time when reason fails us.

An unexpected or protracted illness, the untimely passing of a loved one, a destroyed home, the violence of being too poor and without a right to health.

Trust in life is gone.

Why me? Why now? Who cares? Where to?

Questions that death in all its forms poses to afflicted bodies and that science cannot disappear.

We are not machines after all.

In pain we seek Others. We pray for relief. We want language. We plot a hereafter.

Something that can make us feel human and desired again.

Or so we tell ourselves in order to endure.

Overwhelmed, it finally dawns on us that we hold "dual citizenship, in the kingdom of the well and in the kingdom of the sick," as Susan Sontag poignantly notes in *Illness as Metaphor*.[1] Whether in the flesh or in solidarity, we, too, realize that belonging to the kingdom of the well is not evenly distributed: structural determinants and entrenched markers of difference significantly shape variations in morbidity and mortality.

Here is where the artist comes into the picture.

Consider LaToya Ruby Frazier's powerful diptych *Landscape of the Body (Epilepsy Test)* (figure 11.1)—how she juxtaposes the torn-down community hospital of her hometown, Braddock, Pennsylvania, with her mother's testing in a nearby medical facility in Pittsburgh, "where patients were being sent to justify the closing" of the local hospital.[2] These images are part of the autobiographical project *The Notion of Family*, in which Frazier exposes the environmental predation, state disinvestment, and toxicity—call it "slow violence"—that mark the life chances of generations of African Americans in Braddock surviving America's boom-and-bust cycles.[3]

"Photographs are a means of making 'real' (or 'more real') matters that the privileged and the merely safe might prefer to ignore," Susan Sontag points out in her last book, *Regarding the Pain of Others*.[4] Being a spectator of calamities is, after all, "a quintessential modern experience" through which the other is rendered as someone to be seen, "not someone (who like us) also sees."[5] While such a photographic enactment might occasion a fleeting sense of compassion, it is ultimately depoliticizing in its detachment.

Frazier rips such a reductive mode of nonengagement apart. Hers is "a public account of the private life of a working-class African-American family made by a daughter with a camera, from within, instead of by a sociologist with a camera, from without."[6] By looking "both inwardly and outwardly," the artist brings together the familial and the communal in compositions that thwart disregard and (en)closure. She does so by drawing from her kin's lived "file," composed of artifacts and gestures that defy easy classification as past, present, or future; despairing or hopeful—"My mother did not have to read Roland Barthes to understand death in a photograph"—and her own desire "to move beyond boundaries."[7] Desire in Frazier's scenes of decay and survival appears grim, and care is often an act of frustration, a behind-the-scenes affective grappling by gendered bodies in complicity, love, and aggression, in the face of a battered history.

As life goes on, debris remains unsettled in Frazier's "ethnographic sensorium."[8] Her familial characters keep remaking life, even within the precarious political space that Stefano Harney and Fred Moten call "the in-

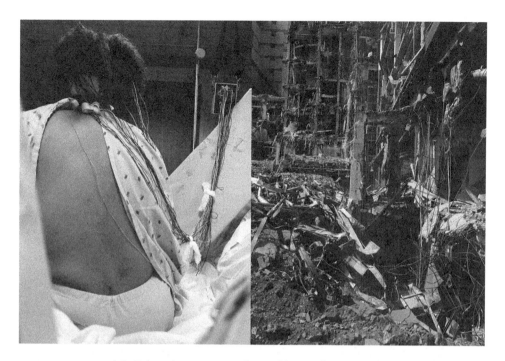

FIGURE 11.1 | LaToya Ruby Frazier, *Landscape of the Body (Epilepsy Test)*, 2011. Gelatin silver print, 61 × 101.6 cm. Princeton University Art Museum. Museum purchase, Hugh Leander Adams, Mary Trumbull Adams, and Hugh Trumbull Adams Princeton Art Fund. © LaToya Ruby Frazier.

determinate."[9] There is thus "a subtle balance of surrealism and realism in each image," the artist says of her work, "a portal or slippage between what is rendered real and not real; the reality of what is physically in front of my camera versus the darkness in the atmosphere that surrounds me."[10]

Fazal Sheikh's arresting image of Qurban Gul in an Afghan refugee village in northern Pakistan (figure 11.2) works as a portal, too: an open passage toward an atmosphere of one's own.

There is so much more than powerlessness in what constitutes the portrait of this grieving mother. She seizes what matters most to her and summons it into focus. As Teju Cole notes, the artist gets it: "A photograph of a face is a photograph, not a face."[11] We are left with a productive absence that exceeds the frame. First, we will never know all Qurban Gul has lived through: "Can't understand, can't imagine."[12] Then, there is her immanent sense that muddles with the intentioned, studied focus of the caring portraitist living with and learning from Gul's displaced community: *a love supreme*.[13] The trace weighs so heavily on Qurban Gul that it takes her place: a cherished image of the child that is no more. The powers of the image—the materiality of the past and its reverberation—are here the very stuff of art.

I am drawn to the unrelenting ways Sheikh's and Frazier's artworks expose brutal political economies undoing lifeworlds and disfiguring peoples'

FIGURE 11.2 | Fazal Sheikh, Qurban Gul, holding a photograph of her son, Mula Awaz, Afghan refugee village, Khairabad, North Pakistan, 1998. Inkjet print, 61 × 61 cm. Princeton University Art Museum. Promised gift of Liana Theodoratou in honor of Eduardo Cadava. © Fazal Sheikh.

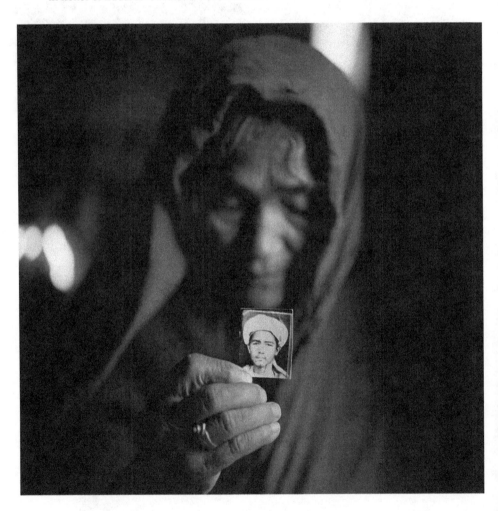

worlding capacities—"the real war" that "will never get in the books," in Walt Whitman's words.[14] All the while, the artists insist on their interlocutors' radical singularities and unfinished stories. In doing so, Sheikh and Frazier approximate peoples' arts of existence, if you will—a vital imaginative force the anthropologist Zora Neale Hurston (who collected folklore from her African American community in Florida in the 1920s) would call "that which the soul lives by."[15]

With their incorporation of the dehumanizing horrors of inequality and war, coupled with their receptiveness to the images and stories "the soul lives by," Frazier's and her mother's and Sheikh's and Qurban Gal's artistic creations (not possible without a relation with each other) challenge the formal boundaries of the artwork and leave us with a probing, unfinished aesthetic excess. Various invisibles lurk behind the reality of these coauthored images: environmental poisoning, economic precarity, familial decay, the war coming home. And underneath it all lurks the presence of time, for it is time that makes poisoning, precarity, decay and the impossibility of love perceptible and mutual becomings sensible. Underlying these aesthetic works are techniques of attunement that retrain our sensorium.

How can peoples' image-survivals (let's keep them plural) become alternative figures of ethical and political thought, holding them open to a distinct futurity?

"Dead alive, dead outside, alive inside."

Come near, Catarina.

The barely literate young woman is writing her "dictionary" in Vita, an asylum in the city of Porto Alegre, in southern Brazil, where the ill and unwanted are left to perish (figure 11.3).[16]

"What I was in the past does not matter."

Abandoned by her family and medics, she invents a new name for herself—Catkine—drawing from the drug Akineton, one of many that mediated her social death and supposed madness.

"Mine is an illness of time," she tells me.

With increasingly poor motor skills, Catarina/Catkine refuses to be reduced to her physical condition and fate. She wants to engage, and I have the gut feeling that something important for sustaining her life and knowledge is going on that I do not want to miss. Her words point to routine abandonment and silencing; yet, in spite of all the disregard she experiences, Catarina conveys an astonishing agency. Once I find myself on her side, we are both

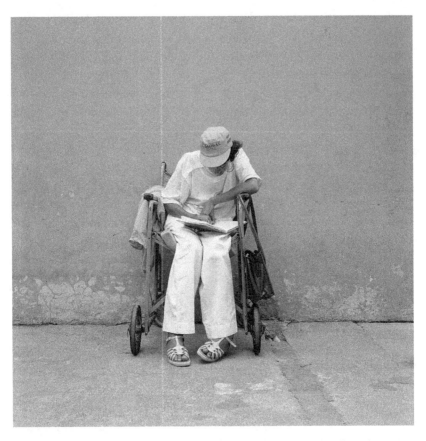

FIGURE 11.3 | *Catarina and Her Dictionary in Vita,* 2001. Photograph by Torben Eskerod.

against the wall of language. Language is not a point of separation but of relation—and comprehension is involved.

This work is not about the person of my thoughts and the impossibility of representation or of becoming a figure for Catarina's psychic forms. It is about human contact enabled by contingency and a disciplined listening that gives each one of us something to look for. "I lived kind of hidden, an animal," Catarina tells me, "but then I began to draw the steps and to disentangle the facts with you." In speaking of herself as an animal, Catarina finds her own way, engaging the human possibilities foreclosed for her: "I began to disentangle the science and the wisdom. It is good to disentangle oneself, and thought, as well."

As for the new letter character she created that resembled a *k* (not part of the Brazilian alphabet at the time), Catarina/Catkine explains, "It is open on both sides. If I wouldn't open the character, my head would explode. . . . I have desire, I have desire."

When the photographer, Torben Eskerod, attempts a close-up, Catarina tilts her head and poses like a model (figure 11.4).

"Try to stay still. No need to smile. Just be natural," Torben says.

"Torben is a portraitist," I add. "He likes to focus on the gaze; he wants to get to the soul of those he portrays."

To which, she replies: "What if in the end he only finds his own?"

Catarina now directs the shooting. "I need my hair comb." I help her open the handbag—her sole property. Catarina takes her cap off and straightens her thick hair. "I am a real woman," she says: "Now photograph me."

At a certain distance, each eye is a freestanding entity: the image of a defiant *multi sighted* subject (figure 11.5).

In her writing, Catarina is herself producing an ethnographic theory of the leftover subject, the *it* she became:

> *Catarina is subjected*
> *To be a nation in poverty*
> *Porto Alegre*
> *Without an heir*
> *Enough*
> *I end*

She places the individual and the collective in the same plane of analysis, just as the country and the city collide in Vita. Subjection has to do with having no money in a nation gone awry. The subject is a body left in Vita without ties to her life with the "ex-husband" who, as she states, now "rules the city" from which she is banished. With nothing to leave behind and no one to leave it to, Catarina's singularity remains—at once the medium through which a collectivity is ordered in terms of lack and an affective state through which she disentangles herself from the killing machine the world has become.

Here she faces the concrete limits of what a human can bear and makes use of polysemy to push against those limits: "I, who am where I go, am who am so." In Catarina/Catkine's words, real and imaginary voyages compose a set of intertwined routes: "I am a free woman, to fly, bionic woman, separated. . . . When men throw me into the air, I am already far away."

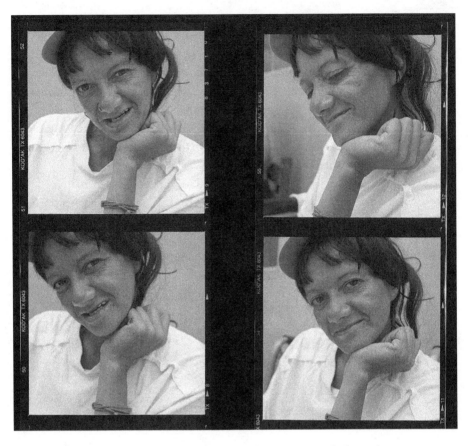

FIGURE 11.4 | *Catarina in Vita, Contact Sheet 1*, 2001. Photographs by Torben Eskerod.

Catarina/Catkine is, in a single instant, both up in the air and entirely elsewhere. We must not hear this as a mere trick or illusion. Amid social erasure and pharmaceuticalized stupor, hers is a hardy if fleeting mode of existence, with its own kind of generativity: a call for as many creatures as possible, human and otherwise, to be wholly engaged yet "already far away."

Like Catarina and the artists, Arthur Kleinman uses his notion of "social and moral experience" to place the individual alongside the collective, the historical, and the macro-structural in the same analytic plane.[17] The anthropologist thinks against dangerously distorted technocratic metrics, as well as

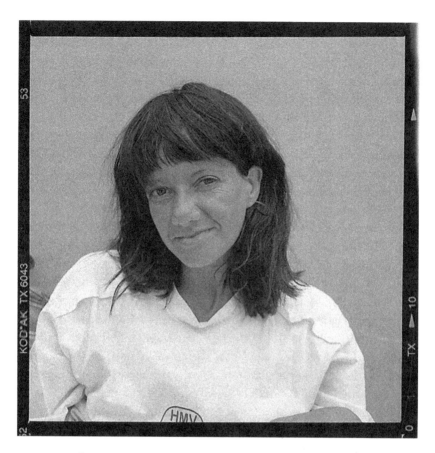

FIGURE 11.5 | *Catarina in Vita, Contact Sheet 2*, 2001. Photograph by Torben Eskerod.

critical theories couched on the total expropriation of experience.[18] Whatever is at stake in a given moment—whether it is an illness, a religious identity, a political project, an economic interest, or a set of relationships—is always embedded in the shifting exigencies of practical, everyday life as it unfolds in particular space-times. In dealing with affliction, peoples are "archivists researching a disorganized file of past experiences."[19] These vast fields of play and techniques of transposition challenge the fixity of the modes of expression with which we are familiar.

Over the years, as part of his efforts to move away from biologically deterministic and atomistic conceptions of the self, as well as the alternatives proposed by posthuman philosophical dead-ends, Kleinman has engaged with artworks to attend to the amalgamation of violence, angst, and solidarity that accompanies "human conditions" in both their disfiguring and their reconfiguring in "local moral worlds."[20] Seen in this light, the anthropologist appears as an "artist manqué" who, against myopic thinking and reductionisms of all kinds, insists on representing the infirmities of the world alongside peoples' life bricolage, their ability to make things anew.

I first met Arthur Kleinman in person in the fall of 1997 at the University of California, Berkeley, where I was carrying out my doctoral studies. After a long flight, generous meetings with students, and fighting symptoms of a cold, Kleinman found himself amid a large audience, talking about the transformations in engagements with pain and suffering that have accompanied the encroachment of technical rationalities and business interests in American medicine. While displaying Pablo Picasso's surreal *Head of the Medical Student* (with a closed eye and an enlarged ear [figure 11.6]), he critiqued biomedical algorithms and bioethical caricatures and reaffirmed unquantifiable values, intense emotional involvement, and sustained listening as crucial building blocks of a moral medical practice.[21] During the heated Q&A that followed, faculty members subjected Kleinman to a barrage of provocative questions—not about what he called "the divided self," but over his "usage of art." Kleinman disarmed every expert trap seeking to theoretically discipline the power of the image by responding on a personal register: "I think I use it because I am an artist manqué."

This statement added a different perspective to my reading of "The Appeal of Experience; the Dismay of Images," which Arthur and Joan Kleinman had just published. In the essay, the Kleinmans examined the South African photographer Kevin Carter's ghastly 1993 image of a collapsed emaciated toddler being stalked by a vulture in the famine-ravaged village of Ayod, in southern Sudan. Published by the *New York Times*, the photograph would be awarded a prestigious Pulitzer Prize. By then the image of the child and the vulture had already become a wrenching case study in the ethics of photojournalistic nonengagement or intervention, as well as in debates about the political work of depictions of calamity and suffering.[22] Shock certainly has its term limits, and compassion can become an abstraction, evincing both one's privileges and one's implication in the reality portrayed.[23]

The Kleinmans thus read Carter's image making (devoid of the forms of reflexivity and relationality enfolded into the photographs of, for example, Frazier, Sheik, and Eskerod) as emblematic of a present-day process of thinning out and commodifying experience—a global phenomenon that, in turn, corroborated a sense of the intractability of human misery and inequality, fostering "moral fatigue, exhaustion of empathy, and political

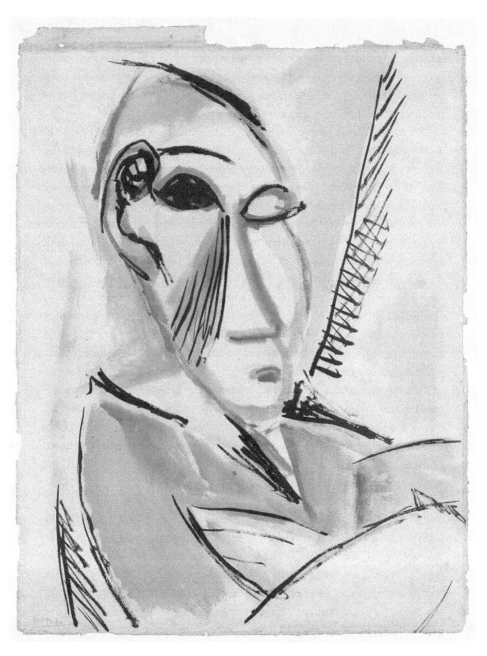

FIGURE 11.6 | Pablo Picasso, *Head of the Medical Student* (Study for *Les Demoiselles d'Avignon*), Paris, spring 1907. Gouache and watercolor on paper, 23 ¾ × 18 ½ in (60.3 × 47 cm). New York, Museum of Modern Art (MoMA). A Conger Goodyear Fund. 00014.52.

despair."[24] Indeed, in July 1994, Carter took his own life. The note he left behind speaks to the toll those "vivid" images took on him, even if his own moral and personal entanglements remained outside the photograph's frame: "I'm really, really sorry. . . . I am haunted by the vivid memories of killings & corpses & anger & pain . . . of starving or wounded children, of trigger-happy madmen, often police, of killer executioners."[25]

But to me, Kleinman's candid utterance—"I think I use it because I am an artist manqué"—also suggested that art is not merely supplemental to the anthropological enterprise. In our engagements with artistic forms of expression, we can amateurishly expand art's institutional boundaries, gatekeeping techniques, and social impacts. The artist and the ethnographer may share an interdependent set of moral, aesthetic, relational, and humanistic commitments. Seen in this light, the Kleinmans' critique of the commodification of suffering (aligned with Sontag's argument in *On Photography*) is not merely a call to obsessively police image making or to halt the quest for representation altogether. For not to try to represent at all, Kleinman continually reminds us, is perhaps the greater failure.[26] The challenge is to articulate a relational, emancipatory reflexivity and to try to ethnographically chart—and then convey—the intricacies of how large-scale forces relate to local histories and biographies, restoring context and particularity to the lived experiences of those represented. Certainly, Kleinman's own ethnographic corpus, colored by his simultaneous commitments as a clinician and an anthropologist, eludes any possible characterization as merely dispassionate representation. Like the families of Frazier and Qurban Gul, Kleinman is challenged to make himself multiple through artistic engagement. He holds the range of his scholarship and practice open.

More than a decade later, in *The Lancet*'s "Perspectives," Kleinman would again draw attention to the attunement that art may conjure, this time vis-à-vis his long-term commitments to resisting the encroachment of technocratic regimes of rationality toward medical practice.[27] In the piece, in which Picasso's watercolor sketch appeared again, Kleinman notes that an engagement with art can help build a "critical, aesthetically alert, and morally responsive" sensibility that is fundamental to the art of care and to the goal of repeopling medicine.[28] That is, the capacity to grow out of oneself, "of making the past and the strange one body with the near and the present"—a plastic power of sorts—enables a distinct human presence amid all kinds of inadequacies and constraints as one seeks "to heal wounds, replace what is lost, repair broken molds."[29] Once again, Kleinman draws us to the primacy of relationality in what art, ethnography, and care are built on: as medical students examine Picasso's depiction of themselves, his interpellation stimulates "a sensibility of critical self-reflection as part of caregiving."[30]

In this rendering, art and caregiving come out of a *mancus* state (Latin for maimed or infirmed). As needed and desirable as technical fixes might be, it is the process of *bricolage* that makes the future healer. In Claude Lévi-Strauss's classical work on the "science of the concrete," a *bricoleur* assembles a "heterogeneous repertoire" from the concreteness of existence. The elements are collected or retained on the principle that "they may always come in handy."[31] "Taking the patient's history is as much art as science," Kleinman adds. "Treatment is pastoral care as well as pharmacological rationality."[32] An artist manqué. "Film, biography, social history, the novel, and ethnography" together cultivate a critical sensibility in the face of the task in hand.[33]

Kleinman's manifold careers as a clinician, ethnographer, and mentor—bringing a humanistic sensibility to an increasingly technical medical practice *and* inspiring academics and activists to dramatically rectify health systems toward equity and quality of care—evinces an awareness that not even art can always fully account for, much less redeem: life's onslaught. Time and again, our sensibilities run up against the brute realities of precarity, structural violence, and situational foreclosure. I vividly recall the occasion when Catarina/Catkine became so enraged that she threw to the ground the dictionary I thought was keeping her alive. I had just told her that I had been unable to convince her family to schedule a visit. Writing, in the end, could not take her back home—what she desired most. And yet . . .

Sharing a critical orientation toward traditional hierarchies, the artist and the anthropologist-cum-artist manqué are after "a strange life in circulation, a vital force," one could say—a voyage and storytelling that evokes particular forms of care and possibilities for what exists and what might exist.[34] The creativity of ethnography arises from our deeply implicated and always incomplete efforts to learn from people's own painstaking arts of living.[35] Life bricolage—what people make, often agonizingly, out of whatever is available to them to endure the terminal force of their realities—is a form of art of its own, "a new language within language."[36]

While struggling to go on and heal, individuals and communities disentangle themselves from the known and establish new relations (or not), negotiate threatening detours and the newly uncertain, and make use of these very realities to craft viable forms of existence and project themselves into a future—or simply remain in suspension amid the collapse of messianic promises. As people face the engineered and the false, the arbitrary and the contingent, they carve out footholds and surprising escapes: if only we can find ways of attending to them.[37] While these openings may ultimately lead nowhere and futurity struggles with futility and a sense of the inevitable, people can simultaneously be stuck and do things—and navigating such contradictions does not amount to nothing. Experimental and radically unpredictable, ethnographic subjects imprint our own doing, thinking, writing and imaging with the indeterminate.

Returns

Ethnographic subjects allow us to return to the place where thought is born.

In what follows, I return to my work with Catarina/Catkine and focus on the unexpected encounters that followed her passing in 2003 to reflect on how fieldwork engagements draw us into an *ethnographic open*. Ethnography is a way of both staying connected to the plasticity of lifeworlds and offsetting the ruse of overdetermination and the foreclosure of knowledge. In other words, ethnography is made of encounters that exceed the conditions of its existence. It uncovers "in the name of who knows what pallid certainties," as Pierre Clastres writes, "a field to which it remains blind . . . one that fails to limit concepts such as mind, soul, body, and ecstasy but at the center of which Death mockingly poses its question."[38]

Moving across immanent fields, questions, relationships, and stories that have animated my work in and out of Vita over time, I am drawn to this ethnographic open—rife with myriad entanglements, double binds, unforeseens, and leakages—and the dialectical flickers engendered therein.[39] These traces carry the suspended imminence of worlds and peoples' creative renderings—"atmospheric attunements," always on the verge of disappearance, as Kathleen Stewart would say—that facilitate the conditions for critical inquiry into how the figure of the human is transformed over time, allowing us to trace the limits and possibilities of "horizoning" and solidarity.[40] The work of ethnography and the returns it propels thus sustain "this event, within the image"—the erratic, interstitial imaging through and beyond the threat of annihilation.[41]

Catarina refused her own erasure and even anticipated an exit from Vita. It was as difficult as it was ethically imperative to sustain this anticipation: to find ways to support Catarina's search for ties to people and the world and her demand for continuity—or, at least, its possibility. Attempting to grasp the intricate infrastructural and intersubjective tensions at the core of Vita and Catarina's life not only revealed the present as embattled and unfinished; it also displaced dominant analytical frameworks, thus marking the ethnographic work as a birthplace of sorts out of which a mode of inquiry, a method of narration, and the possibility of a new and distinct public could take form. I say public, for ours is a practice that also begs for the emergence of a third, as Vincent Crapanzano points out: a reader, a community of sorts, that is neither the character nor the writer, which will manifest and carry forward anthropology's potential to become a mobilizing force in this world.[42]

To put it in more scholarly language, I think I return to Catarina/Catkine much as a field of discourse refers back to its founder or founding moment at each step of its testing and evolution. In his lecture "What Is an Author?" Michel Foucault reminded his audience that "the return to" is not merely a historical supplement or ornament: "On the contrary, it constitutes an effective and necessary task of transforming the discursive practice itself."[43]

I feel that I owe these returns, and the unfinishedness they sustain, to Catarina. For me, this raises the question of what distinguishes the subject of anthropology from that of science. "The fact is that science, if one looks at it closely, has no memory," Jacques Lacan stated. "Once constituted, it forgets the circuitous path by which it came into being."[44] Is it, in part, this form of forgetting that permits the sense of certainty in scientific claims to truth?

In science (and in philosophy, for that matter), human subjects appear, by and large, as sharply bounded, generic, and overdetermined, if they are present at all. But ethnography allows other pathways and potentials for its subjects—and for itself. In our returns to the encounters that shaped us, and the knowledge of human conditions we produced, we can learn from our experiences anew, live them differently, acknowledging an inexhaustible richness and mystery at the core of the people we learn from.

One thinks of what allowed Lévi-Strauss to write *Tristes Tropiques*. "Time, in an unexpected way, has extended its isthmus between life and myself," he recalled. "Twenty years of forgetfulness were required before I could establish communion with my earlier experience, which I had sought the world over without understanding its significance or appreciating its essence."[45]

Lévi-Strauss also spoke of the physical objects and sensations that can help us feel and think through the peoples and worlds that become a part of us. He opened the collection of photographs *Saudades do Brasil* (Nostalgia for Brazil) with this beautiful moment of Proustian precarity, the curious memory of an odor:

When I barely open my notebooks, I still smell the creosote with which, before setting off on an expedition, I used to saturate my canteens to protect them from termites and mildew. . . . Almost undetectable after more than half a century, this trace instantly brings back to me the savannas and forests of Central Brazil, inseparably bound with other smells . . . as well as with sounds and colors. For as faint as it is now, this odor—which for me is a perfume—is the thing itself, still a real part of what I have experienced.[46]

For Lévi-Strauss, photographs did not incite this same return to lived experience. "Photographs leave me with the impression of a void, a lack of something the lens is inherently unable to capture," he lamented.[47] They exhibit the deadly force of modern times, the evisceration of the diversity of humans, animals, plants. And yet the anthropologist presents us both forms of memory together: the hollow clarity of the photographic anthology and the tantalizing whiff of distilled tar inviting anew the imagination of what lies in the interstices between these images.

Ethnography is not just proto-philosophy but a way to stay connected to open-ended, even furtive, social processes and uncertainties—a way to counterbalance certainties and foreclosures produced by other disciplines and a method of illuminating the disavowals needed to sustain those semblances of truth.

There are, of course, many ways to return to our ethnographic sites and subjects or to reengage notes, memories, and visual archives. In my work, I found that physically returning to ethnographic sites and subjects may enable a distinctive longitudinal perspective to emerge, allowing insight not only into how time works on our own senses and sensibilities but also (and perhaps most importantly) into how the world itself shifts—an entry into a worldly arc, if you will, from shifting horizon to shifting horizon. Such returns enable us to trace the tissues that connect then and now, opening up a critical space to examine what happens in the meantime (given a sense of the archness of our work): how a life story transforms, how injury is dodged or passed on, how change actually takes place, and what sustains the intractability of intolerable conditions—as in my own returns to Vita over the years and new entanglements with Catarina's offspring.

Catarina passed away in September 2003, a few weeks after I had last seen her. I was shocked by the news, for when I last talked to Catarina, her physical condition seemed to be improving. Oscar, Vita's chief caretaker, had kept his promise and made sure that she was regularly taken to a genetic medicine clinic for regular checkups on the progression of her ataxia (Machado-Joseph disease) and related speech therapy. She was excited when I told her that, with the medical diagnostic in hand, we would begin procedures to get her a disability pension. Despite much pain in her joints, Catarina kept writing, and she wanted to make sure that I could read her writing—which I barely could. Catarina wanted to get out of the wheelchair, she said, and she began to weep: "I need to go to Novo Hamburgo, to get my documents. Another person cannot get them for me.... I want to go home."

What stayed in my mind as I left that day was Oscar saying: "They don't have the right to be persons." And then Catarina's comment: "I am part of the origins, not just of language, but of people.... I represent the origins of the person." Two weeks later, Oscar called to tell me of her passing. The women in the dorm told Oscar that during the night, Catarina had called for her mother many times and then fallen silent. The next morning, she was found dead.

Laura Jardim, the doctor who was overseeing Catarina's treatment, was positive that she could not have died from complications from Machado-Joseph disease and requested an autopsy. The autopsy revealed that Catarina died as a result of intestinal bleeding—the wear and tear of Vita, the silent work of killing, I still think.

It was eerie to return to southern Brazil in August 2005 knowing that Catarina would not be there.

I wanted to get a headstone for Catarina's grave and decided to visit Vera and Marino, the adoptive parents of her youngest daughter, Andrea. The couple had helped to organize Catarina's burial in Novo Hamburgo's public cemetery. The family, as Oscar had told me, "at least took the dead body home." Andrea was helping at the family's restaurant when I arrived. At thirteen, she had a face and gaze that were indeed extensions of Catarina's, attesting to the continuance of her life story.

Vera did most of the talking. She lambasted every single member of Catarina's family, saying how "fake" they had all behaved during the funeral. Only Nilson, Catarina's ex-husband, had shown "respect," by offering to help defray some of the funeral's costs.

It was striking how Catarina's story continued to shift in the years following her death. In people's recollections, she was no longer seen as "the mad woman." Both Vera and the relatives I saw later that week now spoke of Catarina as having "suffered a lot."

As true as this was, such renderings left unaddressed the everyday practices that had compounded Catarina's intractability—most obviously, the cold detachment that accompanied care conceived solely as pharmaceutical

FIGURE 11.7
Catarina's
Tombstone, 2011.
Photograph
by Torben
Eskerod.

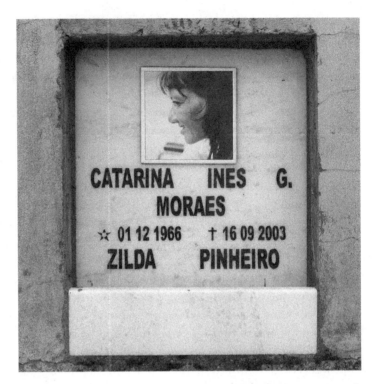

CATARINA INES G. MORAES
☆ 01 12 1966   † 16 09 2003
ZILDA PINHEIRO

intervention rather than as a relational practice that exceeds such rationality. Indeed, the plot of a life story is never securely in the possession of its subject. It is part of the ongoing moral work of those who live on.

The story of a life is always also the story of a death. And it is up to us to project the story into the future, helping shape its afterlife. Catarina had been buried in a crypt together with her mother's remains. I made sure that the crypt was fully paid for so that, in the future, their remains would not be thrown into the mass grave at the edge of the cemetery. And Vera was going to oversee the making of a marble headstone with Catarina's name engraved on it, along with a photo taken by my longtime collaborator and friend Torben Eskerod: a beautiful image of Catarina smiling from that day when we discussed whose soul was going to be held in the portrait (figure 11.7), an image that no one could take away.

That winter I also returned to Vita.

Inside the infirmary, things had only gotten worse. The bedridden were not even brought into the sun's meager warmth. I asked for Iraci, Catarina's good friend. I found him crouched in bed. He said he was happy to see me and began to cry silently. So did I. Yes, Catarina had died "all of a sudden," as had India, the young woman Iraci called his wife and had so dearly looked after. He then asked this simple and piercing question, which still haunts me: "Did you bring the tape recorder?"

I had not. Now it was his time to tell the story.

Iraci—much like Catarina—called on the ethnographer to help give shape to his own life story.

In the lecture "Tell My Story," the literary scholar Stephen Greenblatt follows his "compulsive fascination with the power and pleasure of stories" to explore the human need for life stories through a discussion of the Judeo-Christian origin myth.[48] While the Book of Genesis imagines the origin of life and glosses the lives of Adam and Eve with a few sparse details, Apocryphal texts are concerned with what happened after the fall. "Genesis tells us what it would have been like to be human, but not have human life stories," yet the Apocrypha, Greenblatt says, "grope to supply these details."

Greenblatt is also drawn to Shakespeare's *King Lear* as he reflects on human longevity beyond reproductive life—that is, that which is "least relevant to the biological processes of life history." This endurance "has no claim on the attention of evolutionary biologists. It is . . . a kind of meaningless leftover." Yet for literature, "the leftover is the thing itself," Greenblatt notes. It is precisely here that the human story resides, as does the impulse that propels the Apocrypha to ask not only whether Adam and Eve lived, but how. Whereas for biology, the life story is an "epiphenomenon" (at best, a ruse; at worst, an irrelevance), in literature, Greenblatt asserts, it is "the platform for human experience." Beyond productive and reproductive life, the literary scholar tells us, what matters most to Shakespeare is "what lies just ahead": the rage, grief, madness, and fantasies of a redemption that will never come—the very stuff of stories.

But in asking for "what lies just ahead," Shakespeare seems to suggest something in the future, beyond and in excess of the text already in the archive; is this the space where ethnography affords a privileged path? How, then, does this stuff of our stories continue, drawing our subjects and ourselves into an ethnographic open?

On November 20, 2014, I received an email message from someone I did not immediately recall: Andrea de Lima.

The subject line read: "Mr. João Guilherme [which is how I am addressed in Brazil]—MJD [Machado-Joseph disease]—family case—Vita [where I met

Catarina]." There was much more at work in that composite subject than I could immediately apprehend.

"Good morning, Mr. João Guilherme," she wrote, in a youthful, neighborly, and respectful manner. "It is a great pleasure to be sending you this email."

The message seemed important to her. "I got your contact information from Mr. Magnus at Vita, here in the state of Rio Grande do Sul, Brazil," she informed me. She had gone out of her way and into Vita, searching to establish contact with the anthropologist whom Catarina had known.

"My name is Andrea," she continued.

By then I knew who was writing. In the book *Vita*, I had named her Ana.

A puzzling statement followed: "I'm looking for you for the following. . . . You will remember my case."

How could I not? I felt deeply implicated. The character had acquired a Shakespearean ghostly tone, as in *Hamlet*: "Remember me."

Yet this was not just a call for personal recognition. The memory she invoked was that of her "case"—a broader story of which she was a part. Andrea was looking for the ethnographer of Vita and its peoples. She trusted that the researcher knew of her particular situation and that she was not just an anonymous, floating sample of something occurring in the world: "I am the daughter of Catarina Inês Gomes, who spent years living in Vita with Machado-Joseph disease, and you accompanied her case."

The work with Catarina had unleashed something into the world, something that surfaced all these years later in Andrea. While Catarina had sought to detach herself from the logics that produced her abandonment, her daughter was, in a sense, trying to attach herself to something—to enter into the entanglements that brought kin, biology, and ethnographer together. This time, it was Andrea who was trying to reassemble the dismembered family.

In her email, she wrote: "I was adopted by Vera. So my last name was changed. My siblings stayed with the blood family."

Catarina once told me that she had never signed the adoption papers. Indeed, given her supposed madness and recurrent psychiatric hospitalizations, she never got her day in court to contest her husband's decision to sign away custody of Andrea.

Curiously, twice in the initial message, Andrea invoked the genre of the case, her own and her mother's: "You will remember my case. . . . You accompanied her case." This invocation brought me back to Lauren Berlant's essay "On the Case," in which she argues that cases—whether they are legal, medical, or psychological—are defined by normative power and judgment. Linking the singular to the general, cases express "a relation of expertise to a desire for shared knowledge."[49] So how does ethnography—and the relations it engenders—enter into proximity with a case?

Andrea knew that those who had seen her mother as unproductive, unfit, and mad had closed off Catarina's life. Yet by exploring how Catarina became a case—of psychosis, expert knowledge, and abandonment—ethnographic work had made room for thinking reality and human figures elsewhere. In breaking a case open, ethnography brings crossroads (places where other choices might be made, other paths taken) out of the dustbin of history and illuminates resistances to encased norms—the "leftovers," in Greenblatt's sense, that make up a life. The case is thus not only a form but "an event that takes shape," as Berlant writes.[50] In our probing, there is thus both a refusal of the confines that accompany *encasing* (the values, systems, and experts through which a case is constituted) and a questioning of "precedent and futurity."[51] In this way, ethnography carves out "an opening within realism," suggesting where the case "might travel."[52]

Having found herself in the ethnographic open, Andrea was now using it as means into the unknown. In her email she told me, "I want the genetic test so that I can know whether I am negative or positive" for Machado-Joseph disease.

Part of a dismembered household, Andrea knows that she also belongs to a biological system that exercises its own kind of agency. The knowledge she seeks is life-altering. If she tests positive, she will be diseased, so to speak, and left without a known treatment.

I did not know how to take what I was reading or how to respond to her search, and I was thrown back to the core tension of my fieldwork with Catarina: how to sustain a sense of hope as mortality hovers beneath the surface.

Andrea further wrote to me: "I am very grateful that you attended to my mother and also to Adriano. For I know that some years ago, you helped him."

She was right. A couple of years earlier, I had returned to southern Brazil to work on a visual documentary on the now ubiquitous practice of litigation against the State for access to treatment.[53] Torben had joined me in the field, and at that time we met with Laura Jardim, the doctor who had seen Catarina before her death, to discuss the plight of patients who are filing lawsuits for

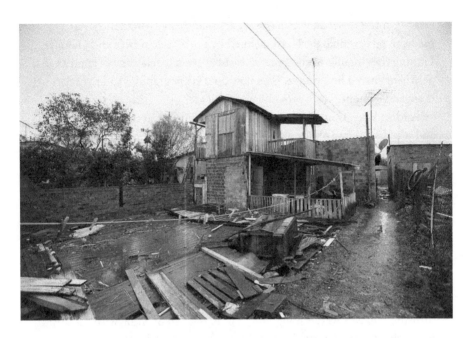

FIGURE 11.8 | *Adriano's Home*, 2011. Photograph by Torben Eskerod.

access to new and high-cost genetic therapies. At the end of the meeting, Laura mentioned that Catarina's son, Adriano, had recently visited her clinic and received the same diagnosis of Machado-Joseph disease as his mother had had. He had been invited to enroll in the first clinical trial for a treatment that, the genetics team hoped, would slow the progression of the disease.

Fieldwork sets often surprising and unforeseeable processes in motion, changing trajectories in the life course of all involved. Between fieldwork's past and future, I was linked indelibly to both Catarina and her offspring. In contrast to the subjects of statistical studies and the figures of philosophy, our ethnographic subjects have a future, and we become part of it in un-expected ways. Their stories become a part of the stories we tell, and we, too, become a part of their life stories.

I found Adriano, his wife, and their two children living in the poorest outskirts of the city of Novo Hamburgo (figure 11.8), not far from where I grew up. The meeting with Adriano and his family taught me much about the dark underside of Brazil's ailing public health-care system. Unable to continue his work at the local steel factory, Adriano was getting by on a disability stipend that he had to reapply for every three months. His son had severe learning disabilities. After a year of trying, the family was still waiting for an appointment with a neurologist. His daughter was tiny, apparently undernourished; she had an umbilical hernia, and they were having trouble making the appointment for her operation.

Living in the brutal stasis of poverty, Adriano and his wife seemed resigned to waiting—a type of waiting "structured and institutionalized" for those relegated to such conditions rather than the "random and contingent" waiting we associate with leisure or idleness.[54] Their situation reveals the broad reality of public health among Brazil's poor: unless they learn to make themselves visible, demand fulfillment of their rights, and make the system care, they are left to live with their conditions and eventually die on their own.

Despite their difficult circumstances, there were traces of Brazilian consumer society in Adriano's remote shack. The children sat on a sofa playing video games. Adriano dreamed of building a house with a yard for the kids to play in, he said, and he had managed to acquire an old Volkswagen Beetle— even though he did not have a driver's license. These possessions and desires helped him maintain a sense of worldliness and worthiness, I thought, as he now fought to escape Catarina's destiny: Vita.

"Onward," he said.

"Please confirm that you received this message," Andrea pleaded in her email to me. "You are very important in my history and in my family. I hope you will remember me or my family that you became a part of."

Besides her entanglement in family, biology, history, and work ("I'm sending this email from work," she said in a postscript), Andrea was part of an ethnographic open constituted by the circuits of fieldwork and the work of time.

"Thank you," Andrea concluded the message.

We began a conversation over email and Skype. Andrea had finished high school, and when she turned eighteen, she said, it was time to leave the home of her adoptive parents: "Vera and Marino gave me a home and education, and I always had everything I needed. I cannot complain. But it was never an affectionate relationship."

Andrea was working as a computing and customer service assistant at a transportation company in Novo Hamburgo, and for the past three years she had been living with her boyfriend, Anderson, and his working-class family. "Not a single day goes by that I don't miss my mother," she told me.

She recalled having seen Catarina only once. Her adoptive parents took her to Vita, and, she said, "I did not know what to say. All that human misery. I regret so much not asking her any questions. I was afraid." She was ten at the time. Vera had told me that they had actually taken Andrea to Vita "for her to see what will happen to her if she does not start behaving."

Through our mutual relation kindled by the ethnographic open, Andrea sought an identification with Catarina. She asked whether I could reach out to the same doctor who had tested and treated her mother and her brother, Adriano—which I did, although I was ambivalent about doing so. If it were me, I would not want to know if I had such a disease. I worried about what would happen to her current life, which seemed well organized and stable, if she was found to have the genetic mutation for Machado-Joseph disease. Yet Andrea was determined to know and went through a long process of evaluation and counseling. It was as if the lethal genetic knowledge would confirm that she was in fact the daughter of the mother who, encased in madness and abandonment, she never had.

A year later, in November 2015, Andrea emailed me again and asked if we could talk.

I thought she wanted to tell me the outcome of the genetic test. But that was not it. She had not yet been called to get the results. I knew from my geneticist colleagues that about half the people who get tested decide not to see their results, and I told her that this option was available to her.

"My sister and I found each other on Facebook," she told me.

That was the story Andrea wanted to tell. She was over the moon with happiness. The last time Andrea had seen her oldest sister Adriana (who had been raised, together with Adriano, by a paternal grandmother) was at Catarina's funeral.

"I saw her message on a Sunday morning when I woke up. The message read: 'Hi Andrea, all good? I think I found the person I sought my entire life, the person I loved my entire life. You are my little sister, right?' Can you imagine? I cried a lot."

Adriana does not have Machado-Joseph disease, Andrea told me. She has two children of her own and works as a supermarket cashier. "And what a coincidence," Andrea continued. "It was the Day of the Dead, and I had already bought flowers to take to my mother's grave." The sisters agreed to meet at the cemetery later that day.

The ethnographic memorial, an out-of-the-way effort to insist on the irreducible truth that a woman named Catarina Inês Gomes Moraes had once walked on the earth, was the site where the characters of the "tragedy generated in life" (in Catarina's own words) reunited (figure 11.9). In spite of all the time and prospects that people and institutions had taken from them, they would continue to tell their family story, to live it a bit differently, and to graft each other anew: "It was there that we found each other, there in front of my mom's remains."

The sisters reached out to Adriano, who was now living by himself on disability benefits. With his disease progressing and conflict in the house, his wife had left him for another man, taking the children with her. Adriano had found solace and support in the evangelical church he attended daily.

Catarina's scattered offspring were now forming the ties that she always imagined and that had sustained her somehow. "To restart a home," she used to say. And now it was Andrea who realized this vision: "This is very important to me. What is happening is the brick that was lacking in my construction."

I told her I would love to meet the reassembling family.

We all met in January 2016 in Novo Hamburgo, the place of my own beginnings and departures.

Andrea was the first to arrive.

FIGURE 11.9 | Andrea's photograph of the ethnographic memorial.

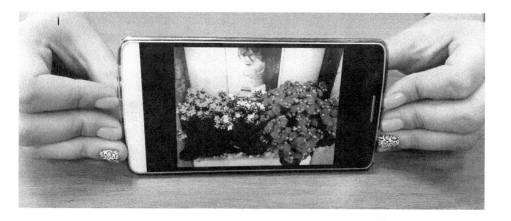

FIGURE 11.10
Catarina and
Andrea, 1992.
Photograph by
João Biehl.

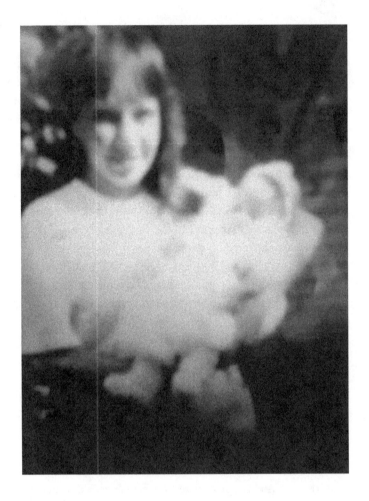

She was eager to show me in her cell phone a photo of herself as a baby in Catarina's arms (figure 11.10). "It's the only image I have of us together. . . . Adriana found it in the middle of our grandma's old stuff and sent it to me."

A surviving image, the persistent trace of care.

And to my continuous surprise, the other thing Andrea wanted show was a neatly assembled folder, with an article on Catarina that I had published in Portuguese.[55] "I found it on the internet. . . . I was happy I could understand most of it," she said with a smile.

A plastic sleeve carefully protected each page. To withstand the test of time.

The image and the ethnographic text kept Catarina's presence alive, I told myself. They allow Andrea to live something she did not live. They mediate the human contact and relationship she so desires. And they serve as a platform to rethink existential and moral orders, for destruction is never absolute, and communities of desire persist.[56]

Andrea was now working as an office assistant at Unimed, a regional private health-care provider. But she added: "I am also following my dream. I just started nursing school."

How striking that the daughter Catarina had been unable to care for and raise was now pursing the art of caregiving. I asked why.

"Just like my mom in Vita, the sick and bedridden have so much to say," Andrea replied. "But so few listen. . . . I like to be attuned to what the person is sensing as she traverses a difficult time."

Catarina's abandonment lay at the core of her vocation, of her sense of presence and purpose, I thought. And I was astounded with the ethics of care she voiced: "Each patient one cares for is the love of someone . . . and this is what I hope had happened to my mother. Caregiving is as if the person were the love of someone."

It was as if Andrea was writing an Apocrypha to Catarina's life story, herself a relational "-n," in Aparecida Vilaça's words, "always pointing to an absent 'other.'"[57]

Before Adriana and Adriano arrived, Andrea still confided—to my great relief—that she had tested negative for Machado-Joseph disease. She asked me not to mention anything to her siblings: "I don't want Adriano to feel bad that he is the only one who has it."

Finally, an uncle dropped Adriano and Adriana off at the sandwich shop Andrea had picked for our meeting. They were both living in the nearby town of Montenegro. With the disease progressing, and unable to perform basic daily routines, Adriano had moved in with the grandmother who had raised him. "[My wife] has left me," he said. Patricia now had the custody of their two children. "*Fazer o quê?*" ("To do what?"), Adriano asked, as if resigned to his fate. The sparkling Adriana said that she was better off without her husband, who had also found another partner. Adriana worked as cashier at a local supermarket and took care of her two children. "And I have fun," she added.

Over lunch, it was quite moving to see how the siblings interacted (figure 11.11), the inside jokes they told, and the way they picked on each other. I brought them copies of the new edition of *Vita* and read parts of Catarina's dictionary to them:

With L I write Love
With R I write Remembrance
Inside your and my heart

To make peace with time
The hours, minutes, and seconds,
With the clock and the calendar
To be well with all
But mainly with the pen

I make love in my mind to scare the cold

My spirit of love nobody can catch

What will become of the world?

"*Our* mom was so intelligent," Andrea said. Catarina/Catkine's own art (of living and poetics) continued to ripple and live beyond her death and persist in a way that memory alone does not. There was one more thing she

FIGURE 11.11 | Adriana, Adriano, and Andrea, 2016. Photograph by João Biehl.

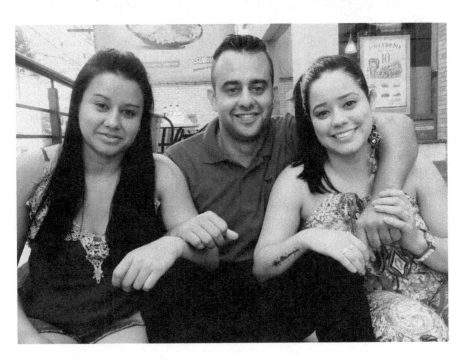

wanted from the anthropologist who had "accompanied" Catarina's case: "Can you, please, tell us: What was her thinking in Vita?"

I immediately recalled Catarina's words: "In my thinking, people forgot me." But I didn't repeat these words, for Andrea was now living (with her siblings, with her partner and his family, with her future patients) Catarina's hereafter. And because her question stoked a desire we shared—that the ethnographic subject might resist enclosure and reappear through the ethnographic open—I chose to read another stanza instead: "I like the ways I am, the ways I know myself."

All possible ways, in her words.

Notes

1 | Sontag, *Illness as Metaphor and AIDS and Its Metaphors*, 3.
2 | "The piece is 2011, and my mother did not get the epilepsy test done at Braddock UPMC [University of Pittsburgh Medical Center], remember they were sending patients to Pittsburgh in order to keep their numbers down to justify closing it": LaToya Ruby Frazier to Laura Giles, art curator, Princeton Museum, personal communication (email, August 28, 2019).
3 | Nixon, *Slow Violence and the Environmentalism of the Poor*, 2.
4 | Sontag, *Regarding the Pain of Others*, 7.
5 | Sontag, *Regarding the Pain of Others*, 72.
6 | Wexler, "A Notion of Photography," 143.
7 | Frazier, *The Notion of Family*, 89, 153.
8 | Biehl and Locke, *Unfinished*, 3.
9 | Harney and Moten, "Politics Surrounded," 20.
10 | Frazier, *The Notion of Family*, 152.
11 | Cole and Sheikh, *Human Archipelago*, 16.
12 | Sontag, *Regarding the Pain of Others*, 126.
13 | *A Love Supreme* is an album recorded in 1964 by the jazz saxophonist John Coltrane. It was released by Impulse! Records in January 1965.
14 | Haraway, *Staying with the Trouble*; Stewart, "In the World That Affect Proposed"; Stewart, *Ordinary Affects*; Whitman, "Specimen Days," 482.
15 | Hurston, "Mules and Men," 10.
16 | Biehl, *Vita*.
17 | Kleinman, *Experience and Its Moral Modes*, 372.
18 | Agamben, *Infancy and History*; Agamben, *Remnants of Auschwitz*.
19 | Kleinman, *The Illness Narratives*, 48.
20 | Kleinman, *What Really Matters*.
21 | Kleinman, "The Art of Medicine."
22 | Carter, *The Vulture and the Little Girl*.
23 | Sontag, *Regarding the Pain of Others*, 79.

24 | Kleinman and Kleinman, "The Appeal of Experience; the Dismay of Images," 9.

25 | MacLeod, "The Life and Death of Kevin Carter."

26 | Kleinman, *The Soul of Care.*

27 | Kleinman, "The Art of Medicine."

28 | Kleinman, "The Art of Medicine," 805.

29 | Nietzsche, *The Use and Abuse of History*, 10, 12.

30 | Kleinman, "The Art of Medicine," 805.

31 | Lévi-Strauss, *The Savage Mind*, 11, 16–18.

32 | Kleinman, "Catastrophe and Caregiving," 22.

33 | Kleinman, "The Art of Medicine," 805.

34 | Deleuze and Foucault, "Cold and Heat," 72.

35 | Biehl and Locke, "The Anthropology of Becoming"; Reynolds, *The Uncaring, Intricate World.*

36 | Deleuze, *Essays*, iv.

37 | Biehl and Locke, *Unfinished*; Dave, "Witness"; Garcia, *The Pastoral Clinic.*

38 | Clastres, "Savage Ethnography (on *Yanoama*)," 89.

39 | Benjamin, *The Arcades Project*, 470, 475; Didi-Huberman, *Survival of the Fireflies.*

40 | Petryna, "Horizoning"; Stewart, "Atmospheric Attunements."

41 | Foucault, "Photogenic Painting," 92.

42 | Crapanzano, "On the Writing of Ethnography," 69.

43 | Foucault, "What Is an Author?" 219.

44 | Lacan, "Science and Truth," 18.

45 | Lévi-Strauss, *Tristes Tropiques*, 44.

46 | Lévi-Strauss, *Saudades do Brasil*, 9.

47 | Lévi-Strauss, *Saudades do Brasil*, 9.

48 | Greenblatt, "Tell My Story."

49 | Berlant, "On the Case," 664.

50 | Berlant, "On the Case," 670.

51 | Berlant, "On the Case," 666.

52 | Berlant, "On the Case," 669.

53 | Biehl, "The Judicialization of Biopolitics."

54 | Hage, "Afterword," 205.

55 | Biehl, "Antropologia do Devir."

56 | Didi-Huberman, *Survival of the Fireflies.*

57 | Vilaça, "A Pagan Arithmetic," 7.

Thinking on Borrowed Time...

About Privileging the Human

IT IS POSSIBLE TO DETECT a sense of foreboding in the vibrant, engaging papers assembled here, an ominous sense of dread as the birds fly off and calamity seems imminent. First written for a conference in the spring of 2017, they convey a mood one might term post millennial, a consciousness of endings and apprehensions—not merely as regards the condition of the late liberal world, or the rise of ever more brazen reminders of fascisms past—almost the same, if not quite. There is also an increasingly audible panic about the future of planetary existence itself. What kind of anthropology, what sort of theory could possibly take the measure of such a moment, could probe the implications of what Adriana Petryna (chapter 3) refers to as "life on borrowed time"? What philosophical, ethical, affective commitments can proffer a plumbline when conventional anchors of truth seem seriously adrift? Might it be, asks Robert Desjarlais (chapter 10), that at the present moment, "to anthropologize is to learn how to die?"

Arthur Kleinman, in whose honor these essays were written, can perhaps be seen as a scholar for whom the hour has always been late. For he has long urged his colleagues, to pause and take stock, to vex themselves with "what really matters," what they should care about amid the clamor of scholarship as usual.[1] "Care" in that sense is a calling, an interpellation, a summons to feel concern. Like Martin Buber's participatory intimacy, it is also a praxis of empathetic engagement, an impetus—in the face of inequality and affliction—to secure, sustain, and heal. In fact, there is an expanding academic preoccupation, at present, with care—"care of the self," "care of the environment," even care as an act of revolution.[2] The word has become almost synonymous with ethical action itself, this at time when older infrastructures of nurture and protection are in question in much of the liberalized world; when "Who cares?" has become a rhetorical question that measures diminishing expectations of welfare, mutuality, kinship, racial equality. Might the renewed preoccupation with care and suffering, phenomena that Kleinman places at the "core of human experience everywhere," provide a means of attunement in precarious times, a focus for political critique, a site where theory-work can find a footing? Can these age-old metaphysical markers—vulnerability, violence, finitude—offer a plumb line when what once served as pivots of truth now seem seriously adrift, and the future of the discipline itself is ever more in peril? When a rising generation is anguished enough to make the "case for letting anthropology burn" (Jobson 2020)?

To be sure, the tangible sense of urgency and unsettlement perceptible in these essays captures the *Zeitgeist* of their day, a time when the yardsticks of sustainable social and environmental order seem increasingly unreadable. But is this feeling something unprecedented? Anthropology, after all, has *long* been preoccupied with human life at its limits, in places where mainstream civil values lose purchase. It has long devised ways of taking the measure of worlds on the wane.[3] In this respect, it has echoed the Romantic strain inherent in Euro modernity itself, its enduring obsession with certainties lost, with time "lapsing," ever receding into history.[4]

In fact, since its inception, anthropology has provided a critical counterdiscourse within mainstream Western thought. It nurtured a deconstructive impetus—a sense of the relative nature of value and truth—a long time before more explicit philosophical debate explored the unstable relation of text and meaning in the 1960s, or urged acknowledgment of the Eurocentrism of Theory and History (all in upper case). It is this inherently subversive potential, perhaps, that has often triggered anxiety about anthropology among authoritarians, early and late.[5] Only recognized as academic discipline in its own right in the early twentieth century, it has exhibited an enduring preoccupation with its own demise, with the challenge of pursuing a method at odds in many respects with the epistemology of the established social sciences.[6] For, like the people it has studied, anthropology has in many ways been out of joint with the dominant telos of modernity, with what Reinhart Koselleck called "*Neuzeit,*" the accelerating forward movement toward progress and possibility.[7] Instead, the discipline has insisted that, at least for "non-Western" societies, the past was not actually past, not definitively behind us. Embodied in "tradition" and the "customary," that past was present in the present—in the "ethnographic present" or the "contemporaneity of the non-contemporaneous."[8] Modernity, by this definition, existed at the intersection of multiple time scales, unevenly empowered. For the temporality of the primitive was other to the telos of World History. From the latter vantage, the kind of "time out" attributed to non-European peoples was a function of the fact that they were actually "out of time," doomed by a relentless rationality that turned difference into sameness. Anthropology struggled to arrive at a perspective capable of viewing such difference less as evolutionary anachronism than a poignant reminder of the frail virtues of human diversity—for the survival of "small-scale" societies seemed already to be at a tipping-point. The discipline nurtured a sense of urgency and elegy, one that long predates our current preoccupation with life on borrowed time, although in truth, its practitioners were more concerned with celebrating the infinite variety of these frail worlds than acknowledging the colonizing forces that already engulfed them—a blindness that has scarred the integrity of discipline from its inception and increasingly threatens to overwhelm it.

This preoccupation with peoples existing in the shadow of doom links anthropology to the sensibility of existentialism, and also to the "rise of the clinic" as described by Michel Foucault. For Foucualt, modern empirical truth found its touchstone in the certainty of death, the body on the slab, the black border that marked the limits of life for those born into a Godless world.[9] In this sense, at least, anthropology has always been "medical"—just as for some, like the nineteenth-century physician and anthropologist Rudolf Virchow, medicine was always a social science.[10] As the "comparative science of non-Western society," anthropology drew, in its early years, on the organic analogy—on the ideas of anatomy and physiology—to imagine the structure and functioning of simple, holistic systems, and the symptoms of social health and pathology.[11] Together, these systems stood in poignant contrast with the war-torn polities of Europe, serving as models of timeless, "pre-modern" order, of an equilibrium lost in the Faustian bargain made, by the West, with the forces of progress.

The homogeneity and order emphasized by functionalist accounts of simple society were idealizations, of course, sustained by suppressing the signs of change, crisis, and engagement with the wider world. The salvage ethnography conduced to document dying languages and vanishing cultures was committed to conserving difference, alive or dead; to that end, its practitioners often quite intentionally excluded the presence of the historical forces that linked "tribal" peoples into more ramifying networks of contact, exchange, and governance. The complex, multidimensional articulations that joined small-scale economies, geographies, and temporalities and more encompassing, rationalizing regimes of value, space, and time, conjunctures that creolized colonial life-worlds, were obscured. Hence the long-standing debate about "time and the other" in anthropological description, and the charge that ethnographers made "schizogenic use of time," that they refused to make their subjects coeval with themselves or accord them of historical agency.[12] Hence, too, the riposte that a commitment to take seriously the temporal understandings of others, the distinct ontological realities they live by, is a cornerstone of the ethnographic method. Claude Lévi-Strauss famously mused on the conundrums this raises: "[E]ither I am a traveler in ancient times, and faced with a prodigious spectacle which would be almost entirely unintelligible to me and might, indeed, provoke me to mockery or disgust; or I am a traveler of my own day, hastening in search of a vanished reality. In either case I am the loser . . . for today, as I go groaning among the shadows, I miss, inevitably, the spectacle that is now taking shape."[13]

Caught between two antithetical dramas, two lived horizons—one "ancient" and one "modern"—the ethnographer can comprehend neither. For if difference is truly other, it resists translation and comparison; and if not, if the traveler is able to comprehend something of the other's enchanted spectacle, it opens the door to the instability of culture, along with the violence of reduction, appropriation, and worse.[14] Faith in the translatability of universal truth goes along with the psychic unity that is a *sine qua non* of anthropological humanism. And Euro centric whiteness: the working assumption was that "people are the same the whole world over, except where they are different," a productive yet irresolvable paradox, at once epistemological and ethical.[15] Vincanne Adams (chapter 1) reminds us of something similar when she ponders the implications of our enduring readiness, as a discipline, to decipher the mysteries held sacred by others, even when they insist that those things are by nature inscrutable.

Many would argue, of course, that Lévi-Strauss's dilemma was a figment of a dualist, ahistorical imagination. The link between the worlds he so lyrically separates is more prosaic, a product of the "storm of progress" that engulfed non-European societies with the onset of capitalism and empire— an onslaught in which the colonized came to figure as primitive foil, as camera obscura to the civilized West.[16] Anthropologists have been the "inside-outsiders" in this process, forever wrangling with the use and abuses of cultural difference: with the would-be virtues of relativism and ontological estrangement, the fact that this position masks subordination and racism. Thus, the critique is leveled by advocates of anthropology as political economy that the failure to include Europe's others within its horizons of modern worldmaking has deprived them of History, eclipsing their enmeshment in the expanding world capitalist order.[17] Yet those approaches have been faulted, in turn, for making history into a commodity; for giving it a phantom objectivity that homogenizes culture and society, suppressing the fragmentation, disruption, and magic that is palpable in human affairs.[18] More castigating still has been the backlash from theorists of culture, their perspective recently radicalized by the so-called ontological turn, who insist that we acknowledge the thoroughgoing otherness of alien worlds as their inhabitants experience them: worlds seen as ensembles in which people, animals, things, powers all hold equitable status. Rather than distinct representations of a single, shared universe—as presumed by an older, comparativist anthropology— such distinct ontologies should be treated as alternative realities *in and of* themselves, challenging Western axioms to the core and disrupting Cartesian ways of knowing, along with anthropocentric understandings of agency. Here ontologists join actor network theorists and posthumanists, who call for the "symmetrical" treatment of human and nonhuman forces alike as actants, thus to "deprivilege" the species whose deluded sense of primacy has endangered planetary life as a whole.[19]

Ironically, one might argue that, in its founding commitment to cultural relativism, to human unity in diversity, anthropology was striving for a kind of symmetry long before the term was invented.[20] As the most humanistic of the social sciences, it was preoccupied with devising a conceptual vocabulary, an analytical horizon capable of grasping all modes of social existence, not least those that lacked the hallmarks of modern "civilization," even humanity. As a consequence, it developed an unusual epistemological awareness, an openness to reflexivity and philosophical argument that lent itself to theory making beyond the grid of scientific positivism.[21] Yet like all modes of knowing the discipline operated from a particular standpoint: the very objectivism of its liberal humanist voice obscured inherent exclusions and obfuscations. The end of colonialism, at least as a formal system, would shake the foundations of the comparativist project, disrupting the framing binaries—West and rest, "hot" and "cold"—and discrediting the models of distinct, self-perpetuating communities and cultures they authorized. Now "old societies" would become "new nations," set on an inevitable trajectory, the quest for development, that would sooner or later converge with the chronos of the modern world system.[22] The Third World, in short, was bequeathed a form of "second-hand time," a telos of modernization borrowed from the First, that required its peoples to fall in step with the international liberal order—just as that order itself was being undermined, at its center, by a new, deregulating political economy that was global in scale.[23]

Indeed, as corporate capitalism has increasingly freed itself from state regulation, it has promoted a division of labor that is ever more translocal, rendering national borders more porous and disrupting the territorial bases of institutional forms in the Keynesian welfarist mode of the mid-century. Whole populations have been ever more forcefully managed by a biopolitics of race, gender, and age, which has disrupted access to the kinds of labor, livelihood, and protection that once bolstered proletarian life, futures, and social belonging. The periodic crises inherent in capitalism—and its disruptive urge to open up new frontiers for extracting value from human and nonhuman sources alike—have been digitally enhanced, accelerated, and ethnicized on an escalating planetary scale. The multiple, intersecting trajectories of production, extraction, and governance that have followed challenge received liberal models of space-time, politics, and history and abet the increasing capacity of corporate power to capture the political process, privatize the commons, and undercut democratic representation and redistribution.[24] Widening disparities of wealth, health, and security erode popular faith in existing political institutions and the plausibility, even in their Western heartlands, of liberal conceptions of community, law, and citizenship. In fact, from the margins those constructs seem little more than the trappings of elite advantage. Disenfranchised populations are forced to seek ways to secure benefits—often by authoritarian, ethnonationalist means—in environments marked by growing scarcity, patronage, demagoguery—all of which mock the promise of global laissez-faire. In popular politics, art, and culture, North and South, darker visions of rogue capitalism and bandit survival spring to life. Fed by social media that offer rapidly mutating channels of communication and transaction, they conjure a cacophony of stimuli that readily conduce to reifying binaries like black and white, we and they, friends and enemy.[25]

How then, *can* anthropology hold itself accountable, in some measure, to such a moment? If, as I have argued, the discipline has long courted estrangement, long grappled with epistemological angst, long sought to conjure meaning against the hard edges of despair, it might be expected to have a special aptitude for such times of challenge, for the "horizoning work" called for as we confront life lived in multiple temporalities, on awkward scales, at the brink of the abyss.[26] To return to a core theme of this collection, can an anthropology explicitly focused on injury and suffering offer a special purchase, a moral compass in history's unceasing storm?

There certainly has been no absence of debate on these issues in recent years. One response has been to focus on issues of crisis and emergency, less as self-evident markers of salience than as complex performative events, always already embedded in historical and geopolitical force fields of varying scale. As is widely noted, the declaration of emergency, like the calling of a state of exception or crisis, is a recurrent feature of the modern condition, drawing attention to points at which disruption—sudden threat to life, health, property, governance, environment—is held to endanger order, normality, and the real (see chapter 4).[27] Emergencies declare imperatives; demand intervention; often call for suspension of normal regulation. They also make claims, in the breach, about whose existence actually matters. Calling the crisis is a communicative act, like proclaiming an "epidemic"—which, as David Jones insists (chapter 5), is always as much a moral and discursive as it is a scientific event. Epidemics carry connotations of acute, contagious diseases (of smallpox, plague, Ebola), an association invoked in polemical talk of epidemics of suicide, gun violence, sexual assault (see chapter 5). To call an emergency is usually to minimize the role of wider antecedent causes and structural entanglements; thus, to prioritize a discrete and urgent problem. This turns on the presumption of a universal register of humane response (Buber's "participatory intimacy") that ensures empathetic resonance and ethical interpolation capable of transcending distance and difference.

In signaling a break in regular routine, a declaration of emergency creates another kind of borrowed time—an interval of suspension in which urgent ends legitimate what are often contentious means, means that mask the play of broader interests and backstage structural causes and effects. Emergencies can enfranchise bold acts of care and healing across otherwise obfuscating borders, but they can also authorize imperious interventions, along with dubious projects of rescue from politically trumped-up dangers. Indeed, the politics of exigency—the effort to transcend the law in the name of crisis and exception—is often a matter of significant political dispute: witness the furor over Donald Trump's declaration of a national emergency on the US southern border in February 2019, putatively "warranted by an invasion of illegal immigrants spreading crime and drugs." "#FakeTrumpEmergency," tweeted his opponents, as sixteen states filed a lawsuit against him in a Northern California federal court, calling his action deceptive and unconstitutional.[28]

The advent of emergency, then, does not offer a direct line to what is salient and important. Many observers choose, instead, to focus on the everyday occurrence of injury and suffering, especially at a time when heightened humanitarian awareness and technical capacity seem to make little dent on growing levels of social, material, and ecological precarity across the globe. Frequently the lives of those who have been the classic focus of anthropological attention are most at risk in postcolonial times, situated as they are on the frontiers of desiccated farmland, plundered commons, disappearing jobs, toxic habitats. In fact, some have suggested that too avid a focus on the symptoms of human hurt risks in turning the discipline into a form of morbid, sentimental witnessing. For Joel Robbins, the suffering subject has come to replace the cultural other as moral alibi for the discipline as a whole, which in the past couple of decades has traded its foundational concern with cultural difference for a paranoid preoccupation with a universally recognizable, empathetic victim.[29] Focusing on documenting such generic abjection, such shared vulnerability, he claims, ignores the thoroughgoing ways in which history and culture *particularize* experiences of distress. It also diverts concern away from the diverse, positive, hopeful features of people's lives, thus limiting the possibility of an "anthropology of the good"—a focus on value, morality, care, gift.[30]

This last claim strikes me as bizarre. Surely an ethnographically based discipline with a commitment to grounded theory making has no place for such evangelism? As if an "anthropology of the good," like the power of positive thinking or the virtues of strategic optimism were a matter of choosing a moral filter, the better to color our pictures of human existence in a more sanguine light; or to cherry-pick what we ourselves judge (on iffy epistemological or philosophical grounds) to be the more hopeful features of often parlous modes of existence. Leaving aside more metaphysical qualms about such generalized notions of the good, along with a naïve, naturalized reading of the affective disposition of others (in what jejune world can one interpret the global spread of Pentecostalism—or like forms of "cruel optimism"[31]—as evidence that "people everywhere are looking for the good"?)[32] one must ask: good for whom? At whose expense? There seems no sense of responsibility, here, to probe the multileveled complexities of actually existing life-worlds, "good", "bad," equivocal. As I have argued, anthropology has long been regarded as "melancholy" by some[33]; or perhaps, more properly, as "critical." The term, as Butler notes, is less negative, less skeptical of emancipatory ideals than concerned to subject those ideals to searching scrutiny—especially where the upliftment of some requires the oppression of others.[34] Processes of betterment call for more than strategic Salvationism. Anthropology, after all, has long insisted that modernity's marginals, those who tend to bear much of the collateral damage of "development," matter. In this sense, the focus on life under threat is hardly a fashionable compromise of the "last two decades." Nor does it become its current practitioners to cringe at the distasteful consequences of imperial rule, racial domination, or material extraction, or dismiss evidence of the disproportionate vulnerability of postcolonial populations as a tedious trafficking suffering.[35]

Such a stance also reveals an alarming failure to appreciate the history of our own discipline, our own precarious epistemology that has drawn, as noted, on the tragic strain both of Romanticism and Existentialism. As Cheryl Mattingly argues in *Moral Laboratories,* the discussion of "virtue ethics" in anthropology reveals the intimate connection of tragedy and suffering to critique, experimentation, and moral possibility, an interplay that is integral, both ethnically and ethnographically to everyday quests for the good life (a liberal philosophical construct far more complex in implication than the 'anthropology of the good).[36] Examination of this interplay has generated some of the discipline's more profound insights about the very issues Robbins sees as comprising an "anthropology of the good"—things such as moral reasoning, or understandings of well-being, empathy, care, transcendence.[37]

Of course the experience of suffering is always mediated by specific personal and cultural values, but it seems too simple to conclude that therefore pain cannot be meaningfully comprehended or shared across social and cultural divides. As if sensory subjects are "so determinately local," as Brian Massumi puts it, that they remain "boxed into [their] site on the cultural map."[38] Claims to the uniqueness of their suffering are often voiced by the victims of historic atrocities, especially in an age sensitive to the need to repair human wrongs through strategies of truth and reconciliation. Yet restorative justice relies precisely on the power of empathy, the capacity—not always limited to *homo sapiens*—to recognize the distress of others. Insistence on the incommensurable nature of suffering (individual or collective) precludes such identification and forestalls the impetus to address the systemic sources of injury. Achille Mbembe has questioned this politics of incommensurable pain that has loomed large in discourses of decolonization in South Africa and elsewhere: "Not only [is it held that] wounds and injuries can't be shared, their interpretation cannot be challenged by any known rational discourse.... This kind of argument is dangerous."[39]

A wealth of testimony bears witness to the fact that affliction, like all acts of violence and wounding, is communicative in nature; that it always signifies beyond the bounds of individual and social specificity (see chapter 1); and that it has a heightened capacity, in the face of difference, alienation, and the disintegration of common trust to prompt affective resonance, fellow feeling, common action.

But can it offer special access to what is essential: to an elementary form of social life in confusing times? Veena Das responds to this question by insisting that, in the abstract, suffering cannot, any more than any other theoretical vantage, alert us to what is "really going on" in particular times or places.[40] It seems clear that human beings are ever more likely to hurt one another in our world and to harm nonhumans, as well. But rather than presuming the nature of such suffering from afar, Das prefers to find its meaning in the framework of what she calls "an ordinary realism," located in the minutiae of everyday life. This is harder than it seems, she cautions, for it is not merely a matter of applying preconceived concepts to a quotidian realm that then reveals itself to our gaze. The challenge is to make that reality appear in the first place—and, with it, the common concepts capable of grasping it in its vibrant complexity. These concepts, like that realism itself, emerge from run-of-the-mill struggles with life's tangible tragedies, such as death, madness, the quest for conception (see chapter 8); dramas in which the protagonists strive to assert a form of normativity in which they, and we, can find a footing. It is this sort of grounding, she suggests, that can provide a yardstick for assessing what actually matters to social investigation.

But does this orientation risk reifying "the everyday" as the "real" horizon of existence? João Biehl (chapter 11) similarly seeks the lodestar of a meaningful anthropology in the micro-dynamics of people's lives, rather than in an "all-knowing" macro theory that he finds nihilistic, dispassionate, and depoliticizing. The task, as he sees it, is not to "fetishize suffering" or to "rescue an essential humanity," but to shine empirical light on affect and on mindful action that produces tears in the fabric, openings in seemingly closed predicaments, in the unfinished business of life on the moral and physical margins of survival. From this perspective, it is the quotidian struggle against the limits of being that is the fundamental drama of existence, the alibi for what is ethical, meaningful, and relevant.

In fact, as the tenor of our times becomes increasingly urgent, increasingly apocalyptic, many scholars find purpose in the tangible substance of ordinary life rather than the more abstract forces and determinations that shape its contours. They seek the real and consequential in ethnographies of the human art of way-finding and self-correction (see chapter 3), the humble, flawed possibilities of care and return (see chapter 11). This is important work, to be sure, but it cannot serve as substitute for the task of probing the less tangible infrastructures that configure everyday possibilities and constraints. For Arthur Kleinman, it is care in its local nexus of value that yields privileged access to those larger abstractions, to the very constitution of the social, sui generis. For him, caregiving is a gift. And following Marcel Mauss, he views care as a total social fact—a core medium of universal sociality, all the more salient in an alienating, technicist age.[41] For our anthropological ancestors, especially those inspired by Émile Durkheim, it was ritual practice that served as the moral engine of fellow feeling—they referred to it as "all-purpose social glue."[42] Kleinman views care likewise as the "special human glue that holds society together." For him, caregiving generates the "presence" that activates the potential of intersubjectivity and "sparks humanness." One might say that caregiving, much of it at the hands of the marginal and exploited, is the unacknowledged labor power, the human infrastructure that reproduces what we term *everyday life*. Caring about care, then, affords a critical entrée to the study of life itself—including the social etiology of affliction, extraction, and the uneven availability of the means of repair and survival.

But our contemporary angst has also given rise to some rather different, avowedly "posthumanist" responses to the conundrum of what really matters. I think here of approaches triggered by the belief that we have entered the Anthropocene, an age in which immoderate human action on the Earth's ecosystems has sparked irreversible processes of species extinction. From this vantage, many insist that it is high time that the existential interdependence of *all* forms of life be given priority over "the foolishness of human exceptionalism."[43] This conviction has engendered a brave new worldview that many find compelling: human nature should be seen as an "interspecies relationship," and what is called for are nonhierarchical alliances among different varieties of life.[44] By treating all species symmetrically, as equally consequential actants in a "pattern of co-becoming," we might succeed in "deprivileging" the human.[45] For having squandered their birthright, mankind must revitalize and reboot through the tutelage that only non-human nature can offer. We should recognize the importance of "listen[ing] to and learn[ing] from other species," exploring the lessons of "nonhuman culture," of insect sociology, and so on.[46]

To be sure, some of the writing in this genre has a decidedly salvific quality.[47] In *Wild Dog Dreaming*, for instance, Deborah Bird Rose offers "a narrative emerging from extinctions," a lesson in relational ethics from wild dingoes and the Aboriginal people who identify with them. "Perhaps voices from the death space *will speak* to us," she writes.[48] Others are less concerned with advocacy than ontology, with the challenge posed to social science by those with radically different understandings of the constitution of life in all its forms. For instance, the thinking of those who extend to all animate beings the capacities we see as characteristic of humans: the ability to signify or to exercise selfhood.[49] Ironically, although they are often termed *posthumanist*, these multispecies ethnographers tend toward an all-purpose anthropomorphism. Rather than denaturing humanist conceptions of subjectivity, affect, or agency, they argue for expanding such qualities as love, "selfing," and learning across the nonhuman world.

How might all this inform our reflections, as anthropologists, on the priorities of life and work on borrowed time? There certainly are lessons, suggestive but also cautionary, to be learned from the horizon opened up by the multispecies turn and the passions it infuses. Few would fault the commitment, shared by the various inflections of this position, to take seriously the increasingly delicate interdependence of humans and nonhumans in the face of ecological fragility. Many would agree, too, that we stand to gain useful insight from searching ethnographies of what it actually means for humans to live with, not merely "think with," other species, especially in ecologically edgy times.[50] But this, too, is inherent in anthropology's genealogy. Nobody can have read *The Nuer* without being made aware, in exquisite detail, of how much those peoples existed in thrall to the demands of their imperious herds, or to their inhospitable physical environment. The multispecies turn, though, pays much more attention to the reciprocal, open-ended, ecologically transforming qualities of such interrelations. It also insists on unsettling the margins between species, broadening the field of actants and significantly decentering the agency and self-determination of human beings.

In one sense, this is a provocative application of anthropology's enduring reflexivity to what has remained its most axiomatic object: humanity itself as discrete species, however diversely conceived. This reflexive stance is not unique to our discipline, of course. The multispecies turn captures a moment in which boundaries between humans and nonhumans have been destabilized in law, biology, ethics, and art; this at precisely the point that *all* forms of life fall under a common cloud of doom.[51] In other respects, though, multispecies perspectives raise serious problems of theory and method. It is certainly suggestive to extend human subjectivity, agency, and affect to all forms of life, at least at the level of allegory; note that the line between storytelling and social analysis is often intentionally blurred in this mode of writing.[52] But how useful *is* it in analytical terms? After all, some much more robust theoretical claims are being made for the multispecies turn. Do we want to tangle, yet again, with problems bequeathed by earlier, colonizing tendencies in anthropology—such as purporting to give voice to the voice-less, to serve as the spokespeople for nonhumans?[53] Do we really want to indulge the dangerous romance that "wild dingoes and Aboriginal peoples" share kindred sensitivities, or that "non-human is like non-white"?[54] Are we ready to reduce notions of culture and society to cross-species common denominators? Or to prefer "culture-as-medium" over "culture-as-meaning?" Or to invoke constructs such as *biosociality* to disinter the kind of models we so objected to in behaviorism and sociobiology?[55] Likewise, is it sensible to respond to the hubris, the wanton destructiveness, of our species by cham-pioning the notion of "symmetrical agency," which radically reduces human power over other forms of life at a moment when our Promethean ambition and greed are propelling the planet to a perilous tipping point? Or when de-grading forms of racism and colorism threaten to turn *homo sapiens* itself into a multispecies category?[56]

True liberal-humanist culture can be faulted for overvaluing the determin-ing power of human beings in the world and for underappreciating the degree to which history is always coproduced, in unintended ways, with nonhu-man forces. Let us recall, here, how Marx complicated human agency—not by giving it indiscriminately to all beings and things, but by showing how concrete abstractions, such as "capital" and "labor power," themselves the unwitting effects of human action, also exercise forceful constraints on the agency of our species. We might make history, goes the cliché, but never as we please; note that elsewhere Marx also remarked the ongoing interdepen-dence of what he termed "organic" and "inorganic" nature.[57] Yet there seems no denying the disproportionate responsibility of human action, albeit some actions more than others, for our current social and environmental predica-ment. As has often been said, approaches that draw on actor network theory point *away* from the ability to judge priorities, to engage in abstraction and theory building, to encourage ethically informed intervention—that is, to permit what we might the art of human interference (*interference*, here, in both its negative and positive senses).[58] For by multiplying the number of putatively symmetrical agents at play in any situation—humans, nonhumans, objects, technologies—and insisting on the contingent, emergent nature of all outcomes, these approaches make it impossible to account for the elements, inequities, and a priori forces that *actually* make a difference in any particular eventuality in the world. They also make it impossible to explain the repetitive, cumulative, nonrandom quality of events and processes, such as those that empower or disempower specific people and species, that configure the field of play and that monopolize or distribute resources that wound or heal. History may not be determined by a single hidden hand or an unvarying unilinear telos. But it is also not lacking in discernible, repetitive vectors of varying scale—politico-economic, psycho-moral, techno-epistemological, biomaterial—of which the Anthropocene is one palpable consequence.

Each of the suggestive essays in this volume provides a different answer to the paradoxes of our time and place, a distinctive mode of engaging the ethical and epistemological challenges that we, collectively, face. As noted, ours is an era at once familiar yet unprecedented in the magnitude of threat it poses to prior social, political, and ecological formations and to the substance of life itself in its myriad incarnations. In one respect, it is the same old story: a tale of capitalist modernity's creative destruction, of the tendency to pile up rubble, to cry wolf, to shore up illusions of permanence on what must clearly be borrowed time. In another sense, we stand on the brink of uncertain biological and geophysical thresholds, of apparently irreversible shifts that exceed existing paradigms, available algorithms, technical capabilities. How, amid forces of such daunting complexity, such transcendent scale, such cosmic adversity, can anthropology deploy its distinctive method, its conjectural style of theory making, so reliant on intersubjective insight, so humanist in its sense of species being, relevance, and scope? As I have tried to suggest here, for all its humanism, the discipline has never taken the durability of the human species for granted—even though it may have classically operated with a naturalized, Eurocentric, neo-evolutionary view of the anthropological subject. It has always been preoccupied with the struggle to reproduce particular forms of life—of person and society, economy and polity, exploitation and care—at the intersection of human and nonhuman being. Whatever determining forces might exist in the wider world, our singular expertise is directed to the manner in which our species acts in, and on, that world—this in ways that, while never simply self-authored, are also never the mere reflex of unmediated, contingent forces, animate or otherwise.

If medical anthropology has taught us one thing, it is that as lived actualities, neither illness nor health—or even death itself—is reducible to biophysical facts that speak for themselves. Yet in observing how social actors intervene in what moves them most, we gain privileged insight into how and what they prioritize; how they, and we, determine what really matters. Anthropologists have shown an acute awareness of the effects, on the phenomena we study, of how we frame our analytical fields, scale our space-time horizons, determine the range of relevant forces in play. Today, amid pressing planetary problems, when many urge us to move beyond anthropocentrism, it might be argued that prioritizing the human is a principled commitment to a vision of the real, the ethical, the politico economic. For these orientations are all in danger of being eclipsed in a world in which, to counter crude Prometheanism or defend the "facts" of life at large, we risk ceding the ground to other postpolitical, posthuman forces, from biodeterminism to technoeconomic rationality. The same might be said of the temptation to give undue weight to poignant allegories of "multispecies love" or stories of natural sociability and agency, doomed, without prosaic human intervention, to waste their sweetness on the desert air. Humanists might still view our species as the stuff of moral self-making—but it is ever more evidently not a project we can make as we please, being enmeshed as it is in an ever more torrid give and take with other beings and forces, animate and inanimate, tangible and otiose. Never has it been more imperative that humankind show a humble awareness of its own limits and interdependencies. But never has it been more necessary, too, to recognize our unique responsibilities and the fact that neither the real nor the human can be taken as ontologically given. Opting for the human in this context, then, is not casual anthropocentrism. It is an ethical and political commitment to the kind of species being that cares, interferes, and makes the very best of borrowed time.

Notes

1 | Kleinman, *What Really Matters.*
2 | Foucault, *The History of Sexuality, Volume 1*; Gulløv, "Welfare and Self Care"; Karakus, "Forms of Governance in Istanbul, Turkey"; Popova, "I and Thou"; Weiss, *Shaping the Future on Haida Gwaii*; Jor-el Carabello, "Self-care as an Act of Revolution When you are Black," *Essence*, June 17, 2020; https://www .essence.com/feature/self-care-is-an-act-of-revolution-when-you-are-black/; accessed July 16, 2022.
3 | Lévi-Strauss, *A World on the Wane.*
4 | Pfau, "Mourning Modernity."
5 | In 2011, Florida's Governor Rick Scott argued that there was no need for more anthropologists in the state and that taxpayers' money would be better spent on giving people science, technology, engineering, and math. And in October 2018, Poland's Minister of Science Jarosław Gowin signed a new law, the Constitution of Science, declaring that ethnology and anthropology

were no longer independent disciplines but part of the study of culture and religion: Goździak and Main, "Erasing Polish Anthropology?"

6 | Jebens and Kohl, *The End of Anthropology*; Leach, *Rethinking Anthropology*, 1; Worsley, "The End of Anthropology."

7 | Koselleck, *Futures Past*.

8 | Koselleck, *Futures Past*, 239.

9 | Foucault, *Madness and Civilization*.

10 | Wilkinson, "Politics and Health Inequalities."

11 | Radcliffe-Brown, *Structure and Function in Primitive Society*.

12 | Fabian, *Time and the Other*, 21.

13 | Lévi-Strauss, *A World on the Wane*, 45.

14 | See also Rachwal, *Precarity and Loss*, 98–99.

15 | On the landmark BBC anthropological series, see Banks-Smith, "Face Values."

16 | Benjamin, "Theses on the Philosophy of History," 261–62.

17 | Wolf, *Europe and the People without History*.

18 | Taussig, "History as Commodity in Some Recent American (Anthropological) Literature."

19 | Haraway, *When Species Meet*; Latour, *We Have Never Been Modern*.

20 | Stocking, "Functionalism Historicized," 4.

21 | Comaroff and Comaroff, "Foreword."

22 | Geertz, *Old Societies and New States*.

23 | Alexievich, *Secondhand Time*.

24 | Comaroff and Comaroff, "Ethnography on an Awkward Scale"; Petryna, "Horizoning."

25 | Ginzburg, *Clues, Myths, and the Historical Method*, 87.

26 | Petryna, "Horizoning."

27 | Agamben, *State of Exception*; Roitman, *Anti-Crisis*.

28 | Mille, "Democrats on Twitter Cry #FakeTrumpEmergency after White House Declaration."

29 | Robbins, "Beyond the Suffering Subject."

30 | Robbins, "Beyond the Suffering Subject," 448.

31 | Berlant, *Cruel Optimism*.

32 | Venkatesan et al., "There Is No Such Thing," 434.

33 | McSweeney, "Tristes Tropiques by Claude Lévy-Strauss—Melancholy Anthropology."

34 | Butler, "The Inorganic Body in the Early Marx: A Limit Concept in Anthropocentrism."

35 | Robbins uses the distasteful image of "the proverbial drunk, searching for his or her lost keys under the streetlight because that is where it is brightest" to describe how "anthropologists" settled on the "suffering subject" to replace the now the discredited "savage slot." Robbins, "Beyond the Suffering Subject," 448, 450.

36 | Mattingly, *Moral Laboratories*.

37 | Evans-Pritchard, *Witchcraft, Oracles, and Magic among the Azande*; Garcia, *The Pastoral Clinic*; Kleinman, "Everything That Really Matters"; Turner, *The Forest of Symbols*.

38 | Massumi, *Parables for the Virtual*, 3.

39 | Mbembe, "The State of South African Political Life."

40 | Das, *Affliction*.

41 | Mauss, *The Gift*.

42 | Horton, "Ritual Man in Africa," 349.

43 | Haraway, *When Species Meet*, 244.

44 | Deleuze and Guattari, *A Thousand Plateaus*; Kirksey and Helmreich, "The Emergence of Multispecies Ethnography"; Tsing, "Unruly Edges."

45 | Latour, *Reassembling the Social*; Van Dooren, *Flight Ways*, 12.

46 | Carlson, "John Hartigan on Multispecies Ethnography."

47 | De Gennaro, "Love Stories, or, Multispecies Ethnography, Comparative Literature, and Their Entanglements."

48 | Rose, *Wild Dog Dreaming*, 146.

49 | Kohn, "How Dogs Dream," 4; Rose, *Wild Dog Dreaming*, 146.

50 | Kirksey and Helmreich, "The Emergence of Multispecies Ethnography."

51 | See De Gennaro, "Love Stories, or, Multispecies Ethnography, Comparative Literature, and Their Entanglements."

52 | Carlson, "John Hartigan on Multispecies Ethnography."

53 | Latour, *Politics of Nature*.

54 | See also Kirksey and Helmreich, "The Emergence of Multispecies Ethnography," 555.

55 | Sahlins, *The Use and Abuse of Biology*.

56 | Anderson, "The Beast Within: Race, Humanity, and Animality."

57 | Butler, "The Inorganic Body in the Early Marx: A Limit Concept in Anthropocentrism."

58 | Bloor, "Anti-Latour"; Chagani, "Critical Political Ecology and the Seductions of Posthumanism."

Lessons Learned from the Ethnography of Care

FROM THE OUTSET OF MY RESEARCH CAREER in the late 1960s, I have worked on caregiving, sometimes in planned and sometimes in unwished ways. I have researched family care in the United States, Taiwan, and China, and professional care in hospitals and clinics. I have read widely and critically in different literatures of caregiving: popular nonfiction and fiction, medical, nursing, and social sciences/humanities.[1] Added to this have been my firsthand clinical experiences as a psychiatrist, clinical teacher, and, most powerfully, though sadly, the primary caregiver for my late wife, who died in 2011 at the close of a ten-year struggle with Alzheimer's disease.[2] I have also had a four-decade-long experience of collaborating with primary care physicians regarding my own self-care in the management of several chronic diseases, including asthma and hypertension. Hence, I have had an extensive and many-sided involvement with this subject, being a long-term observer, caregiver, and recipient of care. No; it is more than this: for me care is irrecusable as the core structure of my life and, I believe, life itself.[3]

Out of this elemental reality (often heartening, at times dispiriting) come distinctive, difficult, incomplete, but eventually secured insights. There are a number, but here I present a few of the ones I feel are most salient both to illustrate that the medical anthropology of caregiving matters and to suggest how it matters:

- Caregiving is a crucial component of everyday life all over the world: medical anthropology shows just how central it is and makes a special contribution to understanding what are the scope, content and consequences of care.
- Ethnography, social theory, and implementable applications of medical anthropology can improve people's responses to pain and suffering and strengthen the quality of caregiving.
- These contributions, in turn, bring something special to anthropology and other social sciences—namely, a deeper understanding of what is at stake in ordinary life and a way of doing research that itself is caring and potentially healing. Notably, medical anthropology has become for some a mode of intervention in global health, social medicine, and domestic health care. This is visible and significant in the COVID-19 pandemic.
- Perhaps most intriguing of all, the ethnography of suffering and care holds the promise of creating a practical wisdom for the art of living (and dying) and for the art of medicine.

What Is Care?

The *Oxford English Dictionary* offers a capacious definition of *care* that creates an availing place to begin. Care is providing what is needed "for the health, welfare, maintenance and protection of someone or something." (This is to care for . . .) The definition is extended even wider to include feelings of concern or anxiety (as in to have cares), as well as those of liking or being serious about doing things the right way to ward off danger and risk (as in to care about and take care). Thus, the contemporary idea of care spans a broad range of experiences from worrying and loving to doing any or all things required to help someone, someone in need.

Defined this way, care is placed at the existential core of human experiences everywhere. Yet this great ambit of care has to be narrowed by ethnographers and theorists into more readily grasped situations and processes for the real significance of care to be fully appreciated. Take feelings, for example. They are the alerting concern to be serious about others and one-self that direct and motivate caregiving acts. Erik Erikson and many child development experts who have followed his pathbreaking work direct our attention to how children, adolescents, and youth, among other things, are socialized first to have certain kinds of cares, then to learn how to take care in real-world cultural contexts always oriented by danger and uncertainty. Erikson and the many others who have followed him in the study of human development also understand old age as a place of life where being generative on behalf of others involves quests for creating certain wisdom out of experience that both is practically useful and contributes to finding meaning and purpose in living.[4] Anthropologists and historians have repeatedly shown that, although this happens differently in distinctive cultural communities, under the pressure of divergent historical and political circumstances and economic realities, and thus prioritizes different values and valued things, when it comes to caregiving itself, it is centered mostly in the experiences of women and girls. This makes understanding gender simply crucial to making sense of care and makes care a centerpiece of gendered approaches to ethics and political theory.[5]

Caregiving in each moral world is constructed out of individual and collective acts such as protecting those who are vulnerable; assisting with grooming, bathing, toileting, eating, ambulating, and so on; and working through the moral emotions that underwrite these actions. By moral emotions and actions, I have in mind such things as acknowledging that others are suffering and in pain; affirming their right to assistance; supporting them by being present for them; and sustaining and enduring the social frustrations, financial and bodily burdens, and psychological toll of caring. The caregiving process, with its moral and emotional dynamics, continues even after death in the caring for memories, which not only makes up much of what bereavement and mourning are about but also constitutes over time that which keeps individuals, families, communities, and even societies going.[6] Those memories are reworked to fit emotional meaning to the life course, with its changing circumstances and challenges. A moral core to social and subjective experience is then realized that enables adaptation (or habituation) even to the inhospitable and unwelcoming and, by preventing alienation and defeat, helps us to endure.[7]

In writing about the "moral" here I have in mind an ethnographic rather than a philosophic ethics approach to ordinary life. We are all grounded in local moral worlds of experience, whether they are actual networks or virtual connections. The local need not be physically local; it can exist as a transnational "local." Acts of care are centered in these local worlds among intimate others and people with whom we may not be intimate but still are engaged and entangled.

The moral, as I understand it, is not necessarily good. It is what is at stake in a local world in the socially shared flow of moral experience and in the individual's always partisan moral life. And what is at stake may be as divided as helping others or hurting them. Collective moral experience and personal moral life may be in concert but often are controverted. This is the case when what matters to a group and to an individual are directly opposed. What is at stake shapes caregiving: whether it is given in a bureaucratic setting with sensitivity or indifference, in a family freely or grudgingly, or professionally as a first thought or afterthought. Ethics, as a quest for what is good and just, comes into play as individuals and groups seek to go beyond what is locally at stake through critical reflection and a search for what is translocally valued.[8] That quest is itself constrained, in this ethnographic perspective, by the socially constructed and politically oriented ethical systems that are religiously, ideologically, and professionally (e.g., bioethics) influential. Vincanne Adams's chapter directly engages with this perspective. In the context of self-immolation in Tibet, she illustrates the limits of clarity and certainty, as well as the significance of contestation in the moral experience of the Tibetan community and in the moral life of her interlocutors. Adams also shows the limits of clarity and certainty in the contrasting ethical systems of Tibetan Buddhism and European science and secular ethics. At the levels of both the moral and the ethical, complexity, ambiguity, and contestation are brought about by the fusion of political and subjective states.

Care itself is one of those things that truly matter. (Hence, it operates on both local moral and ethical levels.) Yet how it matters is an empirical reality that can be ethnographically and historically situated. Seen this way, care is best understood as an action, a relationship, and a process. It can be a presence or an absence. Framing caregiving in stories from ordinary lives and worlds is how we understand the subtleties, contradictions and dynamic trajectories of care as human experience. Such stories also reveal, in keeping with the *Oxford English Dictionary*'s definition, that care can be about aspects of human experience other than broken bodies and minds. Mentoring, nurturing friendships, gardening, maintaining a home, preparing meals and cooking, looking after pets, committing oneself to helping a project flourish, participating in protests advocating for better schools and childcare—all are kinds of care. Viewed this way, care is ordinary life, though it can in its own way be extraordinary or tell us about extraordinary experiences. Hence, studying care offers a way of critically getting at life itself, and doing so in a serious and deep manner.

It is helpful to consider a point Iain Wilkinson and I emphasized in *A Passion for Society* (2016).[9] In settings of danger and uncertainty, such as our current COVID-19 pandemic, that create or intensify social suffering among those most vulnerable and in societies (like our own) that themselves are broken and place huge constraints on what kind of care can be mobilized and implemented, we see most clearly an aspect of care that is present (and absent) everywhere. This is social care and, where present, it is aimed at repairing worlds of social suffering. Its focus is on the recipient of care in societal terms: communities, populations, cities, regions, whole nations, even the planet. Here the plural care receiver is as active as the caregiver in the struggle to realize social care. The problems included are the consequences not only of poverty, racial injustice, and abuse of women and children, but also of famine, earthquake, wars, uprooting and migration, human-generated climate change, and epidemics. Hannah Arendt, following in a grand tradition of social thinkers from Adam Smith, John Stuart Mill, and Voltaire through Max Weber, W. H. R. Rivers, William James, John Dewey, Jane Addams, Franz Boas, C. Wright Mills, W. E. B. Du Bois, Frantz Fanon, and the members of the Combahee River Collective of Black feminists, among many others, identified the "social" as an appropriate level to respond to economic, political, social justice, and, more recently, racial justice problems with *social care*. Scholars have debated its meaning, but Wilkinson and I choose to understand the term as referring not only to an assemblage of individual acts of care for collective problems, though it is certainly partly this, as in the individual effects of the religious admonition to observant Jews to repair the world and the commitment of the African American church that its members should contribute to racial liberation and freedom.

Social care for us is principally about caregiving at the societal level through critical social thinking, social theory, and social research in support of implementation of pro-social policies, programs, and social movements aimed to address concrete problems understood as those at the community and societal level. Of course, the moral emotions needed to mobilize social care may well be based in personal commitments to social justice, repairing the world, or, for that matter, the Chinese cultural emphasis on the embodied intersubjective actions required to cultivate life and make people flourish.[10] Yet it is recognition of the "social" as the level of intervention that defines for us social care, as well as its routine absence.

Medical anthropologists make contributions to global health through critical analysis of cases of epidemics, endemic diseases, floundering and failed health interventions, problematic bioscience, and new ways of incorporating "the social" into how health problems are named and framed, as chapters in this book illustrate. Adriana Petryna's concern with the climate change crisis that is creating, among other things, the truly dangerous forest fires sweeping through the American west and Australia, is an example of caring for the environment and for those whose lives are placed at risk because of global warming. Jean Comaroff's questioning of the centrality of the human in medical anthropology can be read in a similar manner as an affirmation of the inextricable link between the Earth's environmental conditions and people's ways of life. Her defense of privileging humans in part turns on our role in caring for the planet. Hence, in both examples medical anthropologists extend the idea of care to our environmental settings.

David Carrasco's *cri de coeur* calls the reader to attend to how Mexicans have been erased in the Mexico-US borderland. Their quests to survive, flourish, or simply endure represent the failure of social care on both sides of the border. Carrasco, however, offers examples of what that care might look like if the currently hostile response to immigration were remade as social caring. For Salmaan Keshavjee, the lineaments of colonialism, racism, and neoliberalism in global health shape the failure of public health professionals to prioritize care in resource-poor settings. Instead, they treat these "clinical deserts" as if the only practical and ethical approach is the control of disease outbreaks that threaten wealthy societies such as the United States. The absence of care, he insists, invariably undermines public-health actions. In such settings in India, David Jones asks, can the care of patients with cardiac conditions be ethically justified in the face of failing or absent efforts at alleviating poverty and the infections disease burden that results? His answer is to unpack the hidden burden of heart disease and the need for both acute and chronic care systems. Similar concerns run through Marcia Inhorn's chapter on reproductive technologies.

But medical anthropologists have also developed and carried out innovative interventions, so that they have led medical anthropology into direct public-health and social medicine action.[11] These interventions show a new form of global health and humanitarian work—a form that begins with critical review of local situations and application of history and social theory and is followed by ethnographically based interventions featuring great attention to local meanings and practices; involvement of local leaders, change agents, and community workers; and ongoing effort to sustain these implementations and turn them over to communities.[12] This work of critical pragmatism, in my view, has challenged what global health stands for and changed what global health is and does. It brings an ethnographic sensibility to understanding not just why humanitarian assistance breaks down and fails, but why it succeeds, and why it must continue, and how it can be reformed and made more useful to basic human needs.[13]

Care in the context of the family and network, along with self-care by those afflicted, is much more common than professional care. That is to say, most care occurs outside of institutions in domestic spaces. This is true not only for childcare, but also for care of the chronically ill, the disabled, and the elderly. Nonetheless, almost everywhere, with the possible exception of certain social-democratic societies in northern Europe, public resources are inadequate in their support of family care and self-care. And this occurs in the face of impressive evidence that such care reduces substantially the overall economic burden of caregiving for society.[14] Underfunded by society and underappreciated by professionals and policy makers, caregiving turns out to be a special human glue that holds society together. Families and communities require financial assistance and knowledge resources, as well as such supports as home-care services for seniors, home health aides, visiting nurses, physical and occupational therapists, hospice volunteers, and social workers who, especially in America, can help navigate an overly complex, chaotic, and broken health care system. Because the work of caregiving is usually carried out by female family members, it is vulnerable to demographic changes, such as greater numbers of women entering jobs outside the family and thereby being unavailable for caregiving. Men regularly fail to assume responsibility for care; or, as in China, poor peasants attracted to the city to care for the urban elderly find that there are other, less demanding and better remunerated jobs available and leave the health-care field. In the United States and other wealthy societies, immigrant women of color staff caregiving jobs, which most often pay very poorly and are undesirable to all but those on the bottom rung of the ladder. In spite of this, they frequently are found to provide high-quality care. Research also shows that family caregivers get something crucial from the caregiving experience—even when it is stressful, disease causing, and economically and psychologically burdensome—that increases their longevity and shapes lives that feel to those who live them as more meaningful.[15]

Lessons Learned from Caregiving

Care at its most fundamental is about relationships. There is, to begin with, the caregiver–recipient of care relationship. Yet this core arrangement itself is situated in families, networks, communities, markets, and institutions. The anthropological model of exchange offers an appropriate model: gift exchange.[16] The gifts exchanged are practical assistance, emotional responsiveness, human presence, moral solidarity. The relationships are most frequently ongoing, so that care occurs in the trajectory of an arc of conversations and entanglements. Hence, the gift of care may be repaid in the context of balances and imbalances in symbolic capital that constitute the emotional-moral calculus of marriage, friendship, parenthood and childhood, sibling relations, employment, bureaucratic processes, and so on.[17] The ongoing process of exchanging care over time becomes the emotional-moral core of the relationship.

The recipient of care, who is often modeled as passive, is much more likely to be an active partner in the exchange, even in a professional patient-doctor relationship. In family care, the person being cared for is often the most active party. Presence in the relationship is not just that of the caregiver. The recipient of care also carries the responsibility to be spirited, engaged, active, and responsive. The idea of presence means care is a vital performance.[18] Hence, the old-fashioned Parsonian sick role is just that: old-fashioned and off the mark in its definition of care as only a passively legitimated and stereotyped behavior. Think of care in a conjugal or parent-child relationship as part of the exchange of intimacy that is the currency of the relationship overall. Even in cases of disability, serious chronic illness, and care of the fragile—or even terminal—elderly, the recipients of assistance are usually active both in responding to intimate others and in self-care, and often passionately so.

The professional caregiver-recipient of care relationship is also an exchange of practical, emotional, and moral gifts. This can be seen both in the sympathetic responsiveness of the caregiver to the personhood, plight, and lively performance of the care receiver and in the recipient's (and the family's) responsiveness to the professional. Nor is this only in positive terms: ambivalence, frustration, and anger exist in this exchange, as well. It is at times when the emotional-moral legitimacy of the exchange is undermined that we see such negative consequences as physicians or patients alienated and dropping out of care, or legal suits, and in the peculiar current situation of extreme patient-doctor mistrust in China, physical violence.[19] Speak to professional caregivers as I have so very frequently and you learn how important the clinical exchange is to them, too. It is not just time and money that is exchanged, but feelings, values, and memories. Physicians have often told me that caring for certain patients over the long term is among the most significant experiences in their careers and in their lives; it keeps them going in frustrating times when they feel they are burning out and prepared to drop out. Many physicians today blame bureaucratic procedures for getting in the way of the high-quality care they seek to provide, and they reference a thinning out of their relationships with their patients and families as the reason why. Of course, Max Weber would have understood this outcome as the result of the increasing dominance of bureaucratic rationality in professional and lay experience that creates the iron cage of rationality Michael Herzfeld relates to bureaucratic indifference—in caregiving terms, the absence of presence and the dissolution of meaningful relationships.[20]

An impressive recent family caregiving report by the National Academies reviews in detail the crucial role of relationships in caregiving.[21] Family caregivers for Americans older than sixty-five number eighteen million. By 2030, about seventy-three million people (more than one in five US residents) will be older than sixty-five, and the number of family caregivers will go up accordingly. Japan will see its population older than sixty rise to an unprecedented 40 percent by 2040, and China at that time will have between 25 percent and 30 percent of its population older than sixty. These numbers will overwhelm available family caregivers, requiring caregiving relationships with many more home health aides and their equivalents. In the United States, roughly 70 percent of the elderly currently live on their own or with family or friends, and about 30 percent are in institutions. Hence, even a small decline in family care would swamp available facilities. Now add to this family carers for disabled children and adults younger than sixty-five with serious chronic illnesses and you immediately recognize the immense contribution that family carers make. The Caregiver Action Network estimates that more than sixty-five million Americans (29 percent of the population) provide care for twenty hours or more each week, providing $375 billion in free assistance—twice as much as what is spent annually on home care and nursing-home services.[22]

Examining the reality among women caring for children, Anne-Marie Slaughter argues for policies that would support this crucial relationship through the transfer of financial and cognitive resources to such female carers.[23] The same argument could be advanced for family caregivers of the frail elderly and for the active involvement of the elderly themselves in self-care. But what is too often missed is the role of family caregivers in creating high-quality, meaning-infused care. This is why so many elderly want to be cared for by family and friends.

I don't underestimate, of course, the financial, psychological, and other related burdens experienced by family caregivers. I have experienced them firsthand. Caregiving is hard, demanding, and troubling and must be endured under substantial difficulties. In fact, this is the argument for providing greater resources for family carers. What medical anthropology can contribute here are studies of the actual lived experience of caregiving. In the absence of direct measures of the quality of care, which is where we are today, there is an opportunity for ethnography to frame our understanding of quality in light of stories and performances of care that illuminate what really matters to recipients and carers. Quality of care seen this way is about cognitive and emotional communication and relationships that can best be assessed ethnographically. The possibilities for medical anthropology are immense but still largely unrealized.

Janis Jenkins's research with the chronically mentally ill in Mexican American families describes "struggle" as a core experience of patients with psychosis and their families. Jenkins begins to fill in the cultural and interpersonal details of caregiving and care-receiving experiences. Robert Desjarlais's ethnographic engagement with elderly Nepalese approaching death can be considered yet another example of the ethnography of caregiving. This time, the self-care of Buddhist adepts living out their religious commitments in the cultural performance of end-of-life experiences extends the boundaries of care from health and medical to religious and everyday settings. Lawrence Cohen depicts the ultimate bureaucratization of the good death via the Indian government's efforts to use biometric measurement to categorize and control those members of the Indian population who do not easily fall into rational technical slots. Here biopower is the form of governance for the final days of transgendered people who are assaulted by the state's use of control instead of care to handle the marginal and unprotected members of the population. Keshavjee's chapter is yet another illustration of how domestic and global forces join in undermining care of the poorest in favor of lowering the standard of care services on behalf of institutional efficiency.

Caregiving as Presence

Ethnographic studies of presence of the divine in ritual, of the charismatic process through which, following Weber, leaders mobilize followers, and of the infusion of music and art into the ordinary to intensify feeling and meaning reveal how the intersubjective, relational quality of caregiving is created.[24] Presence is that spiritedness, that liveliness, that passion of being that doesn't just reside in a personality. Rather, it is brought out and strengthened in a relationship to which caregiver and care receiver both connect. It is the being there with one another that, put this way, sounds prosaic but is anything but. It is the vital connection, the deeply human openness of a relationship. It is sticking it out, enduring in spite of frustration and failure. Presence is one measure of quality in the caregiving and care-receiving relationship. It is not only in the caregiver but also between the caregiver and care receiver, and at its best it is in all of these, including the recipient of care. Presence is the very soul of care. Not only is it part of the placebo response and a contributor to good outcomes; it is the definition of good clinical relationships.[25] So why is it not measured, and, even though it can be, why is it not taught? Nothing speaks so profoundly to the power of anthropology to reveal the extraordinariness of the ordinary. Yet nothing shows so clearly anthropology's failure to influence health-care experts' understanding of what high-quality care means. The time has come for a major effort to operationalize presence in the education of health professionals and in the everyday experience of care. Presence—cultivating it, sustaining it, and making it count in health policy— will be a lasting contribution of medical anthropology to health care and, quite possibly, to understanding and strengthening life itself.

And this is so also because "presence" occurs in spite of our ordinary limitations and failures. It speaks to something residual yet incandescent within each of us and in our relationships that has the potential to come alive and spark human transformations. It gets at that evidence of mystery that defies social science and the medical taken-for-granted. Presence suggests why biocultural processes that bring relations into subjectivity and project feelings into others' bodies may have the ability to tell us about what terms such as *love, healing,* and *transformation* mean in the lived experiences of all of us who engage in care.[26] But will medical anthropologists find their way from the present fixation on criticism for criticism's sake to the work of care for helping others? I continue to believe we will, we can, we must. Perhaps João Biehl's quest for an ethnography of being and becoming in which life and care remain open and unfinished suggests one direction for such groundbreaking work.

Care amid (and against) Institutions

The ethnography of care also helps clarify the disturbing reality that bureaucratization, runaway technological developments, and destructive neoliberal economic approaches to health care are actually reducing the quality of care and thereby undermine caregiving in unprecedented ways.[27] This is true in the broad health-care system and in medicine and the other health professions. Efficiency, cost control, time limits on direct patient care, bureaucratic indifference, and a sorcerer's apprentice situation of out-of-control obsession with technologies all contribute to the crowding out of human relationships, communication, and presence. There are today many, possibly too many, curriculum reforms in teaching humanistic care to physicians. But no matter what is taught to students, the incentive structure and organization of time in health-care systems militates against the application of humanistic skills by harassed professionals in everyday practice.[28] Ethnographic studies repeatedly have documented this tragedy of history and suggest what the loss of care may mean for human prospects, but more availing still are those studies that also expose the real barriers to improvement and show what can be done to return caregiving to its central place in medicine and health services.[29] When fed back to students as a critical reflection on how to care in a time of crisis, ethnographic understanding has the potential to contribute to a more effective pedagogy that can redeem care. This calls for a critical humanism in the healing professions that not only emphasizes caregiving practices but also revivifies and sustains the emotions and values crucial to keeping those practices central. Such an ethnographically infused, critically pragmatic humanism also can aim to create an effective ecology of care in which policies, programs, and best practices form an alternative reality to the one that has usurped caregiving's mandate. Here we return to the crucial importance of mentored practical caregiving interventions in training that can be scaled up and generalized under more availing systems that reinforce incentives and diminish barriers to high-quality care.[30]

That task makes critical humanities an antidote to the dead hand of traditional bioethics approaches that have become anodyne and ineffective because they fail to challenge narrow and tired professional and institutional values and have allowed bioethics to become a handmaiden of routine professional practice. The established and establishment bioethics continues to limit its pedagogy to high-level abstractions that are usually irrelevant to the complexity of local cases and that lack truly critical reflection. The anthropological approach to moral experience becomes a more relevant means of teaching about values and relating them to actual cases. Here what Weber called "the antinomies of everyday life," as well as the structural violence that the dominant political economy creates for carers, can be the spur for an existential humanism in medicine, nursing, and the other health professions. Medical anthropology is already a leading contributor to the new medical humanities, and it could and should contribute much more.

Caregiving as the Core Structure of Everyday Life

Not only ethics needs to be rethought in light of the ethnography of care; we also need to rethink our understanding of everyday life. Theories of the ordinary have not included nearly enough serious emphasis on caregiving.[31] It is like dark energy in the universe, present everywhere but not well described or understood. Caregiving experiences occupy a huge portion of people's lives, especially those of women, as well as those poor immigrant groups that find work principally at the lowest levels of the health-care system.[32] This absence of presence seriously distorts the pictures we assemble of everyday life in America, in China, and just about everywhere. What happens when we more adequately attend to the omnipresence of caregiving?

The first realization is recognition that social life is largely dependent on the caregiving activities of wives, mothers, grandmothers, daughters, aunts, sisters, and other categories of women.[33] Theirs is the central role of stewarding, cultivating, and deploying human resources. Thus, from this perspective, societal values appear unrepresentative and unjust because of their failure to prioritize this contribution, especially to caregiving, and to compensate it. It also calls into question the already questionable ideology of libertarianism, which has become so popular in our epoch. The idea that individuals receive care only from themselves is preposterous. Almost no one has failed to benefit from the caregiving of others. And few seek out lives where there is no one to care for. Here the individualist mythology of Western (and particularly American) society is especially egregious.[34] Chinese views of the person, who is embedded in families and at the center of their own networks and active in other interpersonal networks, is closer to the truth.[35]

Years ago, my late wife and I conducted a study of the impaired elderly in Shanghai. We found that while their sons happily articulated Confucian principles of revering the elderly and protecting them, it was their daughters-in-law and daughters who did all the exacting work of practical assistance for physically and psychologically dependent elderly. And they bore the greater share of the exhaustion, stress, and frustration. Evidence now exists, however, that associates caregiving with lower mortality rates for caregivers.[36] It also correlates with meaning making in the sense that caregivers, no matter their burden, are more likely to live longer and regard their lives in more positive terms.[37] This image runs against the clichéd view of caregiving as only a burden that dominates the media today. Here again, ethnography can balance the account by showing the varieties of caregiving experiences—from coerced care to care as the unavoidable tax on our relationships: networks of intimate connections that represent the vital constellation that fills life with magic and mystery, pathos and bathos.[38]

Anthropology of (and as) Caregiving

Direct caregiving activities by medical anthropologists include increasing numbers of intervention programs in social development, global health, and humanitarian assistance.[39] The work of the MD-PhD cohort looms large here in the guise of local and regional implementation of interventions for infectious diseases, heart disease, diabetes and other chronic medical conditions, and mental illnesses.[40] Social theory, history, and ethnographic studies ground such interventions in local worlds while, at the same time, biomedical and preventive medicine approaches are leveraged together with community interventions. Examples abound from the development of community projects in poor societies to treat and prevent multidrug-resistant tuberculosis, AIDS, SARS, and Ebola to interventions for heart disease, cancer, depression, schizophrenia, and dementia.[41]

What is notable about these interventions is that they are undertaken with both biomedical and anthropological grounding, often in an explicitly biosocial framework, with great attention to language, culture, and history, on the one side, and ecology, physiology, drugs and vaccines, on the other. The experimentation comes in the way these are interconnected and implemented. Notable in the COVID-19 pandemic is the work of Partners in Health, the international nongovernmental organization founded and still guided by medical anthropologists. Partners in Health has been active in Haiti, Rwanda, and Sierra Leone. But it also has organized and delivered contact tracing, case finding, assistance with isolation and quarantine, and other support for those affected by the SARS-Cov-2 virus in Massachusetts, Illinois, and other states.

Rather than regard such anthropologically directed interventions as anomalous because they are unusual in contemporary anthropology, we need to see them in light of the framing offered by the originators of social science who regarded social knowledge as the basis for improving people's lives and practically reforming society.[42] They believed knowledge should lead to direct action. This development has courted controversy but is likely to increase in scope, substance, and numbers of interventions as anthropology comes to terms with making itself relevant and salient in the current era of reduced support for the humanities and social sciences. Nor should such social action be limited to the health domain; criminal justice reform and racial justice policies and programs can be developed along similar lines, as can the kind of environmental policies required to address environmental disasters such as those rapidly developing and highly destructive forest fires Petryna describes in such terrifying terms in her chapter.

Caregiving's ethnography also demonstrates that research participation, observation, interviewing, life histories, and other methods can be conducted in such a way as to enable research subjects and their communities to benefit from care.[43] Put somewhat differently, care can—and, arguably, should—be a routine way of performing research, making it an activity of human care in which emphasis is placed on the life-embracing and person-empowering aspects of research. Clinicians have long sensed the similarities of ethnographic engagement with interlocutors to their engagement with patients. Communication, personal relationships, and history taking/interviewing should begin with the basic ethical acts of acknowledgment and affirmation of the other. Even questioning about culturally and personally significant issues can be done sensitively and supportively with emphasis on the value of the relationship; protection of the interlocutor; and care for his or her fears, troubles, and preoccupations. Establishment of a trusting relationship with affirmation of the human engagement as being helpful to the research subject means that the ethnographer will be drawn into lives and situations in which he or she needs to feel responsible for their human aspects. In this volume, Adams, Desjarlais, Cohen, and Biehl illustrate this most human of relationships. Numerous other ethnographers, including those who are critical of humanitarian assistance programs, do themselves offer what human solidarity and practical assistance they can to interlocutors who are vulnerable and to communities at risk of things the ethnographer can help contribute to ameliorating or controlling. This happens through the ordinary provision of hard-to-obtain supplies; offering first aid; sharing food; providing protection; and assisting those in need. This is ethnography as care.

For those ethnographers who work on social suffering either in settings of extreme danger and mass violence or in the taken-for-granted tragedy-as-usual life of those experiencing the structural violence of poverty and social deprivation, research interviews and life histories should be conducted in ways that can be healing. For example, providing an affirming and supportive and protected place for people to talk about demoralization, alienation, and what the late songwriter Leonard Cohen called "brokenness" can be a form of emotional revitalization and moral solidarity and thereby beneficial to respondents and their networks.[44] Several years ago I received an unsolicited letter from a Chinese intellectual whom I had interviewed in field research in China more than thirty years before. I had spent several hours intensely listening as he told a terrifying story about abuse during the Cultural Revolution. He wrote that the experience had been liberating and, he thought, therapeutic, because it was the first time he was able to come to terms with and make sense of emotions and moral challenges that he had buried for years and had never before found a safe outlet for expressing—in spite of the fact that they had become such a heavy personal and family burden he felt demoralized and oppressed by these inner demons. My own involvement here had not been directly intended to be therapeutic, yet, surprisingly, it had been just that: healing. Joseph Gone, an American Indian psychologist in the Department of Anthropology at Harvard, explains how such an outcome can occur in the setting of interlocutors' personal crises framed as witnessing historical trauma on behalf of indigenous collective revitalization and individual transformation.[45]

Having care in mind as basic to the research engagement with others holds this potential and, in my long experience, frequently elicits deep and telling responses that provide an extraordinary opportunity to understand what is most at stake for interviewees and why. Once that appreciation is gained, it is awfully hard for the ethnographer not to act on that hard-won knowledge in such a way as to assist people in need. (The current interest in the ontology of interlocutors' being and becoming, as Biehl shows, also entangles the ethnographer in a kind of care for human futures.) There is no reason that such a caring approach can't be taught and learned in ethnographic methods classes and thereafter applied in field research. There is also no reason that such a care-oriented approach can't be applied in other kinds of social-science research to make it more humanly responsive, useful to participants, and ethical in the highest sense.

Ethnography and the Arts of Living

As my final example of the contributions medical anthropology makes to the study of Asian and other societies and, more broadly, to an understanding of human experience and life itself, I want to discuss how ethnography brings researchers, teachers, and students into existential human quests for wisdom: aesthetic, ethical, and religious.[46] Practical wisdom for the art of living (and dying) has been praised by Aristotle, Cicero, and Montaigne, as well as by religious figures and many more recent commentators in the Western tradition, but perhaps even more influentially in Asian ethical and religious traditions, where it could be said to be an outcome of Confucian, Buddhist, and Daoist pathways to cultivation of the self and close others. William James, John Dewey, and Jane Addams felt that it is the obligation of human experience to turn us in the direction of such wisdom.[47] Of course, this is not the explicit or even implicit knowledge created and transmitted in today's universities, with their technology and applied science emphasis. Nonetheless, ethnography's intimate engagement with the deep subjectivity and sociality of colleagues, interlocutors, and students offers a legitimate opportunity to do just this. I feel that the contributions to this volume by Comaroff, Adams, Desjarlais, Jenkins, Cohen, and Inhorn accomplish something akin to this. Carrasco alerts readers to the significance of aesthetic wisdom for the community and the individual in this existential quest.

So what kind of wisdom for the art of living does ethnography put on offer? For the ethnographer herself or himself, it provides an extraordinary opportunity to watch and interpret how people worldwide live: not just at the surface of life, but in their own quests for more profound understandings. Ethnographers learn the hard way that they must attend not just to the words people use but also to their human tone. At its best, ethnography is a great leveler and preventive against hypocrisy and moral superiority. We learn over time the cultural humility and the ethnical ideal that we are all equal in engaging with the trials and tribulations of lived experiences. Ethnography offers no ethical high ground. Existential human conditions are to be found everywhere and are experienced by everyone. Not just uplift, happiness and success, but falling, failure, incompleteness, inadequacy and brokenness are the shared human conditions. It is these conditions that constitute life itself—not so-called human nature, which from the perspective of anthropology is a dangerous fiction. And life itself is so overflowing that ethnography provides the closest nonfiction description.

Ethnographers' privileged position in standing back and interpreting the meanings of others' words and actions does not usually extend into their own life, where the same confusing uncertainty, resistance to making sense, and emotional and moral blindness exist. The ethnographer experiences the collaborationist's misplaced loyalty as much as do his or her research subjects. The ethnographer experiences hubris and creates nemesis too. The ethnographer also misperceives, misapprehends and misbehaves. And, she or he has got to pay bills, face up to distrusting neighbors, deal with resources unequal to what is needed, and respond to racism, homophobia and sexual harassment. This human sharedness in suffering and care is a quintessential ethnographic wisdom, even though most of the time we are much more favorably positioned in life than those whom we study. This wisdom has helped me in my life: not in some heroic way (there are few heroes or heroic moments I have also learned); but at the margins it has made a difference that has helped me to keep going and perhaps to avoid getting into even deeper trouble. Again in Leonard Cohen's discerning words it is the realization of our shared brokenness that lets the light in.[48] And even a little light helps.

Unlike the technical knowledge of policy experts, which leads usually to unrealistic, one-size-fits-all solutions, the ethnographer's task is to understand everyday knowledge creation in all its specificity, messiness, and uncertainty. That sense of inevitable vulnerability is hard to live with, but once balanced with ordinary humor and the little happinesses that make life livable, it is an aid to living—at least for the seasoned anthropologist, here not unlike the seasoned clinician. I find my fellow existentialist anthropologist Michael Jackson's idea of "life within limits" crucial here.[49]

And at times the ethnographer records real transformations: people who change and are changed, in values, practices, relationships, and inner life. And this includes the ethnographer. I have seen this in the field of caregiving, and I believe I have experienced it myself. Nor is this only an individual matter. Engaged ethnographers feel motivated to act together with protest and other social movements of their interlocutors: and these become their commitments and their acts of struggle too. Ethnography in this sense can be and sometimes is a life lived more fully with and through others.

These examples should help point to the kinds of contributions medical anthropology (and social and cultural anthropology more generally) makes that deserve to be better appreciated in wider circles of academic and public discourse. It is a much commented upon fact of contemporary life that professional and academic development leads to ever narrower specialization with intellectual silos that sponsor multiple separate discourses which appear to the public to be alienated from the very real problems ordinary people face. Short of making intellectual and academic discussions irrelevant to the central political, economic and social issues of our time, which to my mind would be an unmitigated disaster for all, it is incumbent on every one of us who has skin in the game, which means all of us, to address a wider audience of educated people. I had this in mind in writing this essay and in organizing the symposium that led to this volume. Readers can see how difficult it is to bring the ideas and findings of an entire field into a broader circle of conversations. There are taken-for-granted debates and substantial research developments behind each of this book's chapters including this one. Summarizing them, smoothing out the differences and complexities so there is coherence, and emphasizing relevance to contemporary questions also has a downside. The conclusions can sound too simple, their sources too confused and confusing to foster policies and programs. Existential doubt can paralyze social action. Professional cynicism leads to just that undesirable outcome. It is unavoidable to try to intervene with proposals or direct acts of solidarity. I believe, if we are to allow ourselves to be human. Moreover, to broaden the audience and overcome the pitfalls of overspecialization and the discomfiting comfort of writing in a professional argot that is off-putting and even unintelligible to the generalist reader, we must try to make our work matter for others.

And there are benefits to a specialized field from doing these things. In the case of medical anthropology, it encourages us to acknowledge what we know that seems secure and what is questionable. It raises useful discussion about the kinds of issues we pursue and why we pursue them. It enables us to ask of the latest theoretical enthusiasm if it is pretentious and hypocritical. It introduces a wider arc of commentators and critics, helping to break down artificial barriers and expose our work to scholars whose approaches we have avoided or simply have not encountered. And, best of all, it exposes our work to those in near and not-so-near fields who need to take account of what we have learned and how we have come at shared questions. All of this is desirable. It is another instance of contributing to an arc of interference that calls into question not only the subjects we study and how we study them, but our own discipline and its humanly constructed preoccupations, prejudices, and pessimism. Medical anthropology, as I have seen and practiced it over nearly half a century, should lead to hope for the betterment of human conditions and the nonhuman world. In that foundational sense, medical anthropology itself is unavoidably a kind of care.

Notes

1 | Gaines, "Culture, Medicine, Psychiatry and Wisdom"; Kleinman, "An Intellectual Journey and Personal Odyssey."
2 | Kleinman, "Forum."
3 | Kleinman, *The Soul of Care*.

4 | Burston, *Erik Erikson and the American Psyche*; Erikson, *Childhood and Society*.

5 | Here I have in mind the work of Gilligan, *In a Different Voice*; Pettersen, *Comprehending Care*; Tronto, *Moral Boundaries*.

6 | Connerton, *How Societies Remember*.

7 | Kleinman, "Caregiving as Moral Experience"; Kleinman, "Caring for Memories"; Kleinman, "How We Endure"; Kleinman, "A Search for Wisdom."

8 | Kleinman, *What Really Matters*.

9 | Wilkinson and Kleinman, *A Passion for Society*.

10 | Farquhar and Zhang, *Ten Thousand Things*.

11 | Farmer et al., *Reimagining Global Health*. See also the large and productive networks of anthropologists who have responded to the Ebola epidemic in West Africa, the HIV/AIDS epidemic in Africa, and the COVID-19 pandemic.

12 | Farmer, *Fevers, Feuds, and Diamonds*.

13 | Wilkinson and Kleinman, *A Passion for Society*.

14 | Kleinman et al., "Time for Mental Health to Come out of the Shadows."

15 | National Academies of Sciences, Engineering, and Medicine, *Families Caring for an Aging America*.

16 | Kleinman, "Caregiving as Moral Experience"; Kleinman, "Caregiving"; Kleinman, "From Illness as Culture to Caregiving as Moral Experience"; Mauss, *The Gift*.

17 | See, for example, the dynamics of symbolic and social capital in Bourdieu, *Distinction*.

18 | Kaufman, *And a Time to Die*.

19 | Tucker et al., "Rebuilding Patient-Physician Trust in China."

20 | Herzfeld, *The Social Production of Indifference*; Weber, *From Max Weber*.

21 | National Academies of Sciences, Engineering, and Medicine, *Families Caring for an Aging America*.

22 | "Caregiver Statistics," Caregiver Action Network website, n.d., https://www.caregiveraction.org/resources/caregiver-statistics.

23 | Slaughter, *Unfinished Business*.

24 | Lienhardt, *Divinity and Experience*; Tambiah, *Leveling Crowds*; Weber, *Economy and Society*. Among other works in ethnomusicology that examine what I have referred to as the socio-somatic processes exemplified by the use of music in ritual and its psychophysiological effects, see Feld, *Sound and Sentiment*; Schieffelin, *The Sorrow of the Lonely and the Burning of the Dancers*.

25 | Guess et al., *The Science of the Placebo*; Hahn and Kleinman, "Belief as Pathogen, Belief as Medicine."

26 | A book that contains various approaches to this question as it relates to pain is Coakley and Shelemay, *Pain and Its Transformations*.

27 | Brodwin, *Everyday Ethics*; Buch, "Anthropology of Aging and Care"; Fadiman, *The Spirit Catches You and You Fall Down*; Katz, *The Scalpel's Edge*; Kaufman, *And a Time to Die*; Keshavjee, *Blind Spot*; Kleinman, *The Illness Narratives*; Luhrmann, *Of Two Minds*; Rapp, *Testing Women, Testing the Fetus*; Wolf-Meyer, *The Slumbering Masses*.

28 | I do not mean to underestimate the value of serious medical humanities pro-
grams such as the outstanding Program in Narrative Medicine at Columbia
University, but I believe their important contributions to medical education
are greatly constrained by the political economy, bureaucratic system, and
professional culture of medical education and practice. The best of these
programs clearly does affect students and practitioners, yet other such programs are very limited in their content and time in the curriculum, and, not
surprisingly, their impact appears transient and superficial.

29 | Berger, *A Fortunate Man*; Biehl, *Vita*; Brodwin, *Everyday Ethics*; Farmer,
AIDS and Accusation; B. Good, *Medicine, Rationality, and Experience*; M. Good,
American Medicine; Kleinman, *Writing at the Margin*; Malkki, *The Need to Help*;
Mattingly, *Healing Dramas and Clinical Plots*; Mattingly, *The Paradox of Hope*;
Stevenson, *Life beside Itself*; Verghese, *My Own Country*.

30 | I have had personal experience with Leiden University's program of placing
beginning medical students in the homes of chronically ill and severely disabled family members where they participate in family caregiving. Graduates
of this program have told me that it was the single most important experience
they had in medical school because it taught them the basics of care and how
they are experienced by families and patients. Such programs also exist in
Germany and Scandinavia, but I am not aware of any in the United States. I
have personally mentored students who undertook experiences as family carers and home health aides, and I have been deeply impressed by the meaning
of these experiences not only for those students but also for some of the care
recipients. Medical students at Harvard Medical School are initiating such an
experience on their own, working with local community organizations.

31 | One scholar who has gone against the grain and produced strong accounts
of ordinary experiences of care is Veena Das: see, e.g., Das, *Affliction*. A
key point Das emphasizes is that trauma poisons the care given by those
enmeshed with the traumatized person(s), because the ordinary experiences
of trauma over time infect the relationships of caregiving with poisonous
knowledge, dangerous emotions, and broken ties that form the very core of
restitution and healing. The outcomes, Das argues, are limited and compromised from the start.

32 | Ulrich, *A Midwife's Tale*; Leavitt, *Women and Health in America*; Noddings,
Caring.

33 | Slaughter, *Unfinished Business*.

34 | Lasch, *Haven in a Heartless World*.

35 | Kleinman et al., *Deep China*.

36 | O'Reilly et al., "Caregiving Reduces Mortality Risk for Most Caregivers";
Roth et al., "Family Caregiving and All-Cause Mortality."

37 | National Academies of Sciences, Engineering, and Medicine, *Families Caring
for an Aging America*.

38 | Able, *The Inevitable Hour*; Gawande, *Being Mortal*; Glenn, *Forced to Care*; Klein-
man, *The Soul of Care*.

39 | Farmer et al., *Reimagining Global Health.*
40 | I use the example of the MD-PhD medical anthropology cohort because I
know it best, having mentored twenty-five MD-PhDs. But clearly MD-MA,
RN-PhD, and other health professionals with anthropology degrees also have
the special orientation to make applied contributions.
41 | Farmer et al., *Reimagining Global Health.*
42 | Wilkinson and Kleinman, *A Passion for Society.*
43 | Biehl, *Vita.*
44 | Leonard Cohen, *You Want It Darker*, Columbia Records, 2016.
45 | Gone, "Redressing First Nations Historical Trauma."
46 | I teach a course with colleagues at Harvard—David Carrasco, Michael
Puett, Stephanie Paulsell—titled Quests for Wisdom: Religious, Moral and
Aesthetic Searches for the Art of Living. It tries to do just this with readings
from different religions, moral worlds, and aesthetic genres. It aims to make
the course transformative for participants.
47 | Richardson, *William James.*
48 | Cohen, *You Want It Darker.*
49 | Jackson, *Life within Limits.*

IN MEMORIAM

Paul Farmer (1959–2022)—our colleague, our friend, and our co-contributor—had become by the moment of his untimely death in February 2022 the very icon of the fields of medical anthropology, global health, social medicine, and humanitarian responses to some of the worst inequities and forms of social suffering in our time. Like so many, we loved him, and we miss his generative and piercing presence deeply. His memory is a blessing to our academic fields, to our lives, and to people all over the world, especially the poorest and those in greatest need, because Paul Farmer stood for the practice of social care as the most fundamental response to structural violence. We, in turn, will persist in caring for his audacious vision. His symbolic presence continues to accompany us with the demand to advocate for social and environmental justice and global health equity.

ACKNOWLEDGMENTS

Arc of Interference is a collective stocktaking of contemporary medical anthropology. It is also a tribute to the work of Arthur Kleinman, whose piercing clarity, caring mentorship, and intellectual energy have been guiding our ethnographic efforts to interfere in pressing issues that range from the climate crisis, immigration, political occupation, and pandemics to the more subtle and enduring problems of premature death, reproductive futurity, and the pharmaceuticalized self. We are deeply grateful to Arthur for his unwavering support throughout the years and for his wonderful engagement with this project since its inception in a symposium held in May 2016 at Harvard University's Asia Center on what medical anthropology brings to our understanding of today's world.

The pathway from that convivial and inspiring symposium to this finished book was quite challenging as we pushed one another at every new turn and revised drafts to forge a coherent volume that could provide a conceptual and ethical toolkit to interfere in our worlds on edge. We thank our contributors for their willingness to do the extra work and for the mutual enrichment along the journey.

Getting to this end point has also entailed heeding the critical advice of four independent reviewers, whose careful engagement with the contributions, individually and as a collection, helped enormously. Special thanks are due to the medical anthropologist Raphael Frankfurter, whose brilliant thinking and sharp editorial support have been crucial to every stage of this project.

We thank two other remarkable scholars who also helped greatly with editing and provided seminal critical feedback on the book's contributions and overall flow: Aaron Su and Onur Günay. We are, as ever, grateful to our visionary editor Ken Wissoker at Duke University Press for his immense wisdom and call to creativity at every step and turn. We also acknowledge the support of Princeton University's Committee on Research in the Humanities and Social Sciences, which provided funds toward the publication of this book.

Finally, we are deeply grateful to the Brazilian Indigenous artist Denilson Baniwa for inspiring us and for allowing us to use the powerful artwork "For Hope Beyond the Horizon" for the cover of *Arc of Interference*.

BIBLIOGRAPHY

Able, Emily. *The Inevitable Hour*. Baltimore: Johns Hopkins University Press, 2016.

Abrahams, Roger D. "Ordinary and Extraordinary Experience." In *The Anthropology of Experience*, edited by Victor Turner and Jerome Bruner, 45–72. Champaign: University of Illinois Press, 1986.

Adams, Vincanne. "Disasters and Capitalism . . . and COVID-19." *Somatosphere*, March 26, 2020. http://somatosphere.net/2020/disaster-capitalism-covid19 .html.

Adams, Vincanne. *Markets of Sorrow, Labors of Faith: New Orleans in the Wake of Katrina*. Durham, NC: Duke University Press, 2013.

Adams, Vincanne. *Metrics: What Counts in Global Health*. Durham, NC: Duke University Press, 2016.

Agamben, Giorgio. *Homo Sacer: Sovereign Power and Bare Life*. Translated by Daniel Heller-Roazen. Stanford, CA: Stanford University Press, 1998. https://doi .org/10.1515/9780804764025.

Agamben, Giorgio. *Infancy and History: The Destruction of Experience*. Translated by Liz Heron. London: Verso, 1993.

Agamben, Giorgio. *Remnants of Auschwitz: The Witness and the Archive*. Translated by Daniel Heller-Roazen. New York: Zone, 2002.

Agamben, Giorgio. *State of Exception*. Translated by Kevin Attell. Chicago: University of Chicago Press, 2003.

Alexievich, Svetlana. *Secondhand Time: The Last of the Soviets*. Translated by Bela Shayevich. Johannesburg: Jonathan Ball, 2016.

Allison, Anne. *Precarious Japan*. Durham, NC: Duke University Press, 2013.

Altstedter, Ari. "The World's Cheapest Hospital Has to Get Even Cheaper," *Bloomberg*, March 2019. https://www.bloomberg.com/news/features/2019-03 -26/the-world-s-cheapest-hospital-has-to-get-even-cheaper.

Anderson, Kay. 2000. "'The Best Within:' Race, Humanity, and Animality." *Environment Planning D: Society and Space* 18 (2000): 301–20.

Anderson, Warwick. *Colonial Pathologies: American Tropical Medicine, Race, and Hygiene in the Philippines*. Durham, NC: Duke University Press, 2006.

Andrews, Ross H., S. Devadatta, W. Fox, S. Radhakrishna, C. V. Ramakrishnan, and S. Velu. "Influence of Segregation to Tuberculous Patients for One Year on the Attack Rate of Tuberculosis in a Two-Year Period in Close Family Contacts in South India." *Bulletin of the World Health Organization* 24 (1961): 463–510.

Andrews, Ross H., S. Devadatta, W. Fox, S. Radhakrishna, C. V. Ramakrishnan, and S. Velu. "Prevalence of Tuberculosis among Close Family Contacts of Tuberculous Patients in South India, and Influence of Segregation of the Patient on Early Attack Rate." *Bulletin of the World Health Organization* 23 (1960): 463–510.

Appadurai, Arjun. *Modernity at Large: Cultural Dimensions of Globalization*. Minneapolis: University of Minnesota Press, 1996.

Arendt, Hannah. *The Human Condition*. Chicago: University of Chicago Press, 1958.

Asad, Talal. "The Concept of Cultural Translation in British Social Anthropology." In *Writing Culture: The Poetics and Politics of Ethnography*, edited by James Clifford and George E. Marcus, 141–64. Berkeley: University of California Press, 1986.

Ash, Lucy. "Why Is Glasgow the UK's Sickest City?" BBC News, June 2014. https://www.bbc.com/news/magazine-27309446.

Aulagnier, Piera. *The Violence of Interpretation: From Pictogram to Statement*. Philadelphia: Brunner-Routledge, 1975.

"Aurangabad Engineer's Heart Give Thane Resident New Life." *Times of India*, June 22, 2016. https://timesofindia.indiatimes.com/city/mumbai/aurangabad-engineers-heart-give-thane-resident-new-life/articleshow/52859039.cms.

Bachelard, Gaston. *The Psychoanalysis of Fire*. Translated by Alan C. M. Ross. New York: Beacon, 1964.

Bakaya, Ravi M. *A. V. Baliga: Surgeon and Patriot*. New Delhi: Patriot, 1991.

Baldwin, James. "The White Man's Guilt." In *Baldwin: Collected Essays*, 722–27. New York: Library of America, 1998.

Banerjee, N. "Cardiac Transplantation." *Journal of the Indian Medical Association* 51 (1968): 539–41.

Banerji, Debabar. *Can There Be a Selective Health Care?* New Delhi: Center of Social Medicine and Community Health, School of Sciences, Jawaharlal Nehru University, 1984.

Banks-Smith, Nancy. "Face Values." *The Guardian*, July 21, 1988. https://todayinsci.com/B/BanksSmith_Nancy/BanksSmithNancy-Quotations.htm.

Basu, A. K. "Origin and Development of the Association of Thoracic and Cardiovascular Surgeons of India." *Indian Journal of Thoracic and Cardiovascular Surgery* 1 (1982): 10–11.

Basu, Helene. "Listening to Disembodied Voices: Anthropological and Psychiatric Challenges." *Anthropology & Medicine* 21, no. 3 (2014): 325–42.

Bateson, Gregory. "Minimal Requirements for a Theory of Schizophrenia." *Archives of General Psychiatry* 2, no. 5 (1960): 477–91.

Bateson, Gregory. *Naven: A Survey of the Problems Suggested by a Composite Picture of the Culture of a New Guinea Tribe Drawn from Three Points of View*. Palo Alto, CA: Stanford University Press, 1936.

Becker, Anne. *Body, Self, and Society: The View from Fiji*. Philadelphia: University of Pennsylvania Press, 1995.

Bell, Charles. *Tibet: Past and Present*. Oxford: Clarendon, 1924.

Benedict, Ruth. "Anthropology and the Abnormal." *Journal of General Psychology* 10, no. 1 (1934): 59–82.

Benedict, Ruth. *The Chrysanthemum and the Sword*. Boston: Houghton Mifflin, 1946.

Benjamin, Walter. *The Arcades Project*. Edited by Rolf Tiedmann. Translated by Howard Eiland and Kevin McLaughlin. Cambridge, MA: Harvard University Press, 1999.

Benjamin, Walter. *Illuminations: Essays and Reflections*. Translated by Harry Zohn. New York: Schocken, 1969.

Benjamin, Walter. "Theses on the Philosophy of History." In *Illuminations*, translated by Harry Zohn, 253–64. New York: Schocken, 1969.

Bennett, Carolyn. "The Budget and First Nations: Opportunity Lost." *iPolitics*, 2013. http://www.ipolitics.ca/(2013)/04/01/the-budget-and-first-nations-opportunity-lost.

Berger, John. *A Fortunate Man: The Story of a Country Doctor*. Edited by Mary-Jo DelVecchio Good. New York: Vintage, 1997.

Berlant, Lauren. *Cruel Optimism*. Durham, NC: Duke University Press, 2011.

Berlant, Lauren. "On the Case." *Critical Inquiry* 33, no. 4 (2007): 663–72.

Berman, P. A. "Selective Primary Health Care: Is Efficient Sufficient?" *Social Science and Medicine* 16, no. 10 (1982): 1054–59.

Betts, Reeve H. "Thoracic Surgery: Investigative Procedures." *Journal of the Christian Medical Association of India, Burma, and Ceylon* 23 (1948): 168–74.

Bhalerao, R. A., and J. S. Patil. "Donor Selection and Management." *Journal of the Indian Medical Association* 51 (1968): 555–56.

Bhattacharya, Sanjoy. *Expunging Variola: The Control and Eradication of Smallpox in India, 1947–1977*. London: Orient Blackswan, 2006.

Bhattacharya, Sayan. "The Transgender Nation and Its Margins: The Many Lives of the Law." *South Asia Multidisciplinary Academic Journal* 20 (2019): 1–19. http://journals.openedition.org/samaj/4930, accessed August 2, 2022.

Biehl, João. "Antropologia do Devir: Psicofármacos—abandono social—desejo." *Revista de Antropologia* 51, no. 2 (2008): 413–49.

Biehl, João. "The Judicialization of Biopolitics." *American Ethnologist* 40, no. 3 (2013): 419–36.

Biehl, João. "Pharmaceuticalization: AIDS Treatment and Global Health Politics." *Anthropological Quarterly* 80, no. 4 (2007): 1083–126.

Biehl, João. "The Pharmaceuticalization and Judicialization of Health: On the Interface of Medical Capitalism and Magical Legalism in Brazil." *Osiris* 36 (2021): 309–27.

Biehl, João. *Vita: Life in a Zone of Social Abandonment.* Berkeley: University of California Press, 2013.

Biehl, João. *Will to Live: AIDS Therapies and the Politics of Survival.* Princeton, NJ: Princeton University Press, 2007.

Biehl, João, Byron Good, and Arthur Kleinman, eds. *Subjectivity: Ethnographic Investigations.* Berkeley: University of California Press, 2007.

Biehl, João, and Onur Günay. "How to Teach Anthropology in a Pandemic?" *Somatosphere,* May 25, 2020. http://somatosphere.net/2020/how-to-teach-anthropology-in-a-pandemic.html.

Biehl, João, and Peter Locke. "The Anthropology of Becoming." In *Unfinished: The Anthropology of Becoming,* edited by João Biehl and Peter Locke, 41–89. Durham, NC: Duke University Press, 2017.

Biehl, João, and Peter Locke. "Ethnographic Sensorium." In *Unfinished: The Anthropology of Becoming,* edited by João Biehl and Peter Locke, 1–38. Durham, NC: Duke University Press, 2017.

Biehl, João, and Peter Locke. *Unfinished: The Anthropology of Becoming.* Durham, NC: Duke University Press, 2017.

Biehl, João, and Federico Neiburg. "Oikography: Ethnographies of House-ing in Critical Times." *Cultural Anthropology* 36, no. 4 (2021): 539–47

Biehl, João, and Adriana Petryna, eds. *When People Come First: Critical Studies in Global Health.* Princeton, NJ: Princeton University Press, 2013.

Binet, Giovanni. "Model Predictive Control Applications for Planetary Rovers," 2012. http://cse.lab.imtlucca.it/bemporad/publications/papers/isairas12-robmpc.pdf.

Biswas, Arpita Phukan. "The Iconography of Hindu(ized) Hijras: Idioms of Hijra Representation in Northern India." In *Gender, Sexuality, Decolonization: South Asia in the World Perspective,* edited by Ahonaa Roy. New Delhi: Routledge India, 2020.

Biswas, Southk. "Why India's Real COVID Toll May Never Be Known." *BBC,* May 5, 2022. https://www.bbc.com/news/world-asia-india-60981318.

Blanchot, Maurice. *The Infinite Conversation.* Translated by Susan Hanson. Minneapolis: University of Minnesota Press, 1992.

Blanchot, Maurice. *The Work of Fire.* Translated by Charlotte Mandell. Stanford, CA: Stanford University Press, 1995.

Blanchot, Maurice. *The Writing of the Disaster.* Translated by Ann Smock. Lincoln: University of Nebraska Press, 1995.

Bloor, David. "Anti-Latour." *Studies in the History and Philosophy of Science* 30, no. 1 (1999): 81–112.

Boas, Franz. *The Mind of Primitive Man.* Norwood, MA: Macmillan, 1911.

Boivin, Jacky. "International Estimates of Infertility Prevalence and Treatment-Seeking: Potential Need and Demand for Infertility Medical Care." *Human Reproduction* 22, no. 6 (2007): 1506–12.

Bonilla, Yarimar, and Marisol LeBrón, eds. *Aftershocks of Disaster: Puerto Rico before and after the Storm.* New York: Haymarket, 2019.

Borovoy, Amy. "Japan's Hidden Youths: Mainstreaming the Emotionally Distressed in Japan." *Culture, Medicine, and Psychiatry* 32 (2008): 552–76.

Boulter, Jonathan. *Beckett: A Guide for the Perplexed*. New York: Continuum, 2008.

Bourdieu, Pierre. *Distinction: A Social Critique of the Judgement of Taste*. Translated by Richard Nice. Cambridge, MA: Harvard University Press, 1987.

Bourgois, Phillippe, and Jeffrey Schonberg. *Righteous Dopefiend*. Berkeley: University of California Press, 2009.

"Boy Missing in Japanese Forest after Parents Kicked Him out of Car as Punishment," ABC News Australia, May 31, 2016. https://www.abc.net.au /news/2016-05-31/boy-missing-in-japan-after-parents-kick-him-out-of-car /7464376.

Briggs, Charles L., and Clara Mantini-Briggs. *Tell Me Why My Children Died: Rabies, Indigenous Knowledge, and Communicative Justice*. Durham, NC: Duke University Press, 2016.

British Medical Research Council. "Emergence of Bacterial Resistance in Pulmonary Tuberculosis under Treatment with Isoniazid, Streptomycin plus PAS, and Streptomycin plus Isoniazid." *The Lancet* 262, no. 6779 (August 1953): 217–23. https://doi.org/10.1016/S0140-6736(53)90160-3.

British Medical Research Council. "Streptomycin Treatment of Pulmonary Tuberculosis." *British Medical Journal* 2, no. 4582 (October 1948): 769–82.

British Medical Research Council. "Treatment of Pulmonary Tuberculosis with Isoniazid." *British Medical Journal* 2, no. 4787 (October 1952): 735–46. https:// www.ncbi.nlm.nih.gov/pmc/articles/PMC2021603/.

British Medical Research Council. "Treatment of Pulmonary Tuberculosis with Streptomycin and Para-Aminosalicylic Acid: A Medical Research Council Investigation." *British Medical Journal* 2, no. 4688 (November 1950): 1073–85.

Brodwin, Paul. *Everyday Ethics: Voices from the Front Line of Community Psychiatry*. Berkeley: University of California Press, 2012.

Brogan, Terry V. F. *Anthimeria*. Edited by Steven Cushman, Clare Cavanagh, Jahan Ramazani, and Paul Rouzer. 4th ed. Princeton, NJ: Princeton University Press, 2012.

Brown, Kate. *Manual for Survival: A Chernobyl Guide to the Future*. New York: W. W. Norton, 2019.

Brown, E. Richard. *Rockefeller Medicine Men: Medicine and Capitalism in America*. Berkeley: University of California Press, 1979.

Buch, Elana. "Anthropology of Aging and Care." *Annual Review of Anthropology* 44 (2015): 277–93.

Bukhman, Gene, Ana Olga Mocumbi, and Richard Horton. "Reframing NCDs and Injuries for the Poorest Billion." *The Lancet* 386 (2015): 1221–22.

Burston, D. *Erik Erikson and the American Psyche: Ego, Ethics, and Evolution*. Lanham, MD: Jason Aronson, 2006.

Butler, Judith. *Frames of War: When Is Life Grievable?* New York: Verso, 2009.

Butler, Judith. "The Inorganic Body in the Early Marx: A Limit Concept in Anthropocentrism." *Radical Philosophy* 206 (Winter 2019): 1–17.

Butler, Judith. *Notes toward a Performative Theory of Assembly*. Cambridge, MA: Harvard University Press, 2015.

Caduff, Carlo. "The Semiotics of Security: Infectious Disease Research and the Biopolitics of Informational Bodies in the United States." *Cultural Anthropology* 27, no. 2 (2012): 333–57.

Callison, Candis. "The Twelve-Year Warning." *Isis* 111, no. 1 (2020): 129–37.

Camarillo, Alberto. "Alambrista and the Historical Context of Mexican Immigration to the United States in the Twentieth Century." In *Alambrista and the US-Mexico Border*, edited by Nicholas Cull and David Carrasco, 13–36. Albuquerque: University of New Mexico Press, 2004.

Campt, Tina. *Listening to Images*. Durham, NC: Duke University Press, 2017.

Canguilhem, Georges. *Knowledge of Life*. Translated by Stephanos Geroulanos and Daniela Ginsburg. New York: Fordham University Press, 2008.

Canguilhem, Georges. *On the Normal and the Pathological*. Translated by Carolyn R. Fawcett. Dordrecht, Netherlands: D. Reidel, 1978.

Carlson, Jennifer. "John Hartigan on Multispecies Ethnography." *Platypus*, August 26, 2014. http://blog.castac.org/2014/08/john-hartigan-on-multispecies-ethnography.

Carothers, J. C. "Frontal Lobe Function and the African." *British Journal of Psychiatry* 97, no. 406 (1951): 12–48.

Carpenter-Song, Elizabeth. "Children's Sense of Self in Relation to Clinical Processes: Portraits of Pharmaceutical Transformation." *Ethos* 37, no. 3 (2009): 257–81.

Carpenter-Song, Elizabeth. "The Kids Were My Drive: Shattered Families, Moral Striving, and the Loss of Parental Selves in the Wake of Homelessness." *Ethos* 47, no. 1 (2019): 54–72.

Carr, Geoffrey. *Bearing Witness: A Brief History of the Indian Residential Schools in Canada*. Morris and Helen Belkin Art Gallery, University of British Columbia, 2013.

Carter, Kevin. *The Vulture and the Little Girl*. Rare Historical Photos, 1993. https://rarehistoricalphotos.com/vulture-little-girl/.

Caudill, William. "Tiny Dramas: Vocal Communication between Mother and Infant in Japanese and American Families." In *Transcultural Research in Mental Health*, edited by William P. Lebra, 25–48. Honolulu: University of Hawai'i Press, 1972.

Cegielski, Peter J. "Extensively Drug-Resistant Tuberculosis: 'There Must Be Some Kind of Way out of Here.'" *Clinical Infectious Diseases* 50 (2010): S195–200.

Chagani, Fayaz. "Critical Political Ecology and the Seductions of Posthumanism." *Journal of Political Ecology* 21 (2014): 424–36.

Chambers, Georgina. "The Economic Impact of Assisted Reproductive Technology: A Review of Selected Developed Countries." *Fertility and Sterility* 91, no. 6 (2009): 2281–94.

Champagne, Frances A. "Epigenetic Mechanisms and the Transgenerational Effects of Maternal Care." *Frontiers in Neuroendocrinology* 29 (2008): 386–97.

Chatterji, Roma. "An Ethnography of Dementia: A Case Study of an Alzheimer's Disease Patient in the Netherlands." *Culture, Medicine, and Psychiatry* 22, no. 3 (1998): 355–82.

Chen, Nancy. *Breathing Spaces: Qigong, Psychiatry, and Healing in China*. New York: Columbia University Press, 2003.

Clark, Rodney. *The Japanese Company*. New Haven, CT: Yale University Press, 1979.

Clarke, Adele E., Laura Mamo, Jennifer R. Fosket, Jennifer R. Fishman, and Janet K. Shim, eds. *Biomedicalization: Technoscience, Health, and Illness in the U.S.* Durham, NC: Duke University Press, 2010.

Clastres, Pierre. "Savage Ethnography (on *Yanoama*)." In *Archeology of Violence*, translated by Jeanine Herman and Ashley Lebner, 81–92. Los Angeles: Semiotext(e), 2010.

Coakley, S., and K. Shelemay, eds. *Pain and Its Transformations: The Interface of Biology and Culture*. Cambridge, MA: Harvard University Press, 2007.

Cohen, Lawrence. "Accusations of Illiteracy and the Medicine of the Organ." *Social Research* 78, no. 1 (2011): 123–42.

Cohen, Lawrence. "The Kothi Wars: AIDS Cosmopolitanism and the Morality of Classification." In *Sex and Development: Science, Sexuality, and Morality in Global Perspective*, edited by Vincanne Adams and Stacey Leigh Pigg, 269–304. Durham, NC: Duke University Press, 2005.

Cohen, Lawrence. "The Nation, De-duplicated." In *Critical Themes in Indian Sociology*, edited by Sanjay Srivastava, Yasmeen Arif, and Janaki Abraham, 107–26. New Delhi: Sage, 2019.

Cohen, Lawrence. *No Aging in India: Alzheimer's, the Bad Family, and Other Modern Things*. Berkeley: University of California Press, 1998.

Cohen, Lawrence. "The Pleasures of Castration: The Postoperative Status of Hijras, Jankhas, and Academics." In *Sexual Nature, Sexual Culture*, edited by Paul Abramson and Steven Pinkerton, 276–304. Chicago: University of Chicago Press, 1995.

Cohen, Lawrence. "Science, Politics, and Dancing Boys: Propositions and Accounts." *Parallax* 14, no. 3 (2008): 35–47.

Cohen, Lawrence. "The Social De-duplicated: On the Aadhaar Platform and the Engineering of Service." *Contemporary South Asia* 42, no. 3 (2019): 482–500.

Cole, Teju, and Fazal Sheikh. *Human Archipelago*. Göttingen, Germany: Steidl Photography International, 2019.

Colen, Shelee. "'Like a Mother to Them': Stratified Reproduction and West Indian Childcare Workers and Employers in New York." In *Conceiving the New World Order: The Global Politics of Reproduction*, edited by Faye D. Ginsburg and Rayna Rapp, 78–102. Berkeley: University of California Press, 1995.

Collins, John A. "An International Survey of the Health Economics of IVF and ICSI." *Human Reproduction Update* 8, no. 3 (2002): 265–77.

Comaroff, Jean, and John L. Comaroff. "Ethnography on an Awkward Scale: Postcolonial Anthropology and the Violence of Abstraction." *Ethnography* 4, no. 2 (2003): 291–324.

Comaroff, Jean, and John L. Comaroff. "Foreword: Thinking Anthropologically about British Anthropology." In *Sage Handbook of Social Anthropology*, edited by Richard Fardon, John Gledhill, Olivia Harris, Trevor Marchand, Mark Nuttall, Chris Shore, Veronica Strang, and Richard Wilson, xxviii–xli. London: Sage, 2012.

Comroe, J. H. "Pay Dirt: The Story of Streptomycin. Part I: From Waksman to Waksman." *American Review of Respiratory Disease* 114, no. 4 (1978): 773–81.

Coninx, R., G. Pfiffer, and C. Mathieu. "Drug Resistant Tuberculosis in Prisons in Azerbaijan: Case Study." *British Medical Journal*, 1998.

Connerton, Paul. *How Societies Remember*. Cambridge: Cambridge University Press, 2010.

Cooper, Theodore S. *Report of the United States Delegation to the World Health Assembly*. Rockville, MD: Public Health Service, 1976.

Crapanzano, Vincent. "On the Writing of Ethnography." *Dialectical Anthropology* 4, no. 3 (1979): 205–54.

Critchley, Simon. *The Book of Dead Philosophers*. New York: Vintage, 2011.

Crofton, J., and D. A. Mitchison. "Streptomycin Resistance in Pulmonary Tuberculosis." *British Medical Journal* 2 (1948): 1009–15.

Crowley-Matoka, Megan. *Domesticating Organ Transplant: Familial Sacrifice and National Aspiration in Mexico*. Durham, NC: Duke University Press, 2016.

Csordas, Thomas J. *Embodiment and Experience: The Existential Ground of Culture and Self*. Cambridge: Cambridge University Press, 1994.

Csordas, Thomas J. "The Navajo Healing Project." *Medical Anthropology Quarterly* 14, no. 4 (2000): 463–75.

Csordas, Thomas J., and Janis H. Jenkins. "Land of a Thousand Cuts: Self-Cutting, Agency, and Mental Illness among Adolescents." *Ethos* 46, no. 2 (2018): 206–29.

Cueto, Marcos. *Cold War, Deadly Fevers: Malaria Eradication in Mexico, 1955–1975*. Baltimore: Johns Hopkins University Press, 2007.

Cueto, Marcos. "The Origins of Primary Health Care and Selective Primary Health Care." *American Journal of Public Heath* 94, no. 11 (2004): 1864–74.

Cull, Nicholas, and Davíd Carrasco. *Alambrista and the US-Mexico Border*. Albuquerque: University of New Mexico Press, 2004.

Curwen, Thomas. "California's Deadliest Wildfires Were Decades in the Making: 'We Have Forgotten What We Need to Do to Prevent It.'" *Los Angeles Times*, October 2017. http://www.latimes.com/local/california/la-me-fire -perspectives-20171022-story.html.

Dahl, Cortland J., Antoine Lutz, and Richard J. Davidson. "Cognitive Processes Are Central in Compassion Meditation." *Trends in Cognitive Sciences* 20, no. 3 (2016): 161–62.

Dalstrom M. "Arthur Kleinman on Caregiving." *Somatosphere*. 2010. http:// somatosphere.net/2010/arthur-kleinman-on-caregiving.html/.

Das, Veena. *Affliction: Health, Disease, Poverty*. New York: Fordham University Press, 2015.

Das, Veena. *Life and Words: Violence and the Descent into the Ordinary*. Berkeley: University of California Press, 2006.

Das, Veena. "Trauma and Testimony: Implications for Political Community." *Anthropological Theory* 3 (2003): 293–307.

Daschuk, James. *Clearing the Plains: Disease, Politics of Starvation, and the Loss of Aboriginal Life*. Regina, SK: University of Regina Press, 2013.

Datey, K. K., P. A. Kale, S. M. Deshmukh, and M. D. Kelkar. "Cardiac Assessment and Selection." *Journal of the Indian Medical Association* 51 (1968): 546–47.

Dave, Naisargi. "Witness." In *Unfinished: The Anthropology of Becoming*, edited by João Biehl and Peter Locke, 151–72. Durham, NC: Duke University Press, 2017.

David-Neel, Alexandra. *Magic and Mystery in Tibet*. New York: Martino Fine Books, 2014 [1932].

David-Neel, Alexandra. *My Journey to Lhasa: The Personal Story of the Only White Woman Who Succeeded in Entering the Forbidden City*. Important Books, 27, 2014 [1932].

Davidson, Richard J. "Mindfulness-Based Cognitive Therapy and the Prevention of Depressive Relapse: Measures, Mechanisms, and Mediators." *Journal of the American Medical Association Psychiatry* 73, no. 6 (June 2016): 547. https://doi.org/10.1001/jamapsychiatry.2016.0135.

Davidson, Richard J. "Well-Being and Affective Style: Neural Substrates and Biobehavioural Correlates." *Philosophical Transactions of the Royal Society B: Biological Sciences* 359, no. 1449 (2004): 1395–1411.

Davidson, Richard J., and Anne Harrington. *Visions of Compassion: Western Scientists and Tibetan Buddhists Examine Human Nature*. Oxford: Oxford University Press, 2002. https://doi.org/10.1093/acprof:oso/9780195130430.001.0001.

Davidson, Richard J., Jon Kabat-Zinn, Jessica Schumacher, and Melissa Rosenkranz, et al. "Alterations in Brain and Immune Function Produced by Mindfulness Meditation." *Psychosomatic Medicine* 65, no. 4 (July 2003): 564–70. https://doi.org/10.1097/01.PSY.0000077505.67574.E3.

Davidson, Richard J., and Alfred W. Kaszniak. "Conceptual and Methodological Issues in Research on Mindfulness and Meditation." *American Psychologist* 70, no. 7 (October 2015): 581–92. https://doi.org/10.1037/a0039512.

Davies, Ian P., and Ryan D. Haugo, James C. Robertson, and Phillip S. Levin. "The Unequal Vulnerability of Communities of Color to Wildfire." *PLOS ONE* (2018). https://doi.org/10.1371/journal.pone.0205825.

Davis, Angela. *Are Prisons Obsolete?* New York: Penguin Random House, 2003.

Davis, Angela. *With My Mind on Freedom: An Autobiography*. New York: Bantam, 1974.

Dawson, J. J., S. Devadatta, W. Fox, and S. Radhakrishna, et al. "A Five-Year Study of Patients with Pulmonary Tuberculosis in a Concurrent Comparison of Home and Sanatorium Treatment for One Year with Isoniazid plus PAS." *Bulletin of the World Health Organization* 34, no. 4 (1966): 533–51.

De Gennaro, Mara. "Love Stories, or, Multispecies Ethnography, Comparative Literature, and Their Entanglements." *State of the Discipline Report*, May 30, 2015. https://stateofthediscipline.acla.org/entry/love-stories-or-multispecies-ethnography-comparative-literature-and-their-entanglements.

De León, Jason. *The Land of Open Graves: Living and Dying on the Migrant Trail*. Berkeley: University of California Press, 2015.

Deleuze, Gilles. *Difference and Repetition*. Translated by Paul Patton. New York: Columbia University Press, 1994.

Deleuze, Gilles. *Essays: Critical and Clinical*. Translated by Daniel W. Smith and Michael A. Greco. Minneapolis: University of Minnesota Press, 1997.

Deleuze, Gilles. *Foucault*. Translated by Sean Hand. Minneapolis: University of Minnesota Press, 1988.

Deleuze, Gilles, and Michel Foucault. "Cold and Heat." In *Revisions 2, Photogenic Painting—Gerard Fromanger*. London: Black Dog, 1999.

Deleuze, Gilles, and Félix Guattari. *A Thousand Plateaus: Capitalism and Schizophrenia*. Translated by Brian Massumi. Minneapolis: University of Minnesota Press, 1987.

Desjarlais, Robert. *The Blind Man: A Phantasmography*. New York City: Fordham University Press, 2019.

Desjarlais, Robert. *Body and Emotion: The Aesthetics of Illness and Healing in the Nepal Himalayas*. Phildelphia: University of Pennsylvania Press, 1992.

Desjarlais, Robert. *Sensory Biographies: Lives and Deaths among Nepal's Yolmo Buddhists*. Berkeley: University of California Press, 2002.

Desjarlais, Robert. *Shelter Blues: Sanity and Selfhood among the Homeless*. Philadelphia: University of Pennsylvania Press, 1997.

Desjarlais, Robert. *Subject to Death: Life and Loss in a Buddhist World*. Chicago: University of Chicago Press, 2016.

Devereux, George. "Normal and Abnormal: The Key Problem of Psychiatric Anthropology." In *Some Uses of Anthropology: Theoretical and Applied*. Washington, DC: Washington Anthropological Society, 1956.

Dhawan, J., and C. L. Bray. "Are Asian Coronary Arteries Smaller Than Caucasian? A Study on Angiographic Coronary Artery Size Estimation during Life." *International Journal of Cardiology* 49 (1995): 267–69.

Didi-Huberman, Georges. *Survival of the Fireflies*. Translated by Lia Swope Mitchell. Minneapolis: University of Minnesota Press, 2018.

"Dr. Sen Does His Second Heart Graft." *Indian Express*, September 16, 1968, 1.

Doi, Takeo. *The Anatomy of Self: The Individual versus Society*. Tokyo: Kodansha International, 1986.

Downey, Clare. "Why Are California's Wildfires So Out of Control?" Video, 2017. https://www.theguardian.com/world/video/2017/dec/08/why-are-californias-wildfires-so-out-of-control-video-explainer.

Du Bois, Cora A. *The People of Alor: A Social-Psychological Study of an East Indian Island*. Minneapolis: University of Minnesota Press, 1944.

Dubos, Rene. "Microbiology." *Annual Review of Biochemistry* 11 (1942): 659–78.

Dubow, Saul. "Smuts, the United Nations and the Rhetoric of Race and Rights." *Journal of Contemporary History* 43, no. 1 (January 2008): 45–74. https://doi.org/10.1177/0022009407084557.

Dumit, Joseph. *Drugs for Life: How Pharmaceutical Companies Define Our Health.* Durham, NC: Duke University Press, 2012.

Duncan, Whitney L. *Transforming Therapy: Mental Health Practice and Cultural Change in Mexico.* Nashville, TN: Vanderbilt University Press, 2018.

Dunn, Frederick L. "Traditional Asian Medicine and Cosmopolitan Medicine as Adaptive Systems." In *Asian Medical Systems: A Comparative Study,* edited by Charles Leslie, 133–58. Berkeley: University of California Press, 1976.

Durand, Jorge, and Douglas S. Massey. *Miracles on the Border: Retablos of Mexican Migrants to the United States.* Tucson: University of Arizona Press, 1995.

Dutta, Aniruddha, Adnan Hossain, and Claire Pamment. "Representing the Hijras of South Asia: Toward Transregional and Global Flows." In *Mapping LGBTQ Spaces and Places: A Changing World,* edited by Marianne Blidon and Stanley D. Brunn, 85–103. Cham, Switzerland: Springer, 2022.

Ecks, Stefan. *Eating Drugs: Psychopharmaceutical Pluralism in India.* New York: New York University Press, 2013.

Engerman, David C. *The Price of Aid: The Economic Cold War in India.* Cambridge, MA: Harvard University Press, 2018.

Erikson, E. *Childhood and Society.* New York: W. W. Norton, 1950.

Evans-Pritchard, E. *Witchcraft, Oracles, and Magic among the Azande.* Oxford: Clarendon, 1937.

Fabian, Johannes. *Time and the Other: How Anthropology Makes Its Object.* New York: Columbia University Press, 2002.

Fadiman, Anne. *The Spirit Catches You and You Fall Down.* New York: Farrar, Straus and Giroux, 2012.

Fanon, Frantz. *The Wretched of the Earth.* Translated by Constance Farrington. Middlesex, UK: Penguin, 1969.

Farley, John. *Brock Chisholm, the World Health Organization, and the Cold War.* Vancouver: University of British Columbia Press, 2008.

Farmer, Paul. *AIDS and Accusation: Haiti and the Geography of Blame.* Berkeley: University of California Press, 1992.

Farmer, Paul. "An Anthropology of Structural Violence." *Current Anthropology* 45, no. 3 (2004): 305–25.

Farmer, Paul. *Fevers, Feuds, and Diamonds: Ebola and the Ravages of History.* New York: Farrar, Straus, and Giroux, 2020.

Farmer, Paul. *Infections and Inequalities: The Modern Plagues.* Berkeley: University of California Press, 2001.

Farmer, Paul. "Never Again? Reflections on Human Values and Human Rights." In *The Tanner Lectures on Human Values,* edited by G. B. Peterson, vol. 26. Salt Lake City: University of Utah Press, 2006.

Farmer, Paul, with Haun Saussy and Tracy Kidder. *Partner to the Poor: A Paul Farmer Reader.* Berkeley: University of California Press, 2010.

Farmer, Paul. *Pathologies of Power: Health, Human Rights, and the New War on the Poor.* Berkeley: University of Calfornia Press, 2003.

Farmer, Paul E., and Jim Yong Kim. "Resurgent TB in Russia: Do We Know
Enough to Act?" *European Journal of Public Health* 10, no. 2 (June 2000):
150–53. https://doi.org/10.1093/eurpub/10.2.150.

Farmer, Paul, Jim Yong Kim, Arthur Kleinman, and Mathew Basilico. *Reimagining
Global Health: An Introduction*. Berkeley: University of California Press, 2013.

Farmer, P. E., A. S. Kononets, S. E. Borisov, and A. Goldfarb, et al. "Recrudescent
Tuberculosis in the Russian Federation." In *The Global Impact of Drug-
Resistant Tuberculosis*, 41–83. Boston: Open Society Institute, Harvard Medi-
cal School, 1999.

Farquhar, Judith, and Qincheng Zhang. *Ten Thousand Things: Nurturing Life in Contemporary Beijing*. New York: Zone, 2012.

Fassin, Didier. "Another Politics of Life Is Possible." *Theory, Culture and Society* 26,
no. 5 (2009): 44–60.

Fassin, Didier. *When Bodies Remember: Experiences and Politics of AIDS in South Africa*.
Translated by Amy Jacobs and Gabrielle Varro. Berkeley: University of
California Press, 2007.

Favret-Saada, Jeanne. *Deadly Words: Witchcraft in the Bocage*. Translated by Catherine Cullen. Cambridge: Cambridge University Press, 1981.

Feld, S. *Sound and Sentiment: Birds, Weeping, Poetics, and Song in Kaluli Expression*.
Philadelphia: University of Pennsylvania Press, 1982.

Ferguson, James. *Give a Man a Fish: Reflections on the New Politics of Distribution*.
Durham, NC: Duke University Press, 2015.

Field, M. J. *Search for Security: An Ethnopsychiatric Study of Rural Ghana*. Evanston,
IL: Northwestern University Press, 1960.

"First-Ever Heart Transplant in India: Patient Dies." *Times of India*, February 20,
1968, 1.

"First Ever Successful Heart Transplant Conducted in Mumbai Thanks to Efforts
of Police." *Daily News and Analysis*, August 3, 2015, 2110832.

Fischer, Michael M. J. *Anthropology in the Meantime: Experimental Ethnography,
Theory, and Method for the Twenty-First Century*. Durham, NC: Duke University Press, 2018.

Foucault, Michel. *The Birth of the Clinic: An Archaeology of Medical Perception*. Translated by A. M. Sheridan Smith. New York: Pantheon, 1994.

Foucault, Michel. "The Birth of Social Medicine." In *The Essential Foucault*, edited
by Paul Rabinow and Nikolas Rose, 134–56. New York: New Press, 1974.

Foucault, Michel. *The History of Sexuality, Volume 1: An Introduction*. Translated by
Robert Hurley. New York: Vintage, 1990.

Foucault, Michel. *Madness and Civilization: On the History of Madness in an Age of
Reason*. Translated by Richard Howard. New York: Vintage, 1973.

Foucault, Michel. "Photogenic Painting." In Gilles Deleuze and Michel Foucault,
Revisions 2, Photogenic Painting—Gerard Fromanger. London: Black Dog, 1999.

Foucault, Michel. "What Is an Author?" In *Aesthetics, Methods and Epistemology*,
edited by James Faubion. New York: New Press, 1999.

Fox, Renée C., and Judith P. Swazey. *The Courage to Fail: A Social View of Organ
Transplants and Dialysis*. Chicago: University of Chicago Press, 1974.

Fox, W., G. A. Ellard, and D. A. Mitchison. "Studies on the Treatment of Tuberculosis Undertaken by the British Medical Research Council Tuberculosis Units, 1946–1986, with Relevant Subsequent Publications." *International Journal of Tuberculosis and Lung Disease* 3, no. 10, supp. 2 (October 1999): S231–79.

Fox, Wallace. "The Medical Research Council Trials of Isoniazid: Recent Results of Combined Chemotherapy." *Bulletin of the International Union against Tuberculosis and Lung Disease* 23 (1953): 292–307.

Fox, Wallace. "The Problem of Self-Administration of Drugs, with Particular Reference to Pulmonary Tuberculosis." *Tubercle* 39, no. 5 (October 1958): 269–74. https://doi.org/10.1016/S0041-3879(58)80088-4.

Fox, Wallace. "Realistic Chemotherapeutic Policies for Tuberculosis in the Developing Countries." *British Medical Journal* 1, no. 5376 (January 1964): 135–42. https://doi.org/10.1136/bmj.1.5376.135.

Fox, Wallace. "Whither Short-Course Chemotherapy?" *British Journal of Diseases of the Chest* 75, no. 4 (October 1981): 331–57. https://doi.org/10.1016/0007 -0971(81)90022-X.

Fox, Wallace, and Ian Sutherland. "A Five-Year Assessment of Patients in a Controlled Trial of Streptomycin, Para-Aminosalicylic Acid, and Streptomycin plus Para-Aminosalicylic Acid, in Pulmonary Tuberculosis." *QJM: An International Journal of Medicine* 25, no. 2 (April 1956): 221–44. https://doi.org/10 .1093/oxfordjournals.qjmed.a066751.

Frankfurter, Raphael. "Conjuring Biosecurity in the Post-Ebola Kissi Triangle: The Magic of Paperwork in a Frontier Clinic." *Medical Anthropology Quarterly* 33 (2019): 517–38.

Franklin, Joshua, and Michelle Munyikwa. "The Thinness of Care: The Promise of Medical Anthropology in MD/PhD Training." *Somatosphere* (2021): n.p. http:// somatosphere.net/2021/care-medical-anthropology-md-phd-training.html.

Frazier, LaToya Ruby. *The Notion of Family*. New York: Aperture Foundation, 2014.

Friesen, Joe. "Widening Education Gap Leaves Aboriginal Canadians Further Behind," *Globe and Mail*, October 7, 2013. https://www.theglobeandmail .com/news/national/education/widening-education-gap-leaves-aboriginal -canadians-further-behind/article14738527.

Gaines, Atwood D. "Culture, Medicine, Psychiatry and Wisdom: Honoring Arthur Kleinman." *Culture, Medicine and Psychiatry* 40, no. 4 (2016): 538–69.

Gangadharam, P. R., A. L. Bhatia, S. Radhakrishna, and J. B. Selkon. "Rate of Inactivation of Isoniazid in South Indian Patients with Pulmonary Tuberculosis: 1. Microbiological Assay of Isoniazid in Serum Following a Standard Intramuscular Dose." *Bulletin of the World Health Organization* 25 (1961): 765–77.

Garcia, Angela. *The Pastoral Clinic: Addiction and Dispossession along the Rio Grande*. Berkeley: University of California Press, 2010.

Garon, Sheldon. *Molding Japanese Minds: The State in Everyday Life*. Princeton, NJ: Princeton University Press, 1997.

Gawande, Atul. *Being Mortal*. New York: Picador, 2015.

Geertz, Clifford. "Common Sense as a Cultural System." In *Local Knowledge: Further Essays in Interpretive Anthropology*, 73–93. New York: Basic Books, 1983.

Geertz, Clifford, ed. *Old Societies and New States: The Quest for Modernity in Asia and Africa*. New York: Free Press, 1963.

Getachew, Adom. *Worldmaking after Empire: The Rise and Fall of Self-Determination*. Princeton, NJ: Princeton University Press, 2019.

Gibbs, W. Wayt. "The Unseen Genome: Gems among the Junk." *Scientific American* 289, no. 5 (November 2003): 46–53. https://doi.org/10.1038/scientificamerican1103-46.

Gilbert, Scott F. "The Reactive Genome." In *Origination and Organismal Form: Beyond the Gene in Developmental and Evolutionary Biology*, edited by Gerd B. Müller and Stuart A. Newman, 87–101. Cambridge, MA: MIT Press, 2003.

Gilligan, Carol. *In a Different Voice*. Cambridge, MA: Harvard University Press, 1982.

Gilmore, Ruth Wilson. *Golden Gulag: Prisons, Surplus, Crisis, and Opposition in Globalizing California*. Berkeley: University of California Press, 2007.

Gilpin, Emilee. "Urgency in Climate Change Advocacy Is Backfiring, Says Citizen Potawatomi Nation Scientist." *National Observer*, February 15, 2019.

Ginzburg, Carlo. *Clues, Myths, and the Historical Method*. Translated by John Tedeschi and Anne C. Tedeschi. Baltimore: Johns Hopkins, 1989.

Gish, Oscar. "Selective Primary Health Care: Old Wine in New Bottles." *Social Science and Medicine* 16, no. 10 (January 1982): 1049–54. https://doi.org/10.1016/0277-9536(82)90177-0.

Glaude, Eddie. *Begin Again: James Baldwin's America and Its Urgent Lessons for Our Own*. New York: Penguin Random House, 2020.

Glenn, Evelyn. *Forced to Care*. Cambridge, MA: Harvard University Press, 2012.

Goldstein, Melvyn C. *A History of Modern Tibet, 1913–1951*. Berkeley: University of California Press, 1989.

Gone, J. P. "Redressing First Nations Historical Trauma: Theorizing Mechanisms for Indigenous Culture as Mental Health Treatment." *Transcultural Psychiatry* 50, no. 5 (2013): 83–706. https://doi.org/10.1177/1363461513487669.

Good, Byron J. "The Complexities of Psychopharmaceutical Hegemonies in Indonesia." In *Pharmaceutical Self: The Global Shaping of Experience in an Age of Psychopharmacology*, edited by Janis H. Jenkins, 117–44. Santa Fe, NM: School for Advanced Research Press, 2010.

Good, Byron J. "Culture and Psychopathology: Directions for Psychiatric Anthropology." In *New Directions in Psychological Anthropology*, edited by Theodore Schwartz, Geoffrey M. White, and Catherine A. Lutz, 181–205. Cambridge: Cambridge University Press, 1992.

Good, Byron J. *Medicine, Rationality, and Experience: An Anthropological Perspective*. Cambridge: Cambridge University Press, 1994.

Good, Mary-Jo DelVecchio. *American Medicine: The Quest for Competence*. Berkeley: University of California Press, 1995.

Good, Mary-Jo DelVecchio, Sarah S. Willen, and Seth Donal Hannah. *Shattering Culture: American Medicine Responds to Cultural Diversity*. Edited by Ken Vickery and Lawrence Taeseng Park. New York: Russell Sage Foundation, 2011.

Goździak, Elżbieta M., and Izabella Main. "Erasing Polish Anthropology?" *Anthropology News*, December 7, 2018. http://www.anthropology-news.org/index.php/2018/12/07/erasing-polish-anthropology.

Green, James. *Beyond the Good Death: The Anthropology of Modern Dying*. Philadelphia: University of Pennsylvania Press, 2008.

Greenblatt, Stephen. "'Tell My Story': The Human Compulsion to Narrate." Lecture given to the Royal Danish Academy of Sciences and Letters, posted June 2, 2014. https://www.youtube.com/watch?v=zvtgLkhij2s&ab_channel=VidenskabernesSelskab.

Greene, Jeremy A., and Dora Vargha. "How Epidemics End." *Boston Review*, June 30, 2020. http://bostonreview.net/science-nature/jeremy-greene-dora-vargha-how-epidemics-end.

Guess, H. A., A. Kleinman, J. W. Kusek, and L. W. Engel, eds. *The Science of the Placebo*. London: British Medical Journal Books, 2002.

Gulløv, Eva. "Welfare and Self Care: Institutionalized Visions for a Good Life in Danish Day-Care Centres." *Anthropology in Action* 18, no. 3 (January 2011): 21–32. https://doi.org/10.3167/aia.2011.180303.

Gyatso, J. "The Authority of Empiricism and the Empiricism of Authority: Medicine and Buddhism in Tibet on the Eve of Modernity." *Comparative Studies of South Asia, Africa and the Middle East* 24, no. 2 (January 2004): 83–96. https://doi.org/10.1215/1089201X-24-2-83.

Gyatso, Janet. *Being Human in a Buddhist World: An Intellectual History of Medicine in Early Modern Tibet*. New York: Columbia University Press, 2015.

Gyatso, Janet. "The Ins and Outs of Self-transformation: Personal and Social Sides of Visionary Practice in Tibetan Buddhism." In *Self and Self-Transformation in the History of Religions*, edited by David Shulman and Guy Stroumsa, 183–94. New York: Oxford University Press, 2002.

Hacking, Ian. *Re-writing the Soul: Multiple Personality and the Sciences of Memory*. Princeton, NJ: Princeton University Press, 1995.

Hage, Ghassan. "Afterword." In *Ethnographies of Waiting*, edited by Manpreet K. Janeja and Andreas Bandak, 203–8. London: Bloomsbury, 2018.

Hahn, Robert A., and Arthur Kleinman. "Belief as Pathogen, Belief as Medicine: 'Voodoo Death' and the 'Placebo Phenomenon' in Anthropological Perspective." *Medical Anthropology Quarterly* 14, no. 4 (August 1983): 3–19. https://doi.org/10.1525/maq.1983.14.4.02a00030.

Hallowell, A. Irving. *Culture and Experience*. Philadelphia: University of Pennsylvania, 1955.

Hansen, Helena. "Pharmaceutical Prosthesis and White Racial Rescue in the Prescription Opioid 'Epidemic.'" *Somatosphere*, December 14, 2015. http://somatosphere.net/2015/pharmaceutical-prosthesis-and-white-racial-rescue-in-the-prescription-opioid-epidemic.html.

Hansen, Helena, and Julie Netherland. "Is the Prescription Opioid Epidemic a White Problem?" *American Journal of Public Health* 106, no. 12 (2016): 2127–29.

Haraway, Donna. *Staying with the Trouble: Making Kin in the Chthulucene*. Durham, NC: Duke University Press, 2016.

Haraway, Donna. *When Species Meet*. Minneapolis: University of Minnesota Press, 2008.

Harney, Stefano, and Fred Moten. "Politics Surrounded." In *The Undercommons: Fugitive Planning and Black Study*, by Stefano Harney and Fred Moten, 14–21. Brooklyn: Autonomedia, 2013.

Harris, Gardiner. "'Superbugs' Kill India's Babies and Pose an Overseas Threat." *New York Times*, December 4, 2014. https://www.nytimes.com/2014/12/04/world/asia/superbugs-kill-indias-babies-and-pose-an-overseas-threat.html.

Harvey, David. *The Condition of Postmodernity: An Enquiry into the Origins of Cultural Change*. Cambridge: Blackwell, 1990.

"Heart Operation in Bombay: Indian Machine Used." *Times of India*, February 18, 1961, 9.

Heelas, John, and Andrew Lock. *Indigenous Psychologies: The Anthropology of the Self*. London: Academic Press, 1981.

Hegel, G. W. F., and T. M. Knox. *Aesthetics, Volume 1*. Oxford: Clarendon, 1975.

Hehir, Patrick. "Angina Pectoris with Post-mortem Examination: Fatty Degeneration of Heart." *Indian Medical Gazette* 26, no. 9 (September 1891): 268–69.

Heidegger, Martin. *The Question Concerning Technology, and Other Essays*. Translated by William Lovitt. New York: Harper Perennial, 1982.

Heijmans, B. T., E. W. Tobi, A. D. Stein, and H. Putter et al. "Persistent Epigenetic Differences Associated with Prenatal Exposure to Famine in Humans." *Proceedings of the National Academy of Sciences* 105, no. 44 (November 2008): 17046–49. https://doi.org/10.1073/pnas.0806560105.

Herzfeld, Michael. *The Social Production of Indifference: Exploring the Symbolic Roots of Western Bureaucracy*. Chicago: University of Chicago Press, 1993.

Hill, Leslie. *Maurice Blanchot and Fragmentary Writing: A Change of Epoch*. London: Continuum, 2012.

Hinton, Devon E., and Byron Good. *Culture and Panic Disorder*. Stanford, CA: Stanford University Press, 2009.

Hinton, Devon E., Alexander L. Hinton, Kok-Thay Eng, and Sophearith Choung. "PTSD and Key Somatic Complaints and Cultural Syndromes among Rural Cambodians: The Results of a Needs Assessment Survey." *Medical Anthropology Quarterly* 26, no. 3 (September 2012): 383–407. https://doi.org/10.1111/j.1548-1387.2012.01224.x.

Holmes, Seth. "Discussing 'Suffering Slot Anthropology' with Migrant Farm Workers." *Society for Medical Anthropology* 57, no. 11 (2016): 254–58.

Holmes, Seth. *Fresh Fruit, Broken Bodies*. Berkeley: University California Press, 2013.

Holthaus, Eric. "The First Wintertime Megafire in California History Is Here." *Grist*, December 8, 2017. https://grist.org/article/the-first-wintertime-megafire-in-california-history-is-here.

Hopper, Kim. "Interrogating the Meaning of 'Culture' in the WHO International Studies of Schizophrenia." In *Schizophrenia, Culture, and Subjectivity: The Edge of Experience*, edited by Janis H. Jenkins and Robert J. Barrett, 62–86. New York: Cambridge University Press, 2004.

Horowitz, Michael D., and Jeffrey A. Rosensweig. "Medical Tourism—Health Care in the Global Economy." *Physician Executive* 33, no. 6 (2007): 24–26, 28–30.

Horton, Robin. "Ritual Man in Africa." *Africa* 34 (1964): 85–104.

Hunt, N. R. "Rewriting the Soul in a Colonial Congo." *Past and Present* 198, no. 1 (February 2008): 185–215. https://doi.org/10.1093/pastj/gtm049.

Hurston, Zora Neale. "Mules and Men." In *Folklore, Memoirs, and Other Writings*, 1–267. New York: Penguin, 1995.

Huth, John. *The Lost Art of Finding Our Way*. Cambridge, MA: Harvard University Press, 2013.

Imamura, Anne E. *Urban Japanese Housewives: At Home and in the Community*. Honolulu: University of Hawai'i Press, 1987.

Ingold, Tim. *Making: Anthropology, Archaeology, Art and Architecture*. London: Routledge, 2013.

Ingold, Tim. "The Textility of Making." *Cambridge Journal of Economics* 34, no. 1 (January 2010): 91–102. https://doi.org/10.1093/cje/bep042.

Inhorn, Marcia C. *Cosmopolitan Conceptions: IVF Sojourns in Global Dubai*. Durham, NC: Duke University Press, 2015.

Inhorn, Marcia C. *Local Babies, Global Science: Gender, Religion, and In Vitro Fertilization in Egypt*. New York: Routledge, 2003.

Inhorn, Marcia C. *The New Arab Man: Emergent Masculinities, Technologies, and Islam in the Middle East*. Princeton, NJ: Princeton University Press, 2012.

Inhorn, Marcia C. *Quest for Conception: Gender, Infertility, and Egyptian Medical Traditions*. Philadelphia: University of Pennsylvania Press, 1994.

Inhorn, Marcia C., and P. Patrizio. "Infertility around the Globe: New Thinking on Gender, Reproductive Technologies and Global Movements in the 21st Century." *Human Reproduction Update* 21, no. 4 (July 2015): 411–26. https://doi.org/10.1093/humupd/dmv016.

Ismail, Manal. "Dubai Healthcare City to Compete for Foreign Patients," *The National*, February 12, 2012. https://www.thenational.ae/business/travel-and-tourism/dubai-healthcare-city-to-compete-for-foreign-patients-1.383181.

Jackson, Michael. *Life within Limits: Well-being in a World of Want*. Durham, NC: Duke University Press, 2011.

Jaffrey, Zia. *The Invisibles*. New York: Pantheon, 1996.

"Jawaharlal Nehru Is Dead: Sudden End Follows a Heart Attack." *Times of India*, May 28, 1964, 1.

Jebens, Holger, and Karl-Heinz Kohl. *The End of Anthropology*. Wantage, UK: Sean Kingston, 2011.

Jenkins, Janis H. *Extraordinary Conditions: Culture and Experience in Mental Illness*. Berkeley: University of California Press, 2015.

Jenkins, Janis H., and Robert J. Barrett. *Schizophrenia, Culture, and Subjective: The Edge of Experience*. New York: Cambridge University Press, 2004.

Jenkins, Janis H., ed. *Pharmaceutical Self: The Global Shaping of Experience in an Age of Psychopharmacology*. Santa Fe, NM: School for Advanced Research Press, 2010.

Jenkins, Janis H. "Schizophrenia as a Paradigm for Understanding Fundamental Human Processes." In *Schizophrenia, Culture, and Subjectivity: The Edge of Experience*, edited by Janis H. Jenkins and Robert J. Barrett, 29–61. New York: Cambridge University Press, 2004.

Jenkins, Janis H. "The State Construction of Affect: Political Ethos and Mental Health among Salvadoran Refugees." *Culture, Medicine, and Psychiatry* 15 (1991): 139–65.

Jenkins, Janis H. "Subjective Experience of Persistent Schizophrenia and Depression among Latinos and Euro-Americans." *British Journal of Psychiatry* 171 (1997): 20–25.

Jenkins, Janis H., and Robert J. Barrett, eds. "Introduction." In *Schizophrenia, Culture, and Subjective: The Edge of Experience*, 1–28. New York: Cambridge University Press, 2004.

Jenkins, Janis H., and Elizabeth Carpenter-Song. "The New Paradigm of Recovery from Schizophrenia: Cultural Conundrums of Improvement without Cure." *Culture, Medicine and Psychiatry* 29, no. 4 (2005): 379–413.

Jenkins, Janis H., and Elizabeth Carpenter-Song. "Stigma Despite Recovery: Strategies for Living in the Aftermath of Psychosis." *Medical Anthropology Quarterly* 22, no. 4 (2008): 381–409.

Jenkins, Janis H., and Thomas Csordas. *Troubled in the Land of Enchantment: Adolescent Experience of Psychiatric Treatment*. Oakland: University of California Press, 2020.

Jenkins, Janis H., and Marvin Karno. "The Meaning of Expressed Emotion: Theoretical Issues Raised by Cross-Cultural Research." *American Journal of Psychiatry* 149, no. 1 (1992): 9–21.

Jenkins, Janis H., and Ellen E. Kozelka. "Global Mental Health and Psychopharmacology in Precarious Ecologies: Anthropological Considerations for Engagement and Efficacy." In *The Palgrave Handbook of Sociocultural Perspectives on Global Mental Health*, edited by R. G. White, 151–68. London: Palgrave Macmillan, 2017.

Jenkins, Janis H., and Marta E. Valiente. "Bodily Transactions of the Passions: El Calor (The Heat) among Salvadoran Women." In *Embodiment and Experience: The Existential Ground of Culture and Self*, edited by Thomas Csordas, 163–82. Cambridge: Cambridge University Press, 1994.

Jobson, Ryan. "The Case for Letting Anthropology Burn: Sociocultural Anthropology in 2020." *American Anthropologist* 12, no. 2 (2020): 259–71.

Joglekar, S. V. "Heart Transplant—Ethical and Legal Aspects." *Journal of the Indian Medical Association* 51 (1968): 557–58.

Jones, David S. *Broken Hearts: The Tangled History of Cardiac Care*. Baltimore: Johns Hopkins University Press, 2013.

Jones, David S., and Jeremy A. Greene. "The Decline and Rise of Coronary Heart Disease: Understanding Public Health Catastrophism." *American Journal of*

Public Health 103, no. 7 (July 2013): 1207–18. https://doi.org/10.2105/AJPH.2013 .301226.

Jones, David S., and Kavita Sivaramakrishnan. "Making Heart-Lung Machines Work in India: Imports, Indigenous Innovation, and the Challenge of Replicating Cardiac Surgery in Bombay, 1952–1962." *Social Studies of Science* 48 (2018): 507–39.

Jones, David S., and Kavita Sivaramakrishnan. "Transplant Buccaneers: P. K. Sen and India's First Heart Transplant, February 1968." *Journal of the History of Medicine and Allied Sciences* 73 (2018): 303–32.

Kahneman, Daniel, and Gary Klein. "Conditions for Intuitive Expertise: A Failure to Disagree." *American Psychologist* 64, no. 6 (2009): 515–26. https://doi.org/10 .1037/a0016755.

Kamat, S. R., J. J. Dawson, S. Devadatta, and W. Fox et al. "A Controlled Study of the Influence of Segregation of Tuberculous Patients for One Year on the Attack Rate of Tuberculosis in a Five-Year Period in Close Family Contacts in South India." *Bulletin of the World Health Organization* 34, no. 4 (1966): 517–32.

Kaplan, G. J., R. I. Fraser, and G. W. Comstock. "Tuberculosis in Alaska, 1970: The Continued Decline of the Tuberculosis Epidemic." *American Review of Respiratory Disease* 105, no. 6 (June 1972): 920–26. https://doi.org/10.1164/arrd .1972.105.6.920.

Karakus, Ilkim. "Forms of Governance in Istanbul, Turkey: State Care, and Urban Marginalization." Proposal for doctoral research, Department of Anthropology, Harvard University, Cambridge, MA, November 2018.

Kardiner, Abram. *The Traumatic Neuroses of War*. Washington, DC: National Research Council, 1941.

Katz, Pearl. *The Scalpel's Edge*. Boston: Allyn and Bacon, 1999.

Kaufman, Sharon R. *The Ageless Self: Sources of Meaning in Late Life*. Life Course Studies. Madison: University of Wisconsin Press, 1986.

Kaufman, Sharon. *And a Time to Die: How American Hospitals Shape the End of Life*. Berkeley: University of California Press, 2006.

Kaufman, Sharon. *Ordinary Medicine: Extraordinary Treatments, Longer Lives, and Where to Draw the Line*. Durham, NC: Duke University Press, 2015.

Keller, Evelyn Fox. "From Gene Action to Reactive Genomes." *Journal of Physiology* 592, no. 11 (June 2014): 2423–29. https://doi.org/10.1113/jphysiol.2014.270991.

Keshavjee, Salmaan. *Blind Spot: How Neoliberalism Infiltrated Global Health*. Berkeley: University of California Press, 2014.

Keshavjee, Salmaan, David Dowdy, and Soumya Swaminathan. "Stopping the Body Count: A Comprehensive Approach to Move towards Zero Tuberculosis Deaths." *The Lancet* 386, no. 10010 (December 2015): e46–47. https://doi .org/10.1016/S0140-6736(15)00320-7.

Kim, Jim Yong, Michael Porter, Joseph Rhatigan, and Rebecca Weintraub et al. "Scaling Up Effective Delivery Models Worldwide." In *Reimagining Global Health: An Introduction*, edited by Paul Farmer, Jim Yong Kim, Arthur Kleinman, and Matthew Basilico, 194–211. Berkeley: University of California Press, 2013.

Kimerling, Michael E. "The Russian Equation: An Evolving Paradigm in Tuberculosis Control." *International Journal of Tuberculosis and Lung Disease* 4 (2000): S160–67.

Kimerling, Michael E., H. Kluge, N. Vezhnina, and T. Iacovazzi et al. "Inadequacy of the Current WHO Re-treatment Regimen in a Central Siberian Prison: Treatment Failure and MDR-TB." *International Journal of Tuberculosis and Lung Disease* 3, no. 5 (May 1999): 451–53.

Kinare, S. G. "Autopsy." *Journal of the Indian Medical Association* 51 (1968): 558–62.

Kirksey, Eben, and Stefan Helmreich. "The Emergence of Multispecies Ethnography." *Cultural Anthropology* 25, no. 4, 2010: 545–76. https://anthropology.mit .edu/sites/default/files/documents/helmreich_multispecies_ethnography .pdf.

Kirmayer, Laurence J., and James M. Robbins. "Three Forms of Somatization in Primary Care: Prevalence, Co-occurrence, and Sociodemographic Characteristics." *Journal of Nervous and Mental Disease* 179, no. 11 (November 1991): 647–55. https://doi.org/10.1097/00005053-199111000-00001.

Kitanaka, Junko. *Depression in Japan: Psychiatric Cures for a Society in Distress*. Princeton, NJ: Princeton University Press, 2012.

Kleinman, Arthur. "The Art of Medicine: The Divided Self, Hidden Values, and Moral Sensibility in Medicine." *The Lancet* 377, no. 9768 (March 2011): 804–5. https://doi.org/10.1016/S0140-6736(11)60295-X.

Kleinman, Arthur. "The Background and Development of Public Health in China." In *Public Health in the People's Republic of China*, edited by M. E. Wegman, T. Y. Lin, and E. F. Purcell, 1–23. New York: Josiah Macy Jr. Foundation, 1973.

Kleinman, Arthur. "Caregiving as Moral Experience." *The Lancet* 380, no. 9853 (2012): 1550–51.

Kleinman, Arthur. "Caregiving: The Odyssey of Becoming More Human." *The Lancet* 373, no. 9660 (2009).

Kleinman, Arthur. "Caring for Memories." *The Lancet* 387, no. 10038 (2016): 2596.

Kleinman, Arthur. "Catastrophe and Caregiving: The Failure of Medicine as an Art." *The Lancet* 371, no. 9606 (January 2008): 22–23. https://doi.org/10.1016 /S0140-6736(08)60057-4.

Kleinman, Arthur. "The Delegitimation and Relegitimation of Local Worlds." In *Pain as Human Experience: An Anthropological Perspective*, edited by Mary-Jo DelVecchio Good, Paul Brodwin, Byron J. Good, and Arthur Kleinman, 169–97. Berkeley: University of California Press, 1994.

Kleinman, Arthur. "Depression, Somatization and the 'New Cross-Cultural Psychiatry.'" *Social Science and Medicine* 11, no. 1 (January 1977): 3–9. https://doi .org/10.1016/0037-7856(77)90138-X.

Kleinman, Arthur. "'Everything That Really Matters': Social Suffering, Subjectivity, and the Remaking of Human Experience in a Disordering World." *Harvard Theological Review* 90, no. 3 (1997): 315–35.

Kleinman, Arthur. *Experience and Its Moral Modes: Culture, Human Conditions, and Disorder*. Stanford, CA: Stanford University Press, 1998.

Kleinman, Arthur. "Forum: On Caregiving." *Harvard Magazine*, July–August 2010. https://harvardmagazine.com/2010/07/on-caregiving.

Kleinman, Arthur. "From Illness as Culture to Caregiving as Moral Experience." *New England Journal of Medicine* 368, no. 15 (2013): 1376–77.

Kleinman, Arthur. "How Rituals and Focus Can Turn Isolation into a Time for Growth." *Wall Street Journal*, April 9, 2020. https://www.wsj.com /articles/how-rituals-and-focus-can-turn-isolation-into-a-time-for-growth -11586445045.

Kleinman, Arthur. "How We Endure." *The Lancet* 383, no. 9912 (2014): 119–20.

Kleinman, Arthur. *The Illness Narratives: Suffering, Healing, and the Human Condition.* New York: Basic, 1988

Kleinman, Arthur. "An Intellectual Journey and Personal Odyssey." *Bulletin of the American Academy of Arts and Sciences* 68, no. 3 (2015): 58–59.

Kleinman, Arthur. "Local Worlds of Suffering: An Interpersonal Focus for Ethnographies of Illness Experience." *Qualitative Health Research* 2, no. 2 (May 1992): 127–34. https://doi.org/10.1177/104973239200200202.

Kleinman, Arthur. "Medicine's Symbolic Reality: A Central Problem in the Philosophy of Medicine." *Inquiry* 16 (1973): 206–13.

Kleinman, Arthur. "Moral Experience and Ethical Reflection: Can Ethnography Reconcile Them? A Quandary for 'The New Bioethics.'" *Daedalus* 128, no. 4 (1999): 69–97.

Kleinman, Arthur. *Patients and Healers in the Context of Culture: An Exploration of the Borderland between Anthropology, Medicine, and Psychiatry.* Berkeley: University of California Press, 1980.

Kleinman, Arthur. *Rethinking Psychiatry: From Cultural Category to Personal Experience.* New York: Free Press, 1988.

Kleinman, Arthur. "A Search for Wisdom." *The Lancet* 378, no. 9803 (November 2011): 1621–22. https://doi.org/10.1016/s0140-6736(11)61688-7.

Kleinman, Arthur. "The Search for Wisdom: Why William James Still Matters." In *The Ground Between*, edited by Veena Das, Michael D. Jackson, Arthur Kleinman, and Bhrigupati Singh, 119–37. Durham, NC: Duke University Press, 2014. https://doi.org/10.1215/9780822376439-006.

Kleinman, Arthur. *Social Origins of Distress and Disease: Depression, Neurasthenia, and Pain in Modern China.* New Haven, CT: Yale University Press, 1986.

Kleinman, Arthur. "Some Issues for a Comparative Study of Medical Healing." *International Journal of Social Psychology* 19 (1973): 159–65.

Kleinman, Arthur. *The Soul of Care: The Moral Education of a Husband and a Doctor.* New York: Penguin, 2019.

Kleinman, Arthur. "Toward a Comparative Study of Medical Systems." *Science, Medicine and Man* 1 (1973): 55–65.

Kleinman, Arthur. *What Really Matters: Living a Moral Life amidst Uncertainty and Danger.* New York: Oxford University Press, 2006.

Kleinman, Arthur. *Writing at the Margin: Discourse between Anthropology and Medicine.* Berkeley: University of California Press, 1995.

Kleinman, Arthur, Veena Das, and Margaret Lock, eds. *Social Suffering*. Berkeley: University of California Press, 1997.

Kleinman, Arthur, Leon Eisenberg, and Byron Good. "Culture, Illness and Care: Clinical Lessons from Anthropological and Cross-Cultural Research." *Annals of Internal Medicine* 88 (1978): 251–58.

Kleinman, Arthur, G. Estrin, S. Usmani, and D. Chisholm et al. "Time for Mental Health to Come out of the Shadows." *The Lancet* 387, no. 10035 (2016): 2274–75.

Kleinman, Arthur, and Byron J. Good, eds. *Culture and Depression: Studies in the Anthropology and Cross-Cultural Psychiatry of Affect and Disorder*. Berkeley: University of California Press, 1985.

Kleinman, Arthur, and Joan Kleinman. "The Appeal of Experience; the Dismay of Images: Cultural Appropriations of Suffering in Our Times." *Daedalus* 125, no. 1 (1996): 1–23.

Kleinman, Arthur, and Joan Kleinman. "Suffering and Its Professional Transformation: Toward an Ethnography of Interpersonal Experience." *Culture, Medicine and Psychiatry* 15, no. 3 (1991): 275–300.

Kleinman, Arthur, and Joan Kleinman. "The Transformation of Everyday Social Experience: What a Mental Health and Social Health Perspective Reveals about Chinese Communities under Global and Local Change." *Culture, Medicine and Psychiatry* 23 (1999): 7–24.

Kleinman, Arthur, Yunxiang Yan, Jing Jun, and Sing Lee et al. *Deep China: The Moral Life of the Person*. Berkeley: University of California Press, 2011.

Knight, Kelly Ray. *Addicted. Pregnant. Poor*. Durham, NC: Duke University Press, 2015.

Kochi, A. "Tuberculosis Control: Is DOTS the Health Breakthrough of the 1990s?" *World Health Forum* 18, nos. 3–4 (1997): 225–47.

Kohn, Eduardo. "How Dogs Dream: Amazonian Natures and the Politics of Transspecies Engagement." *American Ethnologist* 34, no. 1 (2007): 3–24.

Kolk, B. A., and O. Hart. "Pierre Janet and the Breakdown of Adaptation in Psychological Trauma." *American Journal of Psychiatry* 146, no. 12 (1989): 1530–40.

Kondo, Dorinne. *Crafting Selves: Power, Gender, and Discourses of Identity in a Japanese Workplace*. Chicago: University of Chicago Press, 1990.

Kopenawa, Davi. 2013. *The Falling Sky: Words of a Yanomami Shaman*. Cambridge, MA: Belknap Press of Harvard University Press.

Koselleck, Reinhart. *Futures Past: On the Semantics of Historical Time*. Translated by Keith Tribe. New York: Columbia University Press, 2004.

Kozelka, Ellen Elizabeth, and Janis H. Jenkins. "Renaming Non-communicable Diseases." *The Lancet Global Health* 5, no. 7 (July 2017): e655. https://doi.org/10.1016/S2214-109X(17)30211-5.

Kral, Michael J. "Postcolonial Suicide among Inuit in Arctic Canada." *Culture, Medicine, and Society* 36 (2012): 306–25.

Kreiger, Nancy, and George Davey-Smith. "'Bodies Count' and Body Counts: Social Epidemiology and Embodying Inequality." *Epidemiologic Reviews* 26 (2013): 92–103.

Krenak, Ailton. *Ideas to Postpone the End of the World*. Toronto: Anansi International, 2020.

Kring, Ann M., and Sheri L. Johnson. *Abnormal Psychology: The Science and Treatment of Psychological Disorders*, 14th ed. Hoboken, NJ: Wiley, 2018.

Kutumbiah, P. "A Study of the Lesions in Rheumatic Heart Disease in South India." *Indian Journal of Medical Research* 27 (1940): 631–41.

Kyu, Hmwe Hmwe, Emilie R. Maddison, Nathaniel J. Henry, and Jorge R. Ledesma et al. "Global, Regional, and National Burden of Tuberculosis, 1990–2016: Results from the Global Burden of Diseases, Injuries, and Risk Factors 2016 Study." *The Lancet Infectious Diseases* 18, no. 12 (December 2018): 1329–49. https://doi.org/10.1016/S1473-3099(18)30625-X.

Laas, Haida. *Journal of the Haida Nation*. Haida Gwaii, Canada: Council of the Haida Nation, 2009.

Lacan, Jacques. "Science and Truth." *Newsletter of the Freudian Field* 3 (1989): 4–29.

Lakoff, Andrew. *Unprepared: Global Health in a Time of Emergency*. Berkeley: University of California Press, 2017.

Lambek, Michael, ed. *A Reader in the Anthropology of Religion*. New York: Wiley-Blackwell, 2008.

Lasch, Christopher. *Haven in a Heartless World*. New York: W. W. Norton, 1995.

Latour, Bruno. *Politics of Nature*. Cambridge, MA: Harvard University Press, 2004.

Latour, Bruno. *Reassembling the Social: An Introduction to Actor-Network Theory*. Oxford: Oxford University Press, 2005.

Latour, Bruno. *We Have Never Been Modern*. Translated by Catherine Porter. Cambridge, MA: Harvard University Press, 1993.

Latour, Bruno, and Steve Woolgar. *Laboratory Life: The Construction of Scientific Facts*. Princeton, NJ: Princeton University Press, 1986.

Lawrence, Christopher, and Michael Brown. "Quintessentially Modern Heroes: Surgeons, Explorers and Empire, c. 1840–1914." *Journal of Social History* 50 (2016): 148–78.

Lazar, S. W., G. Bush, R. L. Gollub, and G. L. Fricchione et al. "Functional Brain Mapping of the Relaxation Response and Meditation." *Neuroreport* 11, no. 7 (May 2000): 1581–85.

Leach, Edmund R. *Rethinking Anthropology*. London: Athlone, 1961.

Leavitt, J. *Women and Health in America: Historical Readings*, 2d ed. Madison: University of Wisconsin Press, 1999.

Leblanc, Daniel. "List of Missing, Killed Aboriginal Women Involves 1,200 Cases." *Globe and Mail*, May 2014. https://www.theglobeandmail.com/news/national/rcmp-dont-deny-report-of-more-than-1000-murdered-missing-native-women/article18363451.

Lebra, Takie. *Japanese Patterns of Behavior*. Honolulu: University of Hawai'i Press, 1976.

Leslie, Charles, ed. *Asian Medical Systems: A Comparative Study*. Berkeley: University of California Press, 1976.

Levinas, Emmanuelle. *Entre Nous*. New York: Columbia University Press, 2002.

Lévi-Strauss, Claude. *Saudades do Brasil: A Photographic Memoir*. Translated by Sylvia Modelski. Seattle: University of Washington Press, 1994.

Lévi-Strauss, Claude. *The Savage Mind*. Chicago: University of Chicago Press, 1966.

Lévi-Strauss, Claude. *Tristes Tropiques*. Translated by John Russell. New York: Penguin, 1992.

Lévi-Strauss, Claude. *The View from Afar*. Translated by Joachim Neugroschel and Phoebe Hoss. Chicago: University of Chicago Press, 1983.

Lévi-Strauss, Claude. *A World on the Wane*. Translated by John Russell. London: Hutchinson, 1961.

Lewontin, Richard. "It's Even Less in Your Genes." *New York Review of Books*, 2011. https://www.nybooks.com/articles/2011/05/26/its-even-less-your-genes.

Lienhardt, G. *Divinity and Experience*. Oxford: Oxford University Press, 1961.

Light, Sharee N., Zachary D. Moran, Lena Swander, and Van Le et al. "Electromyographically Assessed Empathic Concern and Empathic Happiness Predict Increased Prosocial Behavior in Adults." *Biological Psychology* 104 (January 2015): 116–29. https://doi.org/10.1016/j.biopsycho.2014.11.015.

Litsios, Socrates. "The Christian Medical Commission and the Development of the World Health Organization's Primary Health Care Approach." *American Journal of Public Health* 94, no. 11 (November 2004): 1884–93. https://doi.org/10.2105/AJPH.94.11.1884.

Livingston, Julie. *Improvising Medicine: An African Oncology Ward in an Emerging Cancer Epidemic*. Durham, NC: Duke University Press, 2012.

Lock, Margaret. "Comprehending the Body in the Era of the Epigenome." *Current Anthropology* 56 (2015): 151–77.

Lock, Margaret. *East Asian Medicine in Urban Japan: Varieties of Medical Experience*. Berkeley: University of California Press, 1980.

Lock, Margaret. *Encounters with Aging: Mythologies of Menopause in Japan and North America*. Berkeley: University of California Press, 1993.

Lock, Margaret. "Inventing a New Death and Making It Believable." *Anthropology & Medicine* 9 (2002): 97–115.

Lock, Margaret. "A Nation at Risk: Interpretations of School Refusal in Japan." In *Biomedicine Examined*, edited by Margaret Lock and Deborah Gordon. Dordrecht, Netherlands: Kluwer Academic, 1988.

Lock, Margaret. *Twice Dead: Organ Transplants and the Reinvention of Death*. Berkeley: University of California Press, 2002.

Lopez, Donald S., Jr. *The Madman's Middle Way: Reflections on Reality of the Tibetan Monk Gendun Chopel*. Chicago: University of Chicago Press, 2006.

Lopez, Donald S., Jr. *The Scientific Buddha: His Short and Happy Life*. New Haven, CT: Yale University Press, 2012.

Lovell, Anne. "'The City Is My Mother': Narratives of Schizophrenia and Homelessness." *American Anthropologist* 99, no. 2 (1997): 355–68.

Lovell, Anne. "Tending to the Unseen in Extraordinary Circumstances: On Arendt's Natality and Severe Mental Illness after Hurricane Katrina." *Iride: Filosofiae Discussione Publica* 26, no. 20 (2013): 563–78.

Luhrmann, Tanya. *Of Two Minds*. New York: Knopf, 2000.

Luria, Salvador, and Max Delbrück. "Mutations of Bacteria from Virus Sensitivity to Virus Resistance." *Genetics* 28, no. 6 (November 1943): 491–511.

Lutz, A., J. Brefczynski-Lewis, T. Johnstone, and R. J. Davidson. "Regulation of the Neural Circuitry of Emotion by Compassion Meditation: Effects of Meditative Expertise." *PLoS ONE* 3, no. 3 (2008): 1897.

Lutz, Catherine. *Unnatural Emotions: Everyday Sentiments on a Micronesian Atoll and Their Challenge to Western Theory*. Chicago: University of Chicago Press, 1988.

Lutz, Pierre Eric, and Gustavo Turecki. "DNA Methylation and Childhood Maltreatment: From Animal Models to Human Studies." *Neuroscience* 264 (2014): 142–56.

Maask. *Myths Surrounding Hijra Community* (blog), 2009. http://theoutcasts-maask .blogspot.com.

MacLean, Katherine A., Emilio Ferrer, Stephen R. Aichele, and David A. Bridwell et al. "Intensive Meditation Training Improves Perceptual Discrimination and Sustained Attention." *Psychological Science* 21 (2010): 820–30.

MacLeod, Scott. "The Life and Death of Kevin Carter." *Time Magazine*, July 2001.

Magnuson, J. J. "Long-Term Ecological Research and the Invisible Present." *BioScience* 40, no. 7 (1990): 495–501.

Malabou, Catherine. *Plasticity at the Dusk of Writing: Dialectic, Destruction, Deconstruction*. New York: Columbia University Press, 2005.

Malhotra, R. P., and N. S. Pathania. "Some Aetiological Aspects of Coronary Heart Disease: An Indian Point of View Based on a Study of 867 Cases Seen during 1948–55." *British Medical Journal* 2, no. 5095 (August 1958): 528–31. https://doi.org/10.1136/bmj.2.5095.528.

Malhotra, S. L. "Geographical Aspects of Acute Myocardial Infarction in India with Special Reference to Patterns of Diet and Eating." *British Heart Journal* 29 (1967): 337–44.

Malkki, L. *The Need to Help*. Durham, NC: Duke University Press, 2015.

Mani, Bhagwan J. "Letter to the Editor." *Times of India*, May 17, 1968, 5.

Mann, Michael. *The New Climate War: The Fight to Take Back Our Planet*. New York: PublicAffairs, 2021.

Mantel, Hilary. *Bring up the Bodies*. New York: Henry Holt, 2012.

Manten, A., and L. J. Van Wijngaarden. "Development of Drug-Resistance to Rifampicin." *Chemotherapy* 14, no. 2 (1969): 93–100.

Marcelin, Louis Herns. "A linguagem da casa entre os negros no Recôncavo Baiano." *Estudos de Antropologia Social* 5, no. 2 (1999): 31–60.

Martin, Emily. *Bipolar Expeditions: Mania and Depression in American Culture*. Princeton, NJ: Princeton University Press, 2007.

Martin, Emily. "Sleepless in America." In *Pharmaceutical Self: The Global Shaping of Experience in an Age of Psychopharmacology*, edited by Janis H. Jenkins, 187–207. Santa Fe, NM: School for Advanced Research Press, 2010.

Massumi, Brian. *Parables for the Virtual: Movement, Affect, Sensation.* Durham, NC: Duke University Press, 2002.

Mastana, Sarabjit S. "Unity in Diversity: An Overview of the Genomic Anthropology of India." *Annals of Human Biology* 41 (2014): 287–99.

Mattingly, Cheryl. *Healing Dramas and Clinical Plots: The Narrative Structure of Experience.* Cambridge: Cambridge University Press, 1998.

Mattingly, Cheryl. *Moral Laboratories: Family Peril and the Struggle for the Good Life.* Berkeley: University of California Press, 2014.

Mattingly, C. *The Paradox of Hope: Journeys through a Clinical Borderland.* Berkeley: University of California Press, 2010.

Mauss, Marcel. "Une catégorie de l'esprit humaine: La notion de personne, celle de Moi." Huxley Memorial Lecture. *Journal of the Royal Anthropological Institute of London* (1939): 263–362. (English translation by B. Brewster. "A Category of the Human Mind: The Notion of Person, the Notion of 'Self.'" In Marce Mauss, *Sociology and Psychology: Essays,* 57–94. New York: Routledge and Kegan Paul, 1979.)

Mauss, Marcel. *The Gift: The Form and Reason for Exchange in Archaic Societies.* Translated by W. D. Halls. London: Routledge, 1990.

Mazower, Mark. *No Enchanted Palace: The End of Empire and the Ideological Origins of the United Nations.* Princeton, NJ: Princeton University Press, 2009.

Mbembe, Achille. "Necropolitics." *Public Culture* 15, no. 1 (2003): 11–40.

Mbembe, Achille. *Out of the Dark Night: Essays on Decolonization.* New York: Columbia University Press, 2021.

Mbembe, Achille. "The State of South African Political Life." *Africa Is a Country,* September 19, 2015. https://africasacountry.com/2015/09/achille-mbembe-on -the-state-of-south-african-politics.

McCarthy, Julie. "India's Philanthropist-Surgeon Delivers Cardiac Care Henry Ford Style." National Public Radio, January 5, 2015.

McClintock, Anne. "Monster: A Fugue in Fire and Ice." E-flux Journal, 2020. https://www.e-flux.com/architecture/oceans/331865/monster-a-fugue-in-fire -and-ice/.

McGowan, Patrick O., Aya Sasaki, Ana C D'Alessio, and Sergiy Dymov et al. "Epigenetic Regulation of the Glucocorticoid Receptor in Human Brain Associates with Childhood Abuse." *Nature Neuroscience* 12, no. 3 (March 2009): 342–48. https://doi.org/10.1038/nn.2270.

McGranahan, Carole, and Ralph Litzinger. "Self-Immolation as Protest in Tibet." Hot Spots, Fieldsights, April 9, 2012. https://culanth.org/fieldsights/series /self-immolation-as-protest-in-tibet.

McKay, Alex. *Their Footprints Remain: Biomedical Beginnings across the Indo-Tibetan Frontier.* Amsterdam: Amsterdam University Press, 2007.

McKeigue, P. M., and M. G. Marmot. "Mortality from Coronary Heart Disease in Asian Communities in London." *British Medical Journal* 297 (1988): 903.

McMillen, Christian W. *Discovering Tuberculosis: A Global History 1900 to the Present.* New Haven, CT: Yale University Press, 2015.

McSweeney, R. "Tristes Tropiques by Claude Lévy-Strauss—Melancholy Anthropology." *The Guardian, August 15,* 2015. https://www.theguardian.com/books/booksblog/2015/aug/17/tristes-tropiques-by-claude-levi-strauss-melancholy-anthropology, accessed February 22, 2019.

Meaney, M. J., J. Diorio, Francis D. Widdowson, and J. Laplante et al. "Early Environmental Regulation of Forebrain Glucocorticoid Receptor Gene Expression: Implications for Adrenocortical Responses to Stress." *Development Neurosciences* 18 (1996): 49–72.

Meloni, Maurizio. "How Biology Became Social, and What It Means for Social Theory." *Sociological Review* 62 (2014): 593–614.

Mendenhall, Emily. "The Georgetown Symposium on Global Mental Health: Transdisciplinary Perspectives." *Global Public Health* 13, no. 9 (2017): 1145–51.

Metzl, Jonathan M., and Helena Hansen. "Structural Competency: Theorizing a New Medical Engagement with Stigma and Inequality." *Social Science and Medicine* 103 (2014): 126–33.

Mille, Ryan. "Democrats on Twitter Cry #FakeTrumpEmergency after White House Declaration." *USA Today,* February 15, 2019.

Mitchison, S. A., J. B. Selkon, and A. Weiner. "A Case of Pulmonary Tuberculosis due to Isoniazid-Resistant, Guinea-Pig Attenuated, Mycobacterium Tuberculosis." *Tubercle* (1957): 382–86.

Miyazaki, Hirokazu. *The Method of Hope: Anthropology, Philosophy, and Fijian Knowledge.* Stanford, CA: Stanford University Press, 2004.

Mol, Annemarie. *The Body Multiple: Ontology in Medical Practice.* Durham, NC: Duke University Press, 2002.

Monk, Catherine, Julie Spicer, and Frances A. Champagne. "Linking Prenatal Maternal Adversity to Developmental Outcomes in Infants: The Role of Epigenetic Pathways." *Development and Psychopathology* 24, no. 4 (November 2012): 1361–76. https://doi.org/10.1017/S0954579412000764.

Moon, Claire. "Human Rights, Human Remains: Forensic Humanitarianism and the Human Rights of the Dead." *International Social Science Journal* 65, nos. 215–16 (2014): 49–63.

"More Donors than Recipients for Heart Transplants." *Times of India,* November 20, 1968, 11.

Morehead, J. B. "Transplants in India." *Times of India,* October 12, 1968, 8.

Morrison, Toni. *Beloved.* New York: Alfred A. Knopf, 1987.

Morton, Caitlin. "The Ten Most Popular Cities of 2019." *Condé Nast Traveler,* September 5, 2019.

Moten, Fred. *Black and Blur.* Durham, NC: Duke University Press, 2017.

Mount, F. W., and S. H. Ferebee. "United States Public Health Service Cooperative Investigation of Antimicrobial Therapy of Tuberculosis, V. Report on Thirty-Two-Week Observations on Combinations of Isoniazid, Streptomycin, and Para-Aminosalicylic Acid." *American Review of Tuberculosis* 70, no. 3 (September 1954): 521–26. https://doi.org/10.1164/art.1954.70.3.521.

Murray, Christopher. "Quantifying the Burden of Disease: The Technical Basis for Disability Adjusted Life Years." *Bulletin of the World Health Organization* 72, no. 3 (1994): 429–45.

Muyskens, John, Andrew Ba Tran, Naema Ahmed, and Anna Phillips. "1 in 6 Americans Live in Areas with Significant Wildfire Risk." *Washington Post,* May 17, 2022. https://www.washingtonpost.com/climate-environment /interactive/2022/wildfire-risk-map-us/

Myers, Neely, and Kristin Yarris. "Extraordinary Conditions: Global Psychiatric Care and the Anthropology of Moral Experience." *Ethos* 47, no. 1 (2019): 3–12.

Nadkarni, D. V. "Transplants in India." *Times of India,* October 24, 1968, 10.

Narayan, Kirin. *Storytellers, Saints, and Scoundrels: Folk Narrative in Hindu Religious Teaching.* Philadelphia: University of Pennsylvania Press, 1989.

Nataraj, Shakthi. "Trans-Formations: Projects of Resignification in Tamil Nadu's Transgender Rights Movement." Ph.D. diss., University of California, Berkeley, 2019.

National Academies of Sciences, Engineering, and Medicine. *Families Caring for an Aging America.* Washington, DC: National Academies Press, 2016.

Nichter, Mark. *Global Health: Why Cultural Perceptions, Social Representations, and Biopolitics Matter.* Tucson: University of Arizona Press, 2008.

Nietzsche, Friedrich. *The Use and Abuse of History.* New York: Macmillan, 1955 [1874].

Niezen, Ronald. *Truth and Indignation: Canada's Truth and Reconciliation Commission on Indian Residential Schools.* Toronto: University of Toronto Press, 2013.

Nixon, Rob. *Slow Violence and the Environmentalism of the Poor.* Cambridge, MA: Harvard University Press, 2011.

Noddings, N. *Caring: A Feminine Approach to Ethics and Moral Education.* Berkeley: University of California Press, 1984.

Nordenson, Guy. "Probabilistic Coastal Hazards Mapping for the United States." Princeton Environmental Institute seminar, Princeton, NJ, September 20, 2016.

Normand, Roger, and Sarah Zaidi. *Human Rights at the UN: The Political History of Universal Justice.* Bloomington: Indiana University Press, 2008.

"Obituary: Retired Hyderabad Judge." *Times of India,* February 8, 1926, 13.

Ong, Aihwa, and Stephen J. Collier, eds. *Global Assemblages: Technology, Politics, and Ethics as Anthropological Problems.* Malden, MA: Blackwell, 2005.

O'Reilly, Dermot, Michael Rosato, Aideen Maguire, and David Wright. "Caregiving Reduces Mortality Risk for Most Caregivers: A Census-based Record Linkage Study." *International Journal of Epidemiology* 44, no. 6 (December 2015): 1959–69. https://doi.org/10.1093/ije/dyv172.

Packard, Randall M. *White Plague, Black Labor: Tuberculosis and the Political Economy of Health and Disease in South Africa.* Comparative Studies of Health Systems and Medical Care. Berkeley: University of California Press, 1989.

Padmavati, Sivaramakrishnan. "The Cardiac Patient in Underdeveloped Countries." *American Heart Journal* 58, no. 3 (September 1959): 418–24. https://doi .org/10.1016/0002-8703(59)90159-0.

Pandian, Anand. *A Possible Anthropology: Methods for Uneasy Times*. Durham, NC: Duke University Press, 2019.

Pant, Jaikrishna. "Heart Transplants." *Times of India*, January 16, 1969, 8.

Parulkar, G. B. "Developments in Cardiovascular Surgery in India during Last Five Decades." *Indian Journal of Thoracic and Cardiovascular Surgery* 20 (2004): S24–30.

Pembrey, Marcus, Richard Saffery, and Lars Olov Bygren. ""Human Transgenerational Responses to Early-Life Experience: Potential Impact on Development, Health and Biomedical Research." *Journal of Medical Genetics* 51 (2014): 563–72.

Pennings, G. "International Evolution of Legislation and Guidelines in Medically Assisted Reproduction." *Reproductive BioMedicine Online* 2009, 18 (Suppl. 2): S15–S18.

Perales, Monica. *Smeltertown: Making and Remembering a Southwest Border Community*. Chapel Hill: University of North Carolina Press, 2010.

Petryna, Adriana. "Experimentality: On the Global Mobility and Regulation of Human Subjects Research." *Political and Legal Anthropology Review* 30 (2007): 288–304.

Petryna, Adriana. 2022. *Horizon Work: At the Edges of Knowledge in an Age of Runaway Climate Change*. Princeton, NJ: Princeton University Press.

Petryna, Adriana. "Horizoning." In *Unfinished: The Anthropology of Becoming*, edited by João Biehl and Peter Locke, 243–69. Durham, NC: Duke University Press, 2017.

Petryna, Adriana. *Life Exposed: Biological Citizens after Chernobyl*. Princeton, NJ: Princeton University Press, 2013.

Petryna, Adriana. "What Is a Horizon? Navigating Thresholds in Climate Change Uncertainty." In *Modes of Uncertainty: Anthropological Cases*, edited by Paul Rabinow and Limor Samimian-Darash. Chicago: University of Chicago Press, 2015.

Petryna, Adriana. "Wildfires at the Edges of Science: Horizoning Work amid Runaway Change." *Cultural Anthropology* 33, no. 4 (November 2018): 570–95. https://doi.org/10.14506/ca33.4.06.

Pettersen, Tove. *Comprehending Care*. Boston: Lexington, 2008.

Pfau, Thomas. "Mourning Modernity." In *The Oxford Handbook of the Elegy*, edited by Karen Weisman, 546–64. New York: Oxford University Press, 2010.

Pollock, Anne. *Medicating Race: Heart Disease and Durable Preoccupations with Difference*. Durham, NC: Duke University Press, 2012.

Popova, Maria. "I and Thou: Philosopher Martin Buber on the Art of Relationship and What Makes Us Real to One Another." *Brain Pickings*, March 18, 2018. https://www.brainpickings.org/2018/07/24/martin-buber-i-thou-love.

Povinelli, Elizabeth. "The Will to Be Otherwise/The Effort of Endurance." *South Atlantic Quarterly* 111, no. 3 (2012): 453–75.

Prince, M., et al. "No Health without Mental Health." *The Lancet* 370 (2007): 59–77.

"Proceedings of the XII Annual Conference of the Association of Surgeons in India." *Indian Journal of Surgery* 13 (1951): 1–17.

Quesada, James, Laurie Hart, and Philippe Bourgois. "Structural Vulnerability and Health: Latino Migrant Laborers in the United States." *Medical Anthropology* 30, no. 4 (2011): 339–62.

Rabinow, Paul. *Anthropos Today: Reflections on Modern Equipment.* Princeton, NJ: Princeton University Press, 2009.

Rachwal, Tadeusz. *Precarity and Loss: On Certain and Uncertain Properties of Life and Work.* Wiesbaden, Germany: Springer, 2017.

Radcliffe-Brown, Alfred Reginald. *Structure and Function in Primitive Society: Essays and Addresses.* London: Cohen and West, 1952.

Rajadhyaksha, Ashish, ed. *In The Wake of Aadhaar: The Digital Ecosystem of Governance in India.* Bangalore: Centre for the Study of Culture and Society, 2013.

Ralph, Laurence. *The Torture Letters: Reckoning with Police Violence.* Chicago: University of Chicago Press, 2020.

Ramanathan, Usha. "A Unique Identity Bill." *Economic and Political Weekly* 45, no. 30 (2010). https://www.epw.in/journal/2010/30/commentary/unique-identity-bill.html.

Rapp, Rayna. *Testing Women, Testing the Fetus.* New York: Routledge, 1999.

Read, Ursula. "'I Want the One That Will Heal Me Completely so It Won't Come Back Again': The Limits of Antipsychotic Medication in Rural Ghana." *Transcultural Psychiatry* 49, nos. 3–4 (July 2012): 438–60. https://doi.org/10.1177/1363461512447070.

Read, Ursula, Edward Adiibokah, and Solomon Nyame. "Local Suffering and the Global Discourse of Mental Health and Human Rights: An Ethnographic Study of Responses to Mental Illness in Rural Ghana." *Globalization and Health* 5, no. 13 (2009): 1–16.

Reddy, Gayatri. *With Respect to Sex: Negotiating Hijra Identity in South India.* Chicago: University of Chicago Press, 2005.

Reddy, K. Srinath. "India Wakes Up to the Threat of Cardiovascular Diseases." *Journal of the American College of Cardiology* 50 (2007): 1370–72.

Redfield, Peter. "Doctors, Borders, and Life in Crisis." *Cultural Anthropology* 20, no. 3 (2005): 328–61.

Reyes-Foster, Beatriz M. *Psychiatric Encounters: Madness and Modernity in Yucatan, Mexico.* New Brunswick, NJ: Rutgers University Press, 2018.

Reynolds, Pamela. *The Uncaring, Intricate World: A Field Diary, Zambezi Valley, 1984–1985.* Durham, NC: Duke University Press, 2019.

Rhodes, Lorna A. *Emptying Beds: The Work of an Emergency Psychiatric Unit.* Oakland: University of California Press, 1995.

Rhodes, Lorna A. *Total Confinement: Madness and Reason in the Maximum Security Prison.* Oakland: University of California Press, 2004.

Richardson, Eugene T. "On the Coloniality of Global Public Heath." *Medicine Anthropology Theory* 6, no. 4 (2019): 101–18.

Richardson, Eugene T., Timothy McGinnis, and Raphael Frankfurter. "Ebola and the Nature of Mistrust." *British Medical Journal, Global Health* 4, no. 6 (2019): 001932.

Richardson, R. *William James: In the Maelstrom of American Modernism*. New York: Houghton-Mifflin, 2006.

Rivers, W. H. "The Repression of War Experience." *Proceedings of the Royal Society of Medicine* 11 (1918): 1–20.

Robbins, Joel. "Beyond the Suffering Subject: Toward an Anthropology of the Good." *Journal of the Royal Anthropological Institute* 19, no. 3 (2013): 447–62.

Roebuck, Christopher. *"Workin' It": Trans* Lives in the Age of Epidemic*. Berkeley: University of California Press, 2013.

Rohlen, Thomas. *For Harmony and Strength: Japanese White-Collar Organization in Anthropological Perspective*. Berkeley: University of California Press, 1974.

Rohlen, Thomas. *Japan's High Schools*. Berkeley: University of California Press, 1983.

Roitman, Janet. *Anti-Crisis*. Durham, NC: Duke University Press, 2013.

Rosaldo, Michele. "The Shame of Headhunters and the Autonomy of Self." *Ethos* 11 (1983): 135–51.

Rose, Deborah Bird. *Wild Dog Dreaming: Love and Extinction*. Charlottesville: University Press of Virginia, 2011.

Rose, Nikolas. "Biopolitics in the Twenty-First Century." In *The Politics of Life Itself: Biomedicine, Power, and Subjectivity in the Twenty-First Century*, 9–40. Princeton, NJ: Princeton University Press, 2006.

Rose, Steven. *Lifelines: Life beyond the Gene*. Oxford: Oxford University Press, 1997.

Rosenberg, Charles. "Pathologies of Progress: The Idea of Civilization as Risk." *Bulletin of the History of Medicine* 72 (1998): 714–30.

Rosenberg, Charles. "The Therapeutic Revolution: Medicine, Meaning, and Social Change in Nineteenth Century America." *Perspectives in Biology and Medicine* 20 (1977): 485–506.

Rosenberg, Charles. "What Is an Epidemic? AIDS in Historical Perspective." *Daedalus* 118 (1989): 1–17.

Rosenberger, Nancy. "Productivity, Sexuality, and Ideologies of Menopausal Problems in Japan." In *Health and Medical Care in Japan: Cultural and Social Dimensions*, edited by Edward Norbeck and Margaret Lock, 158–88. Honolulu: University of Hawai'i Press, 1987.

Rosenkranz, Melissa A., Antoine Lutz, David M. Perlman, and David R. W. Bachhuber et al. "Reduced Stress and Inflammatory Responsiveness in Experienced Meditators Compared to a Matched Healthy Control Group." *Psychoneuroendocrinology* 68 (2016): 117–25. https://doi.org/10.1016/j.psyneuen.2016.02.013.

Roth, D. L., W. E. Haley, M. Hovater, and M. Perkins et al. "Family Caregiving and All-Cause Mortality: Findings from a Population-Based Propensity-Matched Analysis." *American Journal of Epidemiology* 178, no. 10 (November 15, 2013): 1571–78. https://doi.org/10.1093/aje/kwt225.

Rouse, Carolyn. *Uncertain Suffering: Racial Health Care Disparities and Sickle Cell Disease*. Berkeley: University of California Press, 2009.

Roy, Arundhati. *The Ministry of Utmost Happiness*. New York: Alfred A. Knopf, 2017.

Roy, Sujoy B., Madan L. Bhatia, Erica Lazaro, and V. Ramalingaswami. "Juvenile Mitral Stenosis in India." *The Lancet* 282 (1960): 1193–95.

Rutstein, S. O., and I. H. Shah. *Infecundity, Infertility, and Childlessness in Developing Countries*. Geneva: World Health Organization, 2004.

Sahlins, Marshall. *The Use and Abuse of Biology: An Anthropological Critique of Sociobiology*. Ann Arbor: University of Michigan Press, 1976.

Sapir, Edward. "Cultural Anthropology and Psychiatry." *Journal of Abnormal* and *Social Psychology* 27 (1932): 229–42.

Sapir, Edward. "Culture, Genuine and Spurious." *American Journal of Sociology* 29, no. 4 (1924): 401–29.

Sapir, Edward. *Culture, Language and Personality: Selected Essays*. Berkeley: University of California Press, 1949.

Saria, Vaibhav. *Hijras, Lovers, Brothers: Surviving Sex and Poverty in Rural India*. New York: Fordham University Press, 2021.

Saria, Vaibhav. "To Be Some Other Name: The Naming Games That Hijras Play." *South Asia Multidisciplinary Academic Journal* 12 (2015): 2–14.

Sartorius, N., W. Gulbinat, G. Harrison, E. Laska, and C. Siegel. "Long-term Follow-up of Schizophrenia in Sixteen Countries." *Social Psychiatry and Psychiatric Epidemiology* 31 (1996): 249–58. https://doi.org/10.1007/BF00787917.

Sartre, Jean-Paul. *Search for a Method*. Translated by Hazel Barnes. New York: Knopf, 1963.

Sassen, Saskia. *The Global City: New York, London, Tokyo*. Princeton, NJ: Princeton University Press, 2001.

Scheper-Hughes, Nancy. "The Primacy of the Ethical: Propositions for a Militant Anthropology." *Current Anthropology* 36, no. 3 (1995): 409–40.

Schieffelin, E. *The Sorrow of the Lonely and the Burning of the Dancers*. London: Palgrave Macmillan, 2005.

Schwartz, Leah N., Jonathan D. Shaffer, and Gene Bukhman. "The Origins of the 4 × 4 Framework for Noncommunicable Disease at the World Health Organization." *SSM–Population Health* 13 (March 2021): 100731. https://doi.org/10.1016/j.ssmph.2021.100731.

Sedgwick, Eve Kosofsky. *Touching Feeling: Affect, Pedagogy, Performativity*. Durham, NC: Duke University Press, 2003.

Selikoff, I. J., E. H. Robitzek, and G. G. Ornstein. "Treatment of Pulmonary Tuberculosis with Hydrazide Derivatives of Isonicotinic Acid." *Journal of the American Medical Association* 150, no. 10 (1952): 973–80.

Selkon, J. B., W. Fox, P. R. J. Gangadharam, K. Ramachandaram, C. V. Ramakrishnan, and S. Velu. "Rate of Inactivation of Isoniazid in South Indian Patients with Pulmonary Tuberculosis 2. Clinical Implications in the Treatment of Pulmonary Tuberculosis with Isoniazid Either Alone or in Combination with PAS." *Bulletin of the World Health Organization* 25, no. 6 (1961): 779–92.

Semeniuk, Ivan. "The Hunt for Humanity." *Globe and Mail*, 2014, F1, F6–7.

Sen, P. K. "Heart Transplantation—The Triumph and the Muddle." *Indian Journal of Chest Disease* 12 (1970): 66–72.

Sen, P. K. "The Present Status of Surgery of the Heart." *The Antiseptic* 51 (1954): 537–47.

Sen, P. K., S. R. Panday, J. Daulatram, and A. P. Chaukar. "The Operation." *Journal of the Indian Medical Association* 51 (1968): 549–50.

Shange, Savannah. *Progressive Dystopia: Abolition, Antiblackness, and Schooling in San Francisco*. Durham, NC: Duke University Press, 2019.

Shannon, Claude. "Prediction and Entropy of Printed English." *Bell Labs Technical Journal* 30, no. 1 (1951): 50–64.

Sharma, Dinesh C. "Panditiji Bled to Death in a Medical Mess." *Mail Today*, January 2008, 1.

Sharp, Lesley. *Strange Harvest: Organ Transplants, Denatured Bodies, and the Transformed Self*. Berkeley: University of California Press, 2006.

Siddiqi, Javed. *World Health and World Politics: The World Health Organization and the UN*. Columbia: University of South Carolina Press, 1995.

Siklenka, K., S. Erkek, M. Godmann, and R. Lambrot et al. "Disruption of Histone Methylation in Developing Sperm Impairs Offspring Health Transgenerationally." *Science* 350 (2015): 651–63.

Simpson, Audra. *Mohawk Interruptus: Political Life across the Borders of Settler States*. Durham, NC: Duke University Press, 2014.

Singer, Merrill. "Critical Medical Anthropology." In *Encyclopedia of Medical Anthropology: Health and Illness in the World's Cultures*, 23–30. New York: Springer, 2004.

Singer, Merrill, Nicola Bulled, Bayla Ostrach, and Emily Mendenhall. "Syndemics and the Biosocial Conception of Health." *The Lancet* 389, no. 10072 (March 4, 2017): 941–50. https://doi.org/10.1016/S0140-6736(17)30003-X.

Singh, Ilina. "Human Development, Nature and Nurture: Working beyond the Divide." *Biosocieties* 7 (2012): 308–21.

Sivaramakrishnan, Kavita. "The Return of Epidemics and the Politics of Global-Local Health." *American Journal of Public Health* 101 (2011): 1032–41.

Slaughter, Anne-Marie. *Unfinished Business: Women, Men, Work, Family*. New York: Random House, 2015.

Smith, Robert. *Japanese Society: Tradition, Self and the Social Order*. Cambridge: Cambridge University Press, 1983.

Sontag, Susan. *Illness as Metaphor and AIDS and Its Metaphors*. New York: Doubleday, 1990.

Sontag, Susan. *Regarding the Pain of Others*. New York: Picador, 2003.

Sophocles. *Oedipus the King*. Translated by David Grene. Chicago: University of Chicago Press, 2010.

Spinoza, Baruch. *The Collected Works of Spinoza*, vol. 1. Edited and translated by Edwin Curley. Princeton, NJ: Princeton University Press, 1985.

Stainova, Yana. "Enchantment as Method." *Anthropology and Humanism* 44, no. 2 (December 2019): 214–30. https://doi.org/10.1111/anhu.12251.

Stein, C. E., C. H. D. Fall, K. Kumaran, C. Osmond, V. Cox, and D. J. P. Barker. "Fetal Growth and Coronary Heart Disease in South India." *The Lancet* 348 (1996): 1269–73.

Stevenson, Lisa. *Life beside Itself: Imagining Care in the Canadian Arctic.* Oakland: University of California Press, 2014.

Stevenson, Lisa. "The Psychic Life of Biopolitics: Survival, Cooperation, and Inuit Community." *American Ethnologist* 39, no. 3 (2012): 592–613.

Stewart, Kathleen. "Atmospheric Attunements." *Environment and Planning D: Society and Space* 29, no. 3 (2011): 445–53.

Stewart, Kathleen. "Cultural Poesis: The Generativity of Emergent Things." In *Handbook of Qualitative Research*, edited by Norman Denzin and Yvonna Lincoln, 3d ed., 1027–42. New York: Sage, 2005.

Stewart, Kathleen. "In the World That Affect Proposed." *Cultural Anthropology* 32, no. 2 (2017): 192–98.

Stewart, Kathleen. *Ordinary Affects.* Durham, NC: Duke University Press, 2007.

Stocking, George, ed. "Functionalism Historicized." In *Functionalism Historicized: Essays on British Anthropology.* History of Anthropology, vol. 2. Madison: University of Wisconsin Press, 1984.

Strong, John. *Relics of the Buddha.* Princeton, NJ: Princeton University Press, 2004.

Subramanian, S. V., Daniel J. Corsi, Malavika A. Subramanyam, and George Davey Smith. "Jumping the Gun: The Problematic Discourse on Socioeconomic Status and Cardiovascular Health in India." *International Journal of Epidemiology* 42, no. 5 (2013): 1410–26.

Summerfield, Derek. "Afterword: Against Global Mental Health." *Transcultural Psychiatry* 49, no. 3 (2012): 519–30.

Suzuki, Tomi. *Narrating the Self: Fictions of Japanese Modernity.* Stanford, CA: Stanford University Press, 1996.

Swanson, Maynard W. "The Sanitation Syndrome: Bubonic Plague and Urban Native Policy in the Cape Colony, 1900–1909." *Journal of African History* 18, no. 3 (July 1977): 387–410. https://doi.org/10.1017/S0021853700027328.

Tambiah, S. *Leveling Crowds: Ethnonationalist Conflicts and Collective Violence in South Asia.* Berkeley: University of California Press, 1996.

Taussig, Michael. "History as Commodity in Some Recent American (Anthropological) Literature." *Critique of Anthropology* 9, no. 1 (n.d.): 7–23. https://doi.org/10.1177/0308275X8900900102.

Taylor, Keeanga-Yamahtta. *From #BlackLivesMatter to Black Liberation.* Chicago: Haymarket, 2016.

Taylor, William B. *Theater of a Thousand Wonders: A History of Miraculous Images and Shrines in New Spain.* Cambridge: Cambridge University Press, 2016.

Thakur, Pallavi. "A Eunuch's Journey: From Life to Death!" *SpeakingTree* (blog), August 16, 2016. http://www.speakingtree.in/allslides/a-eunuchs-journey-from-life-to-death.

Thomas, Deborah. *Political Life in the Wake of the Plantation: Sovereignty, Witnessing, Repair.* Durham, NC: Duke University Press, 2019.

Thomas, Martin. *The Artificial Horizon: Reading a Colonised Landscape*. Melbourne: Melbourne University Press, 2004.

Thompson, Charis. *Making Parents: The Ontological Choreography of Reproductive Technologies*. Cambridge, MA: MIT Press, 2005.

Thompson, Evan. "Is the Brain a Decomposable or Nondecomposable System? Comment on 'Understanding Brain Networks and Brain Organization' by Pesoa." *Physics of Life Reviews* 11 (2014): 458–59.

Thompson, Evan. "Neurophenomenology and Francisco Varela." In *The Dalai Lama at MIT*, edited by Anne Harrington and Arthur Zajonc, 19–26. Cambridge, MA: Harvard University Press, 2003.

Thorat, Nikhil. "17 Things You Didn't Know about Hijras—India's Officially Recognised Third Gender," TOPYAPA, September 30, 2015. http://topyaps.com/journey-of-eunuchs.

Ticktin, Miriam. "Where Ethics and Politics Meet: The Violence of Humanitarianism in France." *American Ethnologist* 33, no. 1 (2006): 33–49.

Traphagan, John W. "Being a Good Rôjin: Senility, Power, and Self-Actualization in Japan." In *Thinking about Dementia: Culture, Loss, and the Anthropology of Senility*, edited by Annette Leibing and Lawrence Cohen, 269–88. New Brunswick, NJ: Rutgers University Press, 2006.

Tronto, J. *Moral Boundaries: A Political Argument for an Ethic of Care*. New York: Routledge, 1993.

Tsing, Anna Lowenhaupt. "On Nonscalability: The Living World Is Not Amenable to Precision-Nested Scales." *Common Knowledge* 18, no. 3 (2012): 505–24.

Tsing, Anna Lowenhaupt. "Unruly Edges: Mushrooms as Companion Species." *Environmental Humanities* 1 (2012): 141–54.

Tuberculosis Chemotherapy Center. "A Concurrent Comparison of Home and Sanatorium Treatment of Pulmonary Tuberculosis in South India." *Bulletin of the World Health Organization* 21, no. 1 (1959): 51–144.

Tuberculosis Chemotherapy Center. "A Concurrent Comparison of Isoniazid plus PAS with Three Regimens of Isoniazid Alone in the Domiciliary Treatment of Tuberculosis in South India." *Bulletin of the World Health Organization* 23, nos. 4–5 (1960): 535–85.

Tucker, J. D., B. Wong, J. Nie, and A. Kleinman. "Rebuilding Patient-Physician Trust in China." *The Lancet* 388, no. 10046 (2016): 755.

Turner, Victor. *Dramas, Fields and Metaphors: Symbolic Action in Human Society*. Ithaca, NY: Cornell University Press, 1975.

Turner, Victor. *The Forest of Symbols*. Ithaca, NY: Cornell University Press, 1967.

Turner, Victor, and Jerome Bruner. *The Anthropology of Experience*. Champaign: University of Illinois Press, 1986.

Tylee, André, and Paul Gandhi. "The Importance of Somatic Symptoms in Depression in Primary Care." *Primary Care Companion Journal of Clinical Psychiatry* 7, no. 4 (2005): 167–76.

Ulrich, Laurel T. A *Midwife's Tale*. New York: Vintage, 1990.

Unger, Jean-Pierre, and James R. Killingsworth. "Selective Primary Health Care: A Critical Review of Methods and Results." *Social Science and Medicine* 22, no. 10 (January 1986): 1001–13. https://doi.org/10.1016/0277-9536(86)90200-5.

Upadhyay, Nishant. "Hindu Nation and Its Queers: Caste, Islamophobia,and De/coloniality in India." *Interventions* 22, no. 4 (2020): 464–80.

US Centers for Disease Control and Prevention. "Primary Multidrug-Resistant Tuberculosis–Ivanova Oblast, Russia, 1999." *Morbidity and Mortality Weekly Report* 48, no. 30 (August 6, 1999): 661–63.

Vakil, Rustom Jal. "Cardiology—Past and Present." *Indian Heart Journal* 8 (1956): 1–14.

Vakil, Rustom Jal. "Modern Approach to Cardiovascular Problems." *Journal of the Indian Medical Association* 25 (1955): 520–23.

Van Dooren, Thom. *Flight Ways: Life and Loss at the Edge of Extinction*. Critical Perspectives on Animals: Theory, Culture, Science, and Law. New York: Columbia University Press, 2014.

Vara, Vauhini. "Heart Disease Snares South Asians." *Wall Street Journal*, March 2011. https://www.wsj.com/articles/SB10001424052748703409304576167003904805530.

Vaughan, Megan. *Curing Their Ills: Colonial Power and African Illness*. Stanford, CA: Stanford University Press, 1991.

Vélez-Ibáñez. *Border Visions: Mexican Cultures of the Southwest United States*. Tucson: University of Arizona Press, 1996.

Venkatanarayanan, Anand. "The Curious Case of the World Bank and Aadhaar Savings." *The Wire*, October 3, 2017. https://thewire.in/economy/the-curious-case-of-the-world-bank-and-aadhaar-savings.

Venkatesan, S., V. Das, H. Al-Mohammad, J. Robbins, C. Stafford, J. Mair. "There Is No Such Thing as the Good. The 2013 Meeting of the Group for Debates in Anthropological Theory." *Critique of Anthropology* 35, no. 4 (2015): 430–80.

Venturi, Frederica. "The Thirteenth Dalai Lama on Warfare, Weapons and the Right to Self-Defense." In *Trails of the Tibetan Tradition: Papers for Eliot Sperling*, edited by Roberto Vitali. Dharamsala, India: Amnye Machen Institute, 2014.

Verghese, A. *My Own Country: A Doctor's Story*. New York: Vintage, 1994.

Vilaça, Aparecida. "A Pagan Arithmetic: Unstable Sets in Indigenous Amazonia." *Interdisciplinary Science Reviews* 46, no. 3 (2021): 304–24.

Vitale, Alex. *The End of Policing*. New York: Verso, 2018.

Vogel, Ezra. *Japan's New Middle Class: The Salary Man and His Family in a Tokyo Suburb*. Berkeley: University of California Press, 1971.

Vogel, Susanne H. "Professional Housewives: The Career of Urban Middle Class Japanese Women." *Japan Interpreter* 12 (1978): 16–43.

Vora, Neha. *Impossible Citizens: Dubai's Indian Diaspora*. Durham, NC: Duke University Press, 2013.

Waddington, Conrad Hal. *The Strategy of the Genes: A Discussion of Some Aspects of Theoretical Biology*. London: George Allen and Unwin, 1957.

Walker, Elizabeth Reisinger, Robin E. McGee, and Benjamin G. Druss. "Mortality in Mental Disorders and Global Disease Burden Implications: A Systematic Review and Meta-analysis." *Journal of the American Medical Association, Psychiatry* 72, no. 4 (2015): 334–41.

Wallace, B. Alan. *Contemplative Science: Where Buddhism and Neuroscience Converge.* New York: Columbia University Press, 2007.

Wallace-Wells, David. "Time to Panic." *New York Times,* February 16, 2019. https://www.nytimes.com/2019/02/16/opinion/sunday/fear-panic-climate-change-warming.html.

Wallace-Wells, David. *The Uninhabitable Earth: Life after Warming.* New York: Tim Duggan, 2019.

Walsh, Julia A., and Kenneth S. Warren. "Selective Primary Health Care: An Interim Strategy for Disease Control in Developing Countries." *New England Journal of Medicine* 301, no. 18 (November 1979): 967–74. https://doi.org/10.1056/NEJM197911013011804.

Webb, Allan. *Pathologia India,* 2d ed. Calcutta: Thacker, 1848.

Weber, M. *Economy and Society: An Outline of Interpretive Sociology.* Edited by Guenther Roth and Claus Wittich. Berkeley: University of California Press, 1978.

Weber, Max. *From Max Weber: Essays in Sociology.* Edited and translated by Charles Wright Mills and Hans Gerth. London: Routledge, 1991.

Weiss, Joseph. *Shaping the Future on Haida Gwaii: Life beyond Settler Colonialism.* Vancouver: University of British Columbia Press, 2018.

Weston, Kath. "Lesbian/Gay Studies in the House of Anthropology." *Annual Review of Anthropology* 22, no. 1 (1993): 339–67.

Wexler, Laura. "A Notion of Photography." In *The Notion of Family,* by LaToya Ruby Frazier, 143–47. New York: Aperture Foundation, 2014.

White, Leslie A. "Culturological versus Psychological Interpretations of Human Behavior." *American Sociological Review* 12, no. 6 (1947): 686–98.

White, Paul Dudley. *Coronary Heart Disease (Heart Attack).* New Delhi: All India Heart Foundation, 1972.

White, Ross, Ursula Read, Sumeet Jain, and David Orr, eds. *The Palgrave Handbook of Sociocultural Perspectives on Global Mental Health.* London: Palgrave, 2017.

Whitman, Walt. "Specimen Days." In *The Portable Walt Whitman,* edited by Mark Van Doren, 482–84. New York: Viking, 1974.

Whittaker, Andrea M. "'Outsourced' Patients and Their Companions: Stories from Forced Medical Travellers." *Global Public Health* 10, no. 4 (2015): 485–500.

Whyte, Kyle Powys. "Our Ancestors' Dystopia Now: Indigenous Conservation and the Anthropocene." In *The Routledge Companion to the Environmental Humanities,* edited by Ursula K. Heise, Jon Christensen, and Michelle Niemann, 206–215. New York: Routledge, 2017.

Whyte, Susan Reynolds. "Family Experiences with Mental Health Problems in Tanzania." *Acta Psychiatrica Scandinavica* 83, no. S364 (1991): 77–111.

Whyte, Susan Reynolds. "Health Identities and Subjectivities." *Medical Anthropology Quarterly* 23, no. 1 (2009): 6–15.

Whyte, Susan Reynolds, ed. *Second Chances: Surviving AIDS in Uganda*. Durham, NC: Duke University Press, 2015.

Whyte, Susan Reynolds, Sjaak Van Geest, and Anita Hardon. *Social Lives of Medicines*. New York: Cambridge University Press, 2003.

Wilkinson, Iain, and Arthur Kleinman. *A Passion for Society: How We Think about Human Suffering*. Berkeley: University of California Press, 2016.

Wilkinson, Richard. "Politics and Health Inequalities." *The Lancet* 368, no. 9543 (October 7, 2006): 1229–30.

Williams, Bianca C. *The Pursuit of Happiness: Black Women, Diasporic Dreams, and the Politics of Emotional Transnationalism*. Durham, NC: Duke University Press, 2018.

Willse, Craig, and Patricia Ticineto Clough, eds. *Beyond Biopolitics: Essays on the Governance of Life and Death*. Durham, NC: Duke University Press, 2011.

Wolf, Eric. *Europe and the People without History*. Berkeley: University of California Press, 1982.

Wolf-Meyer, Matthew. *The Slumbering Masses*. Minneapolis: University of Minnesota Press, 2012.

World Bank. *Health Sector Policy Paper*. Washington, DC: World Bank, 1982.

World Bank, "India's Massive I.D. Program Exemplifies 'Science of Delivery.'" May 2, 2013. https://www.worldbank.org/en/news/feature/2013/05/02/India-8217-s-Massive-I-D-Program-Exemplifies-8216-Science-of-Delivery-8217.

World Bank. *Investing in Health: World Development Report*. New York: Oxford University Press, 1993.

World Health Organization. *Report of the International Pilot Study of Schizophrenia*. WHO Offset Publication no. 2. Geneva: World Health Organization, 1973.

World Health Organization. *Schizophrenia: An International Follow-Up Study*. Chichester: Wiley, 1979.

World Health Organization. *Treatment of Tuberculosis: Guidelines for National Programmes*, 2nd ed. Geneva: World Health Organization, 1997.

World Health Organization. *WHO/IUATLD Global Project on Antituberculosis-Drug Resistance Surveillance, 1994–1997*. Geneva: World Health Organization, 1997.

World Health Organization and United Nations Children's Fund. *Primary Health Care: Report of the International Conference on Primafvry Health Care, Alma-Ata, USSR, 6–12 September 1978*. Geneva: World Health Organization, 1978.

Worsley, Peter. "The End of Anthropology." In *Transactions of the Sixth World Congress of Sociology* (1970): 307–13.

Wynter, Sylvia. "Un-settling the Coloniality of Being/Power/Truth/Freedom: Towards the Human, After Man, Its Overrepresentation." *Coloniality's Persistence*, edited by Greg Thomas. Special Issue of *CR: The New Centennial Review*, 2003, 3(3): 257–338.

Yahalom, Jonathan. *Caring for the People of the Clouds: Aging and Dementia in Oaxaca*. Norman: University of Oklahoma Press, 2019.

Yarris, Kristin. "The Pain of 'Thinking Too Much': Dolor de Cerebro and the Embodiment of Social Hardship among Nicaraguan Women." *Ethos* 39, no. 2 (2011): 226–48.

Young, Allan. *The Harmony of Illusions: Inventing Post-traumatic Stress Disorder.* Princeton, NJ: Princeton University Press, 1995.

CONTRIBUTORS

VINCANNE ADAMS is a professor of medical anthropology in the Department of Anthropology, History, and Social Medicine at the University of California, San Francisco.

JOÃO BIEHL is the Susan Dod Brown Professor and Chair of Anthropology at Princeton University, where he also directs the Brazil LAB .

DAVÍD CARRASCO is the Neil L. Rudenstine Professor of the Study of Latin America at Harvard Divinity School, with a joint appointment with the Department of Anthropology in the Faculty of Arts and Sciences.

LAWRENCE COHEN is a professor of anthropology and South and Southeast Asian studies and the codirector of the Medical Anthropology Program at the University of California, Berkeley.

JEAN COMAROFF is the Alfred North Whitehead Professor of African and African American Studies and of Anthropology, and an Oppenheimer Fellow in African studies at Harvard University.

ROBERT DESJARLAIS is a professor of anthropology at Sarah Lawrence College.

PAUL FARMER (1959–2022) was the Kolokotrones University Professor and chair of the Department of Global Health and Social Medicine at Harvard Medical School at the time he wrote the foreword to Arc of Interference. He was a cofounder and chief strategist of Partners in Health and a professor of medicine and chief of the Division of Global Health Equity at Brigham and Women's Hospital.

MARCIA C. INHORN is the William K. Lanman Jr. Professor of Anthropology and International Affairs at Yale University, where she serves as chair of the Council on Middle East Studies.

JANIS H. JENKINS is a professor of anthropology and a professor of psychiatry at the University of California, San Diego, where she is also a faculty member of the Global Health Program and director of the Center for Global Mental Health.

DAVID S. JONES is the A. Bernard Ackerman Professor of the Culture of Medicine in the Department of the History of Science at Harvard University, a joint position between the Faculty of Arts and Sciences and the Faculty of Medicine.

SALMAAN KESHAVJEE is a professor in the Department of Global Health and Social Medicine and Department of Medicine at Harvard Medical School and the director of Harvard Medical School's Center for Global Health Delivery–Dubai. He also serves as a physician in the Division of Global Health Equity at Brigham and Women's Hospital.

ARTHUR KLEINMAN is the Esther and Sidney Rabb Professor of Anthropology at Harvard University. He is also a professor of medical anthropology in the Department of Global Health and Social Medicine and a professor of psychiatry at Harvard Medical School.

MARGARET LOCK is the Marjorie Bronfman Professor Emerita in Social Studies in Medicine at McGill University, where she is also affiliated with the Department of Social Studies of Medicine and the Department of Anthropology.

ADRIANA PETRYNA is a professor of anthropology at the University of Pennsylvania. She directs the MD-PhD program in anthropology and the undergraduate concentration in medical anthropology and global health.

INDEX

Baldwin, James, 10
Baliga, A. V., 122
bardo, 241
Barnard, Christiaan, 125
Barrientos, Braulio, 59–60
Bateson, Gregory, 136
behavioral epigenetics, 211, 213
behaviorism, 299
being-with, 165
Bell, Charles, 29–30
Beloved (Morrison), 1
Benedict, Ruth, 136, 213
Benjamin, Walter, 12, 38
Benson, Herbert, 34
Berlant, Lauren, 276–77
Betts, Reeve, 122
Bevin, Ernest, 99
Biehl, João, xi, xvi–xvii, xviii, 12, 235–37, 296
Bill and Melinda Gates Foundation, 169, 179
bioethics, 316
biofields, 35
biological determinism, 159
biological psychiatry, 146
biomedical algorithms, 266
biomedical knowledge, 7–8
biomedical reductionism, 222
biomedicine, 69–70, 92, 106, 115, 192, 202; psychiatric, 146
biometrics, 11, 157–58, 161, 166, 170; de-duplication and, 176
biopolitics, 192
biopower, 314
biopsychosocial analyses, 114
biosociality, 299, 318
BioSocieties (journal), 225
biotechnology, 192
bio-techno-social interventions, 157
Black Americans, 2
Blanchot, Maurice, 253–55
Blavatsky, Helena, 31
BMRC (British Medical Research Council), 102–3
Boas, Franz, 210, 212–13, 228, 309
borderlands, 42, 46, 57, 310; as boxcar, 47–50; political forces and, 62
Border Visions (Vélez Ibañez), 51
Borovoy, Amy, 216
Box Car (painting), 47–49
Bracero Era, 50–51
brain death, 126
Brazil, public health systems in, 278–79
bricolage, 269
British Medical Journal, 104
British Medical Research Council (BMRC), 102–3

brokenness, 320
Buber, Martin, 288
Buddhism, 26, 240, 244, 308, 321; European science and, 30–32; funeral rites, 236; moral certainty and, 32; rationalism and, 31; suicide and, 27; Western scientific study of, 33–36
bulimia nervosa, 141
bumping, 51
bureaucratic indifference, 313, 316
bureaucratization, 316
Bureau of Science, 94
Butler, Judith, 182, 295
Bygren, Lars Olov, 224

CAD (coronary artery disease), 113, 116–21
Camarillo, Albert, 50
Camp Fire, 67
Canada, historical trauma in, 228–30
cancer, 252; infectious pathogens and, xix
Canguilhem, Georges, 220
Cape Town, South Africa, 96
capital, 299
capitalism, 2; crises of, 292
capitalist modernity, 300
carceral immigration policies, 135
cardiac surgery, 113, 122, 124–25
cardiomyopathy, 112
cardiovascular disease (CVD), 120
care, 235, 237, 288; amid institutions, 316–17; archipelago of, 249–52; contexts of, 311; defining, 306–11; disease control and, xix; ethics of, 251; as filmmaking, 47–50; moral economies of, 124–29; ordinary life and, 308–9; public health systems and, 310; public resources and, 311; rationalism and, 313; recipients of, 312; relationships in, 312–13; self, 52; social, 309; socialization and, 307; social primacy in, 19
care-ful ethnography, xii, xiv, xviii, 37–38
Caregiver Action Network, 313
caregiver-recipient of care relationship, 312–13, 315
caregiving, xii, 237, 283, 306; anthropology of and as, 318–20; arts of, 8–9; competency and, 165–66; after death, 307; ethnography of, 319; experiences of, 317; Kleinman, A., and, 45–46, 62; lessons learned from, 312–14; moral worlds and, 307; as presence, 315; sources of, 7; as structure of everyday life, 317–18
"Caregiving as Moral Experience" (Kleinman), 46
Carothers, J. C., 142
Carrasco, Davíd, xii, xvi, xviii, 10, 20, 310
Carrasco, Miguel, 44
Carter, Kevin, 266, 268

Dakshin, 161–62, 167, 169
Dalai Lama, 29–30, 32, 34
DALY (disability-adjusted life year), 105
Daoism, 321
Das, Veena, 176, 296
Dastur, Kersi, 123–24
databases, 166
data convergence, 175
data federation, 175
Davidson, Richard, 34
Davis, Angela, 4
dead reckoning, 82
death impurity, 246
death with dignity, 240
decision making: for IVF treatment, 194–95;
    pattern recognition in, 66
"Declaration by United Nations," 98
declarations of emergency, 293
decolonization, 88, 296
de-duplication, 167, 174–76
definitive truth, 40n19
De León, Jason, 42, 53–54, 56, 62
Deleuze, Gilles, 203, 243
dementia, 217–18
Demihkov, V. P., 122
demise writing, xiv, 240, 252–55
demoralization, 320
depression, 134–35, 138, 140–41, 144, 199; ethno-
    graphic studies and, 142
Desjarlais, Robert, xiv, xvi, xviii, 12, 235–37, 287, 314
desocialization, xiii
Devereux, George, 136
devotional *retablos*, 20
Dewey, John, 309, 321
Dharmapala, Anagarika, 33
diabetes, 198
Diagnostic and Statistical Manual of Mental Disorders,
    Fourth Edition (*DSM*-IV), 140
diagnostic categories: cultural validity and, 134;
    social construction of, 11, 88
diligent insanity, 78
directly observed therapy short course (DOTS),
    105–6
disability-adjusted life year (DALY), 105
disappearance, 181–82
disease: biomedical reductionism in concepts
    of, 222; colonization and spread of, 228;
    communicable-noncommunicable distinctions,
    xviii; comorbid, 126; control of, xix, 168, 310;
    cultural construction of, 93; disproportionate
    burdens of, 227; erasure of, 88–89; global burden
    of, 129; narratives of, 115–21; pulmonary, 127; seg-
    regation and, 95–97; technology and defining,

94; unequal burdens of, 87.
    See also epidemics
disinformation, 2
DNA expression, signals modifying, 223
DNA methylation, 223
Doi, Takeo, 214
Dome Fire, 72–73
DOTS (directly observed therapy short course),
    105–6
drug-resistant TB, 102, 104, 318
DSM-IV (Diagnostic and Statistical Manual of
    Mental Disorders, Fourth Edition), 140
Dubai, 190–93, 196
Dubai Healthcare City, 190
Du Bois, Cora, 136
Du Bois, W. E. B., 99, 309
Dubos, René, 102
Dumbarton Oaks, 99
Dunn, Frederick, 192
duplication, 166–67
Durand, Jorge, 56, 58
Durkheim, Émile, 212, 297
Dutch Hunger Winter, 225–26
dying: archipelago of care and, 249–52;
    poiesis in, 241–47; ritual poiesis and, 247–49;
    writing about, 252–55

Ebola, xix, 318
ecological fragility, 298
economics, xii
economic supremacy, 101
effacement, 248
efficiency, 316
effigies, 248–49
Eisenhower, Dwight, 100, 116
El Paso, Texas, xviii, 43, 45, 51, 54, 57; PTD and, 53;
    Segundo Barrio, 44
El Paso Job Corps Center, 44–45
embryo couriers, 205
embryonic pluripotent stem cells, 220
emergencies, 293–94
emotional blindness, 321
emotional dysregulation, 224, 226
emotions: expressed, 145; moral, 307
endometriosis, 200
entropy, 166
environmental conditions, 310
environmental destruction, 10
environmental epigenetics, 223
environmental imperialism, 3
environments: epigenetics and, 211; people and,
    211–13; selves and, 218–21
Environments and Mutable Selves, 210

EPIC, 177
epidemics, 240, 293; assumptions in designations
    of, 89; meanings of, 115, 129
epigenetic landscape, 222
epigenetics, xvi, 11, 157–59, 220, 230; behavioral,
    211, 213; environmental, 223; life course and,
    224–28; molecular, 221–24; origins of term, 219;
    transgenerational effects, 224
erasure, 42–43, 88–89
Erikson, Erik, 307
Eskerod, Torben, 263, 274, 277–78
ethambutol, 102
ethical immanence, 12
ethics, 308
ethics of care, 251
ethionamide, 102
ethnographic care, 5
ethnographic memorial, 281
ethnographic open, xvii, 4, 12–13, 236; fieldwork
    engagements and, 270, 275, 277
ethnographic-psychiatric projects, 136
ethnographic sensorium, 2, 236, 258
ethnography of caregiving, 319
Euro-American domination, 101
European science: Buddhism and, 30–32; Tibet
    and, 29–33
existential experience, 143–44
existentialism, 289, 295, 322
experience, xiv; caregiving, 317; Chernobyl as
    natural, 80; ethnographic value of studying,
    139; existential, 143–44; local moral worlds and,
    188–89; moral, 264–66, 308; primacy of, 137–39;
    schizophrenia and, 137–38; social, 143–44,
    264–66; somatic, 142; of suffering, 295; UIDAI
    as, 167
experiment: moral economies of, 124–29; in resi-
    dential schools, 229
Expert Committee on Tuberculosis, 104
expert intuition, 66
expertise, 70, 77; climate change and, 67–68
expressed emotion, 145
extraordinary conditions, 135–36

Facebook, 174, 280
family care, 311, 313–14
family caregivers, 313–14
family relations, 7
Fanon, Frantz, xiii, xix, 309
Farmer, Paul, 92, 108, 113, 115, 128–29
fast thinking, 66
Favret-Saada, Jeanne, 179
federation, 175–76
feelings, 306–7

Ferguson, Jim, 174, 178
Field, M. J., 142
filiation, 180–81
filmmaking, 164; caring as, 47–50
Finney, Mark, 76
Fire (film), 164
fire behavior analysts, 71
fire entrapment, 75, 77
Fire Lab, 74
fire seasons, 71–72
fire shelters, 75–76, 78
fire suppression, 68, 78
First Nations, 228–30
Floyd, George, xviii, 2
food embargoes, 225–26
forced migration, 20
forensic humanitarianism, 54–56
Fortis Hospital, 128–29
Foucault, Michel, 143, 192, 203, 271, 289
Four Families (film), 214
Fox, Wallace, 103, 106
Framingham Heart Study, 118
Frazier, LaToya Ruby, 258–59, 261, 268
free zones, 190
Fukushima nuclear disaster, 80
functionalist accounts, 290
funeral rites, 236, 247–48
futuring, xv

Gandhi, Mahatma, 99
gender-nonbinary persons, 174
genes, 221
genetic reductionism, 222
genome: reactive, 221–24; task of, 222
genomic medicine, 222
Ghana, 142, 146
Gibbon, John, 124
Gibbs, Wayt, 221
Gilbert, Scott, 222
Glasgow effect, 227
global AIDS care, 114, 128
Global Assemblages (Ong and Collier), 203
global cultural economy, 204
global flows, 204
global health, 11, 107–8; COVID-19 as test case for,
    14n12
globalization, 204
Global Mental Health (GMH), 144–49
global mobiles, 193–99
global reproductive assemblage, 203
GMH (Global Mental Health), 144–49
Gomes, Catarina Inês, 276, 281
Gone, Joseph, 320

intracytoplasmic sperm injection (ICSI), 195–96, 199

invisibilization, 5

in vitro fertilization (IVF), 158, 187, 189, 191, 193–95, 200–206

IPSS (International Pilot Studies of Schizophrenia), 145

isoniazid, 102–3

isonicotinic hydrazide (isoniazid), 102

IUATLD (International Union against Tuberculosis and Lung Disease), 104

Ivanivna, Maria, 66–67

IVF (in vitro fertilization), 158, 187, 189, 191, 193–95, 200–206

Jackson, Michael D., 243, 322

jamaat, 170, 184n14

James, William, 33, 309, 321

Janet, Pierre, 144

Jangba, 27–28

Japan: alienation in, 215, 217–18; dementia in, 217–18; punishment in, 214; relational selves and, 213–18; suicide in, 217

Jardim, Laura, 273, 277

Jenkins, Janis H., xvii–xviii, 11, 87, 89, 314, 321

jibun, 210–11, 213, 218

Job Corps, 44–45

Joglekar, S. V., 126–27

Johannsen, Wilhelm, 212

Jolly, Matt, 74

Jones, David S., xvii–xix, 11, 87–89, 293, 310

Journal of the Indian Medical Association, 112, 123

junk DNA, 221

kabarstan, 170–71, 179

Kabat Zin, Jon, 34

Kafka, 37

kakugo no jisatsu (suicide of resolve), 217

Kardiner, Abram, 136

Kaufman, Sharon, 246

Kaur, Amrit, 121

Keshavjee, Salmaan, xvi, xix, 11, 87–88, 310

Keynesian welfarist mode, 292

ki, 218

KID-SCID, 140

King Lear (Shakespeare), 275

kinnars, 162–63, 168, 170–72, 183n4, 184n14, 185n21

Kitanaka, Junko, 217

Klee, Paul, 37–38

Kleinman, Arthur, xii–xxi, 6–12, 113–14, 235, 237, 287–88, 297; caregiving and, 45–46, 62; category fallacy and, 88, 93, 139, 163, 165; on commodification of suffering, 268; depression and, 142,

144; illness narratives and, 189; on interference, 157, 168; interference and, 168, 178; local moral worlds and, 208; on local worlds, 188; mental illness myths challenged by, 147; on moral certainty, 24; on moral as critical problem-space, 184n20; primacy of experience and, 137; primacy of social and, 19–20; reductionism and, 115; on significance of caregiving, 250; on social and moral experience, 264–66; technology and, 157; transcultural psychiatry critiques, 87, 136

Kleinman, Joan, xiii, xx, 12, 237, 266; primacy of experience and, 137

knowledge: baselines of, 81; biomedical, 7–8; Chopel on, 30, 40n19; hybrid crossover, 5, 52

Koch, Robert, 106

kokoro, 218

Kondo, Dorinne, 215

Kopenawa, Davi, 79

Korean War, 51

Koselleck, Reinhart, 289

kothis, 168–69

Kreiger, Nancy, 227

Krenak, Ailton, 1

Kroeber, Alfred, 212

Kwakiutl, 211

kyphoscoliosis, 125

labor power, 299

Lacan, Jacques, 271

The Lancet (journal), 268

The Land of Open Graves (De León), 53–54

Landscape of the Body (diptych), 258–59

Las Conchas fire, 73

laundas, 180

League of Nations, 98, 100

Lebra, Takie, 214

Leslie, Charles, 192

Levinas, Emmanuel, 251

Lévi-Strauss, Claude, 269, 271–72, 290

Lewontin, Richard, 220

libertarianism, 317

life course, epigenetics and, 224–28

lifelines, 222

life of the mind, 8

life within limits, 322

lifeworlds, 10

lived actualities, 300

local knowledge, 167

local moral worlds, 208; grounding in, 307–8

local worlds, 188, 208

"Local Worlds of Suffering" (Kleinman, A.), 188

Lock, Margaret, xiii, xvi, 11, 157–59

necroviolence, 20, 42, 53, 62, 63n20
Nehru, Jawaharlal, 118
neo-Darwinism, xiii, 212
neoliberalism, 101, 310, 316
Nepal, xvi
neurogenesis, 249
Neuzeit, 289
New Deal, 98
NGOs (nongovernmental organizations), 161–63, 169
Nikshay, 175
Nilekani, Nandan, 166, 175–77
Nizam, H. H., 117
non-coding RNA (ncRNA), 222
nongovernmental organizations (NGOs), 161–63, 169
nonprofessional healing, 7
nonscalability, 179
normative baseline, 140
North American Free Trade Agreement (NAFTA), 53
The Notion of Family (Frazier), 258
NR3C1 gene, 226
The Nuer, 298

Oedipus the King (Sophocles), 1
Office International d'Hygiène Publique (OIHP), 100
Omote to Ura (Outside and Inside) (Doi), 214
Ong, Aihwa, 203
"On the Case" (Berlant), 277
ontological turn, 291
open-heart surgery, 123–25
organ donors, 126
Ornstein, George, 102

Packard, Randall, 93–97
Padmavati, Sivaramakrishnan, 117
Pan American Sanitary Bureau (PASB), 100
PAN card, 173
pandemic-industrial complex, 5
para-aminosalicylic acid (PAS), 102
Paradise Lost (Milton), 69
participatory intimacy, 288
Partners in Health, 318
PASB (Pan American Sanitary Bureau), 100
A Passion for Society (Kleinman and Wilkinson), 8, 309
Patel, Vikram, 148
Pathania, N. S., 121
Patients and Healers in the Context of Culture (Kleinman), xx, 7
pattern recognition, 66

patterns: critical thresholds and, 72; of fire, 66, 73–74, 77; models creating misleading, 77; personality, 213; *retablo*, 46; tidal, 82–83; trust in, 74
PCOS (polycystic ovary syndrome), 198, 201
Pehchan (film), 181
Pembrey, Marcus, 224
people, environments and, 211–13
personal agency, 245
personality patterns, 213
personal values, 295
Petrilli, Tony, 75–76
petro-states, 81
Petryna, Adriana, xv–xvi, 4, 10, 20–21, 287, 310
phantasmography, 254
pharmaceuticalized pandemic-industrial complex, 5
Phem Phuti, 25, 27
phenomenology, 57
phenotypic plasticity, 158, 220
philanthrocapitalism, 162
the Philippines, 93–95, 101
photographs, 272
Picasso, Pablo, 266–68
plague, 116
Plato, 239, 242
plume-dominated fires, 72–73
pluripotent stem cells, 220
poiesis, 236, 251; on behalf of another, 245; cultural, 243; forms of, 243–44; in living and dying, 241–47; ritual, 247–49
police violence, 2, 13
political economy, 291
political forces, 4; borderlands and, 62; moral certainty and, 20; personal agency and, 245
polycystic ovary syndrome (PCOS), 198, 201
populism, 2
posthumanism, 297–98
posttraumatic stress disorder, 141
pragmatism, 128
Prasad, Harinath, 164, 173, 180–81
predictive horizons, 68–69
presence, 312, 315
Prevention through Deterrence (PTD), 42, 50, 53–54
primacy of experience, 137–39
progressive cardiomyopathy, 112
proof, identity and, 178–79
provisional truth, 40n19
psychiatric biomedicine, 146; reliability of, 140
psychiatric diagnoses, 141–42
psychiatric diagnostic categories, cultural validity and, 134
psychic trauma, 135

The White Annals (Chopel), 30
white bodies, dominance of, 93-97
white supremacy, 2
Whitman, Walt, 261
WHO. See World Health Organization
Whyte, Kyle, 71
Wild Dog Dreaming (Rose), 298
wildfire fighters, 69, 72, 76; horizoning and, 68; proximity to fire, 74-75
wildfires, 67-69, 71, 77; safety zones, 75
wildland firefighters, 72
Wilkinson, Iain, 8, 309
Williams, Tyrone, 47
Wipro, 162, 170
withdrawal (hikikomori), 216
World Bank, 105-6, 113, 120, 147, 176, 178-79

World Development Report (World Bank), 105
World Health Organization (WHO), 100-101, 103, 105-6, 112; Expert Committee on Tuberculosis, 104; GMH and, 147; IPSS and, 145
worldviews, 57
World War II, 51-52, 98
Writing at the Margins (Kleinman), xx

Yarnell Hill Fire, 75
Yepes, George, 47-48, 51
Young, Robert M., 48
Younghusband expedition, 29, 33

Zen meditation, 215
zone of indistinction, 246
Zuni, 133-34, 211; ritual healing, 141